T0215533

Clinical Consultation Skills in Medicine

This book follows the revised format of the Practical Assessment Clinical Examination Skills (PACES) exam conducted by the Royal College of Physicians in the UK, where 'clinical consultation skills' will be tested twice in two separate stations. Thus, coming closest to what doctors do in real life: obtain a structured history, perform a focussed examination and explain the problem to the patient in lay terms. This book takes readers through a rational approach to 63 common presenting symptoms or laboratory abnormalities in medicine. It is aimed at improving the clinical consultation skills of young doctors and preparing them for the new format of MRCP PACES. Readers will learn:

1. The approaches to common presenting symptoms and blood test abnormalities.
2. What questions to ask the patient and why.
3. What to check when they examine the patient.
4. What to tell the patient and how to convey this information in lay terms without jargon.
5. How to investigate the problem, how to manage and when to refer to a specialist.

Key Features

- This book follows a narrative style with each case being discussed in a story-like manner, helping readers understand the process of narrowing the differential diagnosis, just like solving a crime!
- It includes a 'What to tell the patient' section, where the main points to convey to the patient are highlighted, and fully dialogued to help readers understand how complex medical jargon should be conveyed in layperson's terms.
- It simplifies several complex and difficult-to-understand topics like haematological malignancies, thrombotic microangiopathy, glomerulonephritis, systemic vasculitis and eosinophilia.

MasterPass Series

For more information about this series please visit: https://www.routledge.com/MasterPass/book-series/CRCMASPASS

Clinical Consultation Skills in Medicine
A Primer for MRCP PACES

Ernest Suresh
MD, FRCP (London)

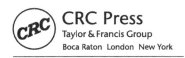

CRC Press
Taylor & Francis Group
Boca Raton London New York

CRC Press is an imprint of the
Taylor & Francis Group, an **informa** business

Contents

Foreword

Our interactions with patients at the bedside or the clinic, delivered in a focussed yet thorough manner, remain the bedrock of clinical practice even today. It involves the skilful interweaving of clinical knowledge and evidence, mental models and algorithms, heuristics and intuition. Needing years of deliberate and thoughtful practice to attain mastery, it is nonetheless a learnable and teachable art and science.

To this end, I commend to you this book. This is a must-read, not only for junior doctors preparing for the MRCP PACES examination but also for those embarking on the learning curve of general clinical medicine. The book is elegant in its simplicity and logic, yet impactful in its practicality and breadth. It is a window into the author's decades of clinical experience and wisdom of practice.

It has been my privilege to have journeyed alongside the author in his roles as a physician and teacher. The book is the distillation of both the roles elegantly crafted as one.

Gerald Chua
Chairman of Medical Board
Ng Teng Fong General Hospital, Singapore

Preface

This book takes you through a rational approach to 63 common presenting symptoms or laboratory abnormalities in medicine. Although it is primarily targeted at those sitting for MRCP PACES, it should also appeal to senior undergraduate medical students and trainees in internal medicine and general practice at all levels. In the two 'clinical consultations' stations, examiners will test your ability to obtain a structured history, perform a focussed examination, explain the problem to the patient in lay terms, construct a differential diagnosis and come up with a management plan. Preparing well for clinical consultations will therefore not only increase your chance of passing PACES but also help you practice high-quality medicine for the rest of your life.

The list of cases included is by no means exhaustive, as it is impossible for any book to cover all possible scenarios. I have included several cases that are unlikely to appear in PACES in the hope that they will provide you with the breadth of knowledge needed to apply in similar scenarios. It is better to be well prepared, as the longer time that is available in the new format broadens the range of scenarios that can be included. For example, although it is unlikely that you will see someone with acutely swollen joints in the exam, reading Case 3 (*The 26-Year-Old Man Who Is Struggling to Walk*) will help you understand the concepts of seronegative spondylarthritis and apply this knowledge to a patient with back pain due to possible ankylosing spondylitis. Likewise, you may not see someone with acute hepatitis or motor neurone disease, but these cases will help you learn the approach to jaundice or neurological weakness. For acute medicine scenarios, I have presented the patients in a stable state to closely match the exam setting (e.g. paroxysmal atrial fibrillation, transient ischaemic attack, seizures, thrombocytopenia, haematemesis).

Each case in this book starts with a stem that outlines the presenting problem. You will be given 5 minutes to read the stem and plan your consultation before you enter the station. It is best to construct a differential diagnosis during this time. I have kept the stem very brief for most cases and only stated the presenting symptoms, but in the exam, you may be given a lot more information, including vital signs.

You should probably spend about 7–9 minutes to obtain the history. History taking is like solving a crime! After some initial standard questions, your subsequent interview should be based on responses to the initial questions. The aim is to narrow the differential diagnosis as the story unfolds. It should not be a box-ticking exercise where you shoot a standard set of questions. Remember to respond appropriately (e.g. If a patient says that she is struggling with her daily chores because of pain, you should respond with 'I am sorry to hear that. I'll try my best to help', not move to the next question without showing any emotion or concern). Patients chosen for the exam may be well trained unlike the ones we see in real life, so as long as you ask the right questions, the answers should keep coming. You should focus on the main symptom or problem (e.g. If your opinion is sought about thrombocytopenia in a woman with menorrhagia, you should focus on thrombocytopenia, not her menorrhagia, however passionate you are about gynaecology!). While obtaining the history, remember to make a mental note of the issues to address later (e.g. If the patient with chronic kidney disease tells you that he regularly takes the naproxen prescribed for his wife to alleviate his gout attacks, you should not forget to address this later).

Physical examination should be focussed and completed within 3–5 minutes. You should plan the examination based on the history. Do not attempt to perform a detailed examination of individual systems. For example, if you have deduced from the history that the patient's weakness is most likely due to myopathy, it should be sufficient to check the power in the limbs, look for the rash of dermatomyositis and listen to the base of the lungs to detect signs of interstitial lung disease. You may then offer to perform a thorough examination to check for possible signs of cancer. In a patient who says he is bumping into objects on his sides, you should remember to check the visual fields. If the visual fields are not examined, you will miss the bitemporal hemianopia and fail to advise the patient to stop driving. This would result in an unsatisfactory mark for physical examination, physical signs, addressing concerns and clinical judgement. For some patients, you should set aside more time to complete the examination (e.g. suspected valvular heart disease, Marfan syndrome), while in others, it may not take much time (e.g. primary headache, osteoporosis). Unlike in stations 1 and 3, you can be more certain about the signs in 'clinical consultations' stations as you would have obtained a history (e.g. If you feel a mass on the left side of the abdomen in a patient with haematuria, you can be confident that it is an enlarged kidney and not the spleen). Most importantly, never make up signs to fit a diagnosis.

Once you have obtained a history and examined the patient, you should have an idea of what the problem is and how the patient should be evaluated or managed. This should be explained to the patient in layman's terms. Keep this brief and to the point. As long as you ask the patient to stop smoking, you will get points. There isn't time for a 2-minute lecture on the ill effects of smoking. I have provided some guidance on how the diagnosis or management plan should be explained in layman's terms under 'What Should You Tell the Patient', but readers can develop their own approach. It is important not to use jargon. Consider the following example: "I suspect you had a transient ischemic attack. We will arrange some imaging investigations and ask a neurologist to see you". Unless the patient is medically trained, they may find it hard to understand what you said. A better way to convey that would be: "I suspect your arm and leg became weak this morning because of a temporary reduction in the blood flow to a part of your brain. We call this a mini stroke. I will arrange a scan of your brain and ask the brain specialist to see you". The manner in which you communicate would largely depend on the education level of the patient and how much they want to know but in general, make sure you clearly tell the patient (a) what you suspect the problem is, (b) what investigations you plan to organise, (c) what treatments you plan to start and (d) who you intend to refer the patient to. Leave at least 2–3 minutes to explain the problem and address the concerns. Never forget the key points (e.g. warning the patient with Transient Ischaemic Attack [TIA] that "it could happen again" or asking the patient with seizures to "stop driving"). The patient may be trained to ask you a couple of questions, which are usually the same kind of questions that they ask you in real life (e.g. "Why do I feel weak?" "Will I get better?" "Could this be cancer?").

Each case in this book has been moved in a certain direction to make it read like a story. I have discussed my thought process and analysis of the case throughout, which should help you answer any questions on differential diagnosis or clinical judgement. If you can piece together all the details to come up with a sensible differential diagnosis and management plan, you should be able to comfortably pass these two skills. If you missed vital information in the history and did not pick up important signs, you will fail the differential diagnosis and clinical judgement skills, no matter how strong your medical knowledge. Remember the most common or important diagnoses for each presentation. For example, in a patient presenting with dyspepsia, the most important differentials to remember are peptic ulcer due to non-steroidal anti-inflammatory drugs (NSAIDs) or *Helicobacter pylori*, cancer (sinister) and functional dyspepsia (common). Remember that a nephrologist might be testing you on the approach to chronic diarrhoea and a gastroenterologist on headaches, so just stick to the basics!

Last but certainly not least, do not hurt the patient, not only physically but also emotionally. This would lead to an unsatisfactory marking for 'patient welfare'. Always be tactful when you ask for sensitive information. Start with "I hope you won't mind if I ask you a sensitive question, as it will help me find out what is wrong". Do not obtain a sexual history from an elderly patient unless necessary. These patients have kindly agreed to volunteer for the exam and the last thing they want is to be embarrassed by a doctor half their age in front of the two examiners! If a patient tells you that he visited a commercial sex worker and asks you not to tell anyone about this, it would be inappropriate and insensitive if you advised an HIV test for him as well as his wife (you should encourage him to tell his wife only if he is found to be positive). Physical roughness can be avoided by checking with the patient if they are in pain. Never expose a patient without obtaining permission first. If you inadvertently hurt a patient, remember to apologise.

At the end of the day, the important question that all examiners will have in mind is 'Would I be happy to have this doctor as my registrar?' If the answer is yes, you deserve to pass the PACES! Luck plays a part indeed, but there is no substitute for hard work and good preparation.

About the Author

Dr Suresh is currently the head of medicine at Ng Teng Fong General Hospital in Singapore. Over the last three decades, he has worked in three different countries with contrasting healthcare systems and cultures. He has been teaching MRCP candidates for over two decades and received more than a dozen teaching excellence awards in the last ten years alone. He has regularly published educational review articles on a wide range of topics in peer-reviewed internal medicine journals and written an acute medicine handbook to guide the junior doctors in his hospital.

He believes that all doctors, regardless of their speciality, should practice holistically and learn to treat the person who has the illness and not just the illness that the person has. He considers himself an 'old-fashioned clinician' and pays a lot of attention to bedside clinical skills and communication, the essential traits that the Royal College expects PACES candidates to possess.

What his junior doctors say about his teaching skills:

'He is a teacher par excellence. I have never met anyone before who could make even the most complex things simple for the juniors. I learnt a lot just by observing his thought processes while approaching a case. MRCP tutorials are a special mention with excellent simulation type tutorials and honest feedback'.

'He teaches the science as well as art of medicine'.

'A mentor knowledgeable vastly beyond his field, a mentor dedicated to both his patients and students, and a mentor who happens to take on the form of a story teller'.

'He has amazing communication skills and ability to speak to even the most difficult of patients'.

The 46-Year-Old Woman with Pain in Multiple Joints

Case 1

A 46-year-old woman presents with pain in her hands, wrists, shoulders and feet.

HOW SHOULD THIS PROBLEM BE APPROACHED?

*When you greet her, you note the presence of **joint deformities in both hands**.*

The differential diagnosis for deforming polyarthritis includes rheumatoid arthritis (RA), psoriatic arthritis (PsA), osteoarthritis (OA), chronic tophaceous gout and systemic lupus erythematosus (SLE).

There are four key questions to ask to narrow down the differential diagnosis in patients presenting with polyarticular joint pain.

- **Question 1: What is the extent and distribution of joint symptoms?**

Ask **which joints are painful**. Even if she only mentions the hands, wrists, shoulders and feet, you should screen for the involvement of other peripheral joints, neck and back.

Note: Knowledge of the distribution of joint symptoms helps to narrow down the differential diagnosis. For example, RA predominantly affects synovial joints, whereas PsA also targets entheses (sites of insertion of tendons, ligaments or capsules on the bone). Thus, patients with PsA may present with inflammatory back pain because of inflammation at the sites of attachment of ligaments that connect the vertebrae, but not those with RA, as there are no synovial joints in the thoracic or lumbar spine (which means if a patient with RA presents with back pain, other causes should be considered).

OA tends to affect weight-bearing joints and those that are subjected to excessive usage, so it should be considered in patients with hip, neck or low back pain. Gout, on the other hand, is rare in the girdle joints or spine because the higher temperatures in these joints (compared to those that are further away from the trunk) are not conducive to uric acid crystal formation.

- **Question 2: Is this an inflammatory or a mechanical problem?**

Ask if [a] the joints are **swollen**, [b] the joints feel **stiff in the morning** (*'How do you feel first thing in the morning?'* is better than directly asking *'Do you feel stiff in the mornings?'*) and [c] she has any **systemic symptoms** like weight loss, fatigue or fever. Although not specific, a **good response to anti-inflammatory medication** would also favour an inflammatory problem.

Note: Patients with OA too may report inflammatory symptoms, but the swelling is usually hard (as it is caused by bony proliferation) and morning stiffness generally lasts less than 30 minutes.

■ *Question 3: What is the sequence of development of various features?*

Ask about the ***onset and progression of symptoms***.

Note: An explosive onset, followed by gradual improvement, would suggest a self-limiting arthritis like viral infection, whereas an insidious onset, followed by evolution of symptoms in an *additive* manner (involvement of new joints while previously affected joints remain symptomatic), is typical of RA.

Other possible patterns of evolution are *flitting or migratory pattern*, which refers to the development of new joint symptoms, while previously affected joints are improving (e.g. rheumatic fever, bacterial endocarditis, gonococcal arthritis) and *intermittent pattern*, which refers to brief episodes of joint symptoms with asymptomatic intervals in between (e.g. gout).

■ *Question 4: Are there any extra-articular features?*

A ***review of systems*** is essential to uncover any extra-articular manifestations.

Note: In patients with inflammatory arthritis, you should look for features that may result from the immune system targeting other organ systems (e.g. skin rashes, Raynaud's phenomenon, dry eyes and mouth, muscle weakness, breathlessness) *or* those that suggest seronegative spondylarthritis (e.g. psoriasis, inflammatory bowel symptoms, ocular inflammation).

*She tells you that her **hands, wrists, shoulders and feet have been painful**. She has no pain in the rest of her joints, neck or back. When her **symptoms first began about two years ago**, she remembers waking in the mornings with pain and stiffness in her fingers. Shortly afterwards, the pain spread to her shoulders and then to the feet over the course of a few weeks.*

*She saw a private GP at the time, and he prescribed diclofenac and referred her to a specialist. She did not attend her appointment with the specialist, as her **symptoms improved with diclofenac**, and she was also very busy at work. She now buys ibuprofen across the counter and takes it up to two to three times a day. She also takes one to two tablets of paracetamol whenever the joints hurt more. Her **hands and wrists do swell up from time to time**, and she **feels stiff in the mornings for the first hour or two**, but she says her symptoms are now nowhere near as bad as how they were two years ago. Review of systems is unremarkable.*

In summary, there is involvement of the large and small joints in a symmetrical fashion (small joints refer to those in the hands and feet). The axial skeleton is spared. The (a) history of swelling of her hands and wrists, (b) prolonged early morning stiffness (>30 minutes) and (c) improvement with non-steroidal anti-inflammatory drug point to an inflammatory form of arthritis. Her symptoms have evolved in an additive manner and lasted two years. There are no extra-articular symptoms. The diagnosis is most likely RA, which is essentially the label that is applied to patients with persistent inflammatory arthritis that has the potential to cause joint damage in the long term (*see Figure 1.1*).

Among the other causes of deforming arthritis, gout can be excluded because it is rare in pre-menopausal women (oestrogens promote renal excretion of urate), and it would not persist for this long or involve the shoulders. An additive pattern of development of symptoms and involvement of wrists and shoulders are not typical of OA. Although the arthritis can sometimes precede psoriasis, there are no other features to suggest PsA. SLE causes Jaccoud's arthropathy, which may present with 'rheumatoid-like' deformities. Although SLE can present with joint symptoms alone, the absence of extra-articular symptoms even after 18 months is somewhat unusual.

It is concerning that she did not see the rheumatologist to commence disease-modifying drug therapy early. She is at risk of developing progressive joint damage if disease activity is not suppressed.

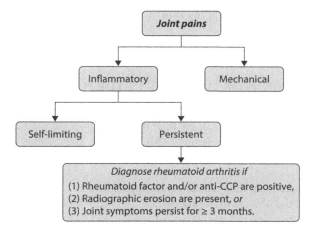

FIGURE 1.1 Simple approach to polyarticular joint pain.

Further questions to ask:

■ Ask about her ***other medical problems***.

Note: Knowledge of co-morbid illnesses is useful to tailor drug therapy accordingly (e.g. methotrexate should be avoided in patients with severe liver disease, prednisolone is not ideal in patients with poorly controlled diabetes, gastroprotection should be used in patients at risk of upper gastrointestinal side effects with NSAID).

■ Complete the ***rest of the history***.

Ask about her regular medications, family history, occupation, smoking habit and alcohol consumption, and obstetric and menstrual history.

■ Ask how these symptoms are ***affecting her function***.
■ Ask if ***she has been told why her joints are painful***.

She was well until two years ago but has never undergone health screening. She does not take any medication apart from ibuprofen and paracetamol. She denies heartburn or indigestion. Her family history is unremarkable. She has never smoked and seldom drinks alcohol. She is single and not sexually active. She has never been pregnant. She thinks she is approaching the menopause, as her menses are getting irregular and scanty. Her last menstrual period was ten days ago. She is a finance consultant. She ***struggles with her household chores*** *but says she somehow manages. She* ***thinks she has developed 'arthritis', which is common in people over the age of 40***.

WHAT SIGNS SHOULD YOU LOOK FOR ON EXAMINATION?

You should

■ Examine ***the joints*** to check for synovitis (*see Box 1.1*) and study the joint deformities.
■ Perform a ***focussed general examination***.

This might help to uncover psoriasis in the skin or nails, cutaneous vasculitis, subcutaneous nodules of RA or signs of interstitial lung disease.

BOX 1.1   SIGNS OF SYNOVITIS IN THE HANDS AND FEET

- Spindled appearance of proximal interphalangeal (PIP) joints (the spindled appearance is caused by distension of the capsule by fluid that collects in the joint cavity).
- Swelling across metacarpophalangeal (MCP) joints, which may be seen as loss of the valleys between the heads of metacarpal bones when the patient is asked to make a fist.
- Tenderness on squeezing the metacarpophalangeal joints.
- Swelling around the ulnar styloid process.
- Tenderness on squeezing the metatarsophalangeal (MTP) joints.

---

*There is **symmetrical deforming arthropathy**, with ulnar deviation of both hands, and subluxation of metacarpophalangeal (MCP) joints. Her **right middle proximal interphalangeal joint (PIP) is swollen**. The **range of movements is restricted in both wrists**. There is **tenderness on squeezing the metatarsophalangeal (MTP) joints**. The rest of her joints are normal. There is no evidence of psoriasis or subcutaneous nodules. Her lungs are clear.*

 The symmetrical deforming arthropathy and active synovitis are in keeping with RA. Persistent synovitis in RA causes hypertrophy of synovial tissue. The hypertrophied synovium (pannus) invades cartilage and bone, leading to destruction of joints. Chemical mediators like tumour necrosis factor and interleukins play a role in mediating joint destruction. The bare area of the bone (bone that is not covered by cartilage at the margins of joints) is eroded first. Laxity of the ligaments follows, leading to subluxation and deformity.

HOW SHOULD THIS PATIENT BE INVESTIGATED?

You should request

- ***Blood tests,*** including full blood count, erythrocyte sedimentation rate (ESR) or C-reactive protein (CRP), liver function tests, serum creatinine and vitamin D.
- ***Autoantibodies***, including rheumatoid factor (RF), cyclic citrullinated peptide antibody (anti-CCP) and anti-nuclear antibody (ANA).
- ***Plain X-rays of hands and feet*** may reveal soft tissue swelling and periarticular osteoporosis in the early stages, and erosions later.
- ***Ultrasound scan*** is useful to demonstrate synovitis and detect erosions earlier.

Other investigations that may be requested are ***chest X-ray, screening tests for hepatitis B and C*** (in anticipation of commencing disease-modifying drug therapy), ***fasting glucose, HbA₁c, lipid panel*** (as RA is associated with increased cardiovascular risk and she has not been tested before) and ***bone density scan*** (as RA increases the risk of osteoporosis and she is approaching menopause).

WHAT SHOULD YOU TELL THE PATIENT?

You should tell her that

- She has developed RA.

'Your joints are painful because they are inflamed. Inflammation causes fluid to collect in the joints and makes them stiff and swollen. If the inflammation remains persistent, as in your case, it can eventually damage the joints. The change in the shape of your fingers is because of this damage. We call this rheumatoid arthritis. This is different from the arthritis that people develop as they get older'.

- RA is an autoimmune disease.

'This type of arthritis occurs when the immune system mistakenly attacks the joints. We do not know why the immune system makes this mistake in some people'.

- You would refer her to the rheumatologist (*'joints specialist'*).
- The rheumatologist will discuss the treatments for RA.

'Ibuprofen only takes the pain away and does nothing to control the underlying arthritis that causes pain. Controlling the underlying arthritis is crucial to stop further damage to the joints. There are medications available to control the arthritis, which the specialist will discuss with you. I would strongly advise you see the specialist this time without fail'.

- You would arrange some blood tests and X-rays in the meantime.

'I'll ask for some blood tests and X-rays in the meantime. You should fast overnight before the blood tests because I would like to check your blood sugar and cholesterol as well'.

- You would prescribe a stronger anti-inflammatory medication, as she is still symptomatic despite taking ibuprofen regularly.

'If your blood counts and kidney function are normal, I'll prescribe a stronger anti-inflammatory medication to take instead of ibuprofen. That will hopefully afford better control of your pain'.

- You will get in touch with her when the test results are available.

OUTCOME

Her results are as follows:

- **Haemoglobin 118 g/L**, mean corpuscular volume 84, white cell count 9.2 × 10⁹/L and **platelet count 434 × 10⁹/L**.
- **ESR 76 mm/hour** and **CRP 58 mg/L**.
- Liver function tests and serum creatinine normal.
- **Serum vitamin D 22 ng/mL** (normal > 30).
- **RF and anti-CCP strongly positive**. ANA negative.

- Fasting glucose 5.2 mmol/L and HbA$_1$c 32 mmol/mol (normal 20–42).
- Low-density lipoprotein 2.2 mmol/L (target <2.7), high-density lipoprotein 1.4 mmol/L (target >1.0) and triglycerides 1.5 mmol/L (target <1.7).
- Plain radiographs show **erosive changes in both wrists and right second and third MCP joints**. There are no erosions in her feet.

The normocytic anaemia, thrombocytosis, and the elevated ESR and CRP are in keeping with chronic inflammation. The anaemia is most likely due to her RA, but serum ferritin, B$_{12}$ and folate should be requested. The radiographic erosions, and positive RF and anti-CCP, support the diagnosis of RA. However, negative RF and/or anti-CCP would not have helped to exclude RA because of their low sensitivity of around 60–70%. SLE can be excluded, as her ANA is negative (sensitivity of more than 98%). The results have excluded diabetes, and lipid panel results are satisfactory.

She should be commenced on disease-modifying drug therapy at the earliest opportunity in order to control the underlying arthritis and limit further damage. Methotrexate and sulphasalazine are the standard drugs used as initial therapy. Her vitamin D should be replaced. She should be referred to a physiotherapist and occupational therapist so that she can receive advice on exercises and her difficulties with activities of daily living could be addressed.

*She is seen by the rheumatologist, who arranges further tests. Chest X-ray is normal. Hepatitis B surface antigen, anti-hepatitis B core antibody and hepatitis C antibody are negative. Bone mineral density scan shows **mild osteopenia**, with T scores of −1.2 and −1.3 in her lumbar spine and femoral neck, respectively.*

He starts her on weekly methotrexate along with folic acid and vitamin D and refers her to a physiotherapist and occupational therapist. He arranges for her to receive influenza and pneumococcal vaccines. He plans to monitor her closely and gradually increase the dose of methotrexate to fully suppress the synovitis and prevent further joint damage.

The 49-Year-Old Man with Recurrent Joint Pain

Case 2

A 49-year-old man presents with a history of recurrent attacks of pain in various joints.

HOW SHOULD THIS PROBLEM BE APPROACHED?

Start with an open-ended question and explore his main complaint.

- ***Which joints*** have been painful?
- Do the joints look ***red or swollen*** during those episodes?

Ask if he has ***photographs of his joints*** taken during an acute episode.

- ***How long*** does each episode last? Does he become asymptomatic between these episodes?
- When did this problem begin and ***how often*** does he get these episodes? When was the last time he had an attack?
- Are there any specific ***triggers***?

*He says he gets **recurrent attacks of painful joints**. Only one joint is affected at a time, usually either the **big toe, ankle or wrist**. The joint would look **red and swollen** at the time, and the **attacks usually last about four to five days**. He is completely pain-free between the attacks. His GP once checked his blood tests more than two years ago and told him that his **uric acid level was high**. He gave him colchicine, but he prefers to take either ibuprofen, which he buys across the counter, or the naproxen prescribed for his wife's back pain, as they are both more effective than colchicine.*

*This problem started about four years ago. He was only getting one or two attacks a year for the first three years, but he has already had **three attacks in the last six months** this year. The last time he had an attack was three weeks ago. He is not sure what triggers these attacks.*

His presentation is in keeping with gout because (a) the attacks are self-limiting and recurrent, (b) joints that are further away from the trunk are involved, including the first metatarsophalangeal joint, and (c) his serum uric acid level was high two years ago (*see Box 2.1*).

He should be asked if any of his joints has ever been aspirated because demonstration of urate crystals in synovial fluid is the best way to confirm the diagnosis of gout. Gout attacks are often triggered by alcohol, meat, seafood, beans, or nuts, but not all patients may report this. The frequency of gout attacks is important to elicit, as it would help with the decision to commence prophylactic treatment.

DOI: 10.1201/9781003430230-2

BOX 2.1   HYPERURICAEMIA AND GOUT

Hyperuricemia is defined based on the urate concentration above which serum saturation occurs (>360 μmol/L). It results from the overproduction and/or renal underexcretion of uric acid. Both genetic and acquired factors such as rich foods, alcohol, insulin resistance and drugs (e.g. diuretics, cyclosporine, low dose aspirin) play a role in the development of hyperuricaemia.

Hyperuricemia is not the same as gout. Gout occurs only when subjects with hyperuricemia progress through the following additional steps:

- Formation of monosodium urate (MSU) crystals from hyperuricaemic serum.

When serum urate is consistently above 360 μmol/L, the propensity to form crystals is increased. MSU crystal formation generally occurs in the cooler, peripheral joints that are further away from the trunk, explaining why gout almost never occurs in girdle joints or the spine. Serum urate levels surge at the time of puberty in men, while, in women, this is delayed until after menopause, as oestrogens increase renal urate excretion. Because crystallisation is a slow process that takes many years, gout occurs from the age of 25 in men, but seldom before 50 in women.

- Interaction between MSU crystals and the inflammatory system.

Once formed, MSU crystals interact with leucocytes and cause synovial inflammation. As this is an intermittent and self-limiting process, patients suffer recurrent episodes of joint inflammation, tenosynovitis or bursitis (acute gout).

Some patients with chronic uncontrolled hyperuricemia accumulate macroscopic aggregates of MSU in soft tissues (chronic tophaceous gout). Clinical effects of tophi depend on the site of formation. Those that form over the pinnae or Heberden's nodes may be 'silent', whereas those that form adjacent to bones could cause 'gouty erosions' and joint deformities.

A vast majority of subjects with hyperuricemia remain asymptomatic because they do not form MSU crystals and, therefore, interaction between MSU and inflammatory system never occurs ('asymptomatic hyperuricemia'). In the absence of a history of recurrent episodes of self-limiting synovitis *or* evidence of tophi, the temptation to label such patients as gout should be resisted.

Pseudogout is a differential diagnosis for recurrent acute arthritis, but it is rare in someone of his age unless there is an underlying metabolic problem like hemochromatosis or hyperparathyroidism. The joints most affected in pseudogout are wrists and knees.

Further questions to ask:

- Ask about his *other medical problems*.

Particularly check for the presence of cardiovascular risk factors, as they often co-exist with gout.

- Ask what *medications* he takes, and if he has ever been prescribed prophylactic treatment (*'pills to take every day to prevent gout attacks'*).
- Ask if he has suffered with *kidney stones*.
- Complete the *rest of the history*. Ask about smoking habit and alcohol consumption, drug allergies, family history of gout and his occupation.

*None of his joints has ever been aspirated. He was diagnosed with **high blood pressure** and **high cholesterol** about five years ago. He was also told at the time that his **kidneys were slightly damaged**. His blood sugar was normal when it was last checked two years ago. He has never suffered with kidney stones.*

*He takes lisinopril and atorvastatin. He **tried allopurinol once before** but stopped it a fortnight later when he developed an attack of gout. He did not experience any side effects with allopurinol. He is not sure what the difference is, between allopurinol and naproxen or colchicine. He **smokes about 20 cigarettes/day** and **drinks two cans of beer most evenings**. He has no known drug allergies. His **father has gout**. He is a self-employed plumber.*

The presence of cardiovascular risk factors is not surprising, given that insulin resistance is a risk factor for gout. He might possibly have diabetes or impaired glucose tolerance as well and should be tested for this. It is useful to remember that a diagnosis of gout in an otherwise 'healthy' patient should prompt a search for cardiovascular risk factors.

It is quite common for patients to get acute attacks of gout when they begin prophylactic treatment with allopurinol, hence the recommendation to start with a smaller dose and increase gradually. He clearly needs to be educated about this and the need to continue taking allopurinol long term. He should be discouraged from taking an non-steroidal anti-inflammatory drug (NSAID). as his renal function was found to be impaired.

WHAT SHOULD YOU LOOK FOR ON EXAMINATION?

You should

- Examine his *joints* for evidence of deformities.
- Look for *tophi*.

The usual sites for tophi are the pinnae, hands, feet and extensor aspect of elbows and knees.

- Ask for his *body mass index* and *blood pressure*.

*His **body mass index is 29**. His joints look normal, with no evidence of synovitis or damage. There is no clinical evidence of tophi.*

HOW SHOULD THIS PATIENT BE INVESTIGATED?

You should request

- ***Blood tests***, including full blood count, liver function tests, creatinine, uric acid, fasting glucose and HbA_1c.

Note: Serum uric acid may be falsely low during an acute attack of gout in many patients (IL-6, which is produced during an acute episode, promotes renal excretion of urate).

Other investigations that may be requested in selected patients are as follows:

- ***HLA B58-01***.

This allele is associated with a 2% risk of severe hypersensitivity reaction during treatment with allopurinol. It is most common among individuals of Hans Chinese, Thai or Korean descent and African Americans. Testing is conditionally recommended for patients in the above ethnic groups, if they have risk factors for allopurinol hypersensitivity, such as older age (>60 years) and renal impairment (GFR <60).

Negative HLA B58-01 does not eliminate the risk, as non-genetic factors are also involved in allopurinol hypersensitivity.

- *Plain radiographs* in patients with chronic gout (to look for erosions).
- *Synovial fluid aspiration* in patients with acute presentation.

Note: Monosodium urate crystals are negatively birefringent on polarising microscopy. The absence of crystals would not exclude acute gout. Conversely, the presence of crystals would not exclude septic arthritis, as gout and infection could co-exist. Crystals may be seen during the asymptomatic inter-critical phase as well.

WHAT SHOULD YOU TELL THE PATIENT?

You should tell him that

- The attacks of joint pain are due to gout.

'Your description of the attacks of joint pain is in keeping with gout. Gout is caused by high uric acid'.

- For acute attacks, he should try colchicine or prednisolone.

'When you get an attack of gout, you should try colchicine first. Colchicine works best if you take it as soon as you know that an attack is coming on. The sooner you start, better the response. You should remember to stop the statin for a few days when you take colchicine because there is a higher chance of getting side effects if you take them together. If colchicine is not helpful or the attack is severe, you can try steroid pills'.

- He should avoid taking NSAIDs, as his renal function is impaired.

'You should avoid taking ibuprofen or naproxen, as they can affect your kidneys'.

- You would recommend pharmacological prophylaxis.

'Colchicine, steroid pills and naproxen only reduce the inflammation during an attack of gout. They do not reduce the uric acid level. Allopurinol, on the other hand, reduces uric acid. If uric acid is brought down to normal, you will stop getting gout attacks, but allopurinol should be taken daily and long-term'.

- Allopurinol may cause an allergic reaction, and acute attacks may be more frequent during the early phase of treatment.

'Allopurinol can occasionally cause an allergic reaction. If you notice a rash, itching or swelling of the lips or eyes, you should stop taking allopurinol straightaway and seek medical advice. During the first few months of treatment, you may get more attacks of gout. We can reduce this risk by starting with a small dose. I will check your uric acid every few weeks and gradually increase the dose'.

- He should stop smoking, reduce his alcohol consumption, eat healthily (*'cut down the sugars and fats'*) and exercise on a regular basis.

If there are specific foods that trigger the attacks, he should avoid them.

- If his gout is difficult to manage, you would refer him to a specialist.

OUTCOME

His blood test results are as follows:

- Full blood count normal.
- **Serum creatinine 122 μmmol/L** and **estimated GFR 56 mL/minute**.
- **Serum uric acid 602 mmol/L**.
- **Fasting glucose 6.4 mmol/L** and **HbA₁c 48 mmol/mol** (normal 20–42).
- An oral glucose tolerance test is arranged, which shows **impaired glucose tolerance**.

He is commenced on 100 mg of allopurinol and given a supply of colchicine and prednisolone to take during an acute attack. The plan is to gradually increase the dose of allopurinol in increments of 100 mg every four to six weeks until the serum urate is brought down to below 360 μmol/L. He is given advice on healthy lifestyle measures.

Prophylactic treatment is indicated in patients with (a) tophaceous gout, (b) erosive disease and (c) frequent gout attacks (at least 2 attacks in 12 months). For patients with chronic kidney disease (stage 3 or worse), prophylaxis is recommended even after one attack of gout.

Allopurinol works by inhibiting xanthine oxidase, which converts xanthine and hypoxanthine to uric acid. It is the drug of choice in nearly all patients who need pharmacological prophylaxis. The aim is to lower the serum uric acid to below the solubility limit, which is 360 μmol/L. For patients with tophi, the target is <300 μmol/L. Patients are likely to develop acute attacks soon after commencing allopurinol, as it mobilises urate stores. This can be reduced by using regular colchicine, but this may be challenging in this patient because of the need to stop the statin for that duration. NSAIDs are contraindicated because of his chronic kidney disease, and prednisolone may not be ideal because of his hypertension. The best strategy might be to start with a small dose of allopurinol to prevent a large drop in serum urate and gradually increase the dose in increments of 100 mg every four to six weeks.

Allergic reactions with allopurinol could potentially be serious, with Stevens-Johnson syndrome or toxic epidermal necrolysis occurring in about 0.4% of patients. For patients who develop allergic reactions with allopurinol, febuxostat, which also acts by inhibiting xanthine oxidase, is an option. Uricosuric drugs like probenecid, sulphinpyrazone and benzbromarone, which work by increasing renal urate excretion, are seldom used these days. Losartan and fenofibrate also have uricosuric properties, but if the blood pressure and lipids are well controlled on lisinopril and statin, he should be left on this regime.

The 26-Year-Old Man Who Is Struggling to Walk

Case 3

A 26-year-old man presents with pain in his knee, ankle and foot. He is struggling to walk because of this pain.

HOW SHOULD THIS PROBLEM BE APPROACHED?

You should

- Establish the **distribution of joint symptoms**.
- Ask about **inflammatory symptoms**, like swelling and stiffness, and **constitutional symptoms** like fever.
- Ask about the **duration of symptoms**, **onset** and **progression**.

*He tells you that his **right ankle, left knee and left middle toe are painful and swollen**. The pain started in the right ankle about four weeks ago and then spread to the left middle toe and left knee a couple of weeks later. He has been **struggling to walk** because of this pain. He has no pain from the rest of his joints.*

*He has been troubled with **pain in the lower part of his back** for the last two-to-three years, but this was put down to the nature of his job, which involves long distance driving and lifting heavy objects. He has no neck pain or systemic symptoms like fever and weight loss.*

- Explore his complaint of **back pain** and ask if [a] the pain is worse with resting or inactivity, [b] his back feels stiff in the mornings and [c] the pain disturbs his sleep at night.

*He says the pain is localised to the **lower part of his back and bottom**. The pain does not radiate down his legs, and there are no neurological symptoms like weakness or numbness. There was no trauma to the back prior to the onset of this pain. The pain often **wakes him from sleep**, especially during the early hours of the morning. His **back feels very stiff in the mornings** for the first 1–2 hours and **gets better when he starts moving about**, so he was surprised when his GP attributed the back pain to the nature of his work.*

There is involvement of the axial as well as appendicular skeleton. In the appendicular skeleton, the distribution is asymmetrical and only involves the lower limbs. The history of joint swelling suggests that this is an inflammatory problem. Because there is involvement of three peripheral joints, this is oligoarthritis (involvement of one joint is *monoarthritis*, while involvement of two-to-four joints is *oligoarthritis*, and involvement of more than four joints or the small joints of the hands and feet is *polyarthritis*).

DOI: 10.1201/9781003430230-3

It appears that the back pain and peripheral joint symptoms are connected, as his description of the back pain is also in keeping with an inflammatory problem. This is inflammatory back pain because [a] it is associated with prolonged early morning stiffness, [b] it gets worse after rest and improves with exercise and [c] it disturbs his sleep, especially during the second half of the night. The gluteal pain is most likely due to sacroiliitis. All these features point to a diagnosis of seronegative spondyloarthropathy (SpA, *see Box 3.1*).

BOX 3.1   SERONEGATIVE SPONDYLOARTHROPATHY EXPLAINED

The central feature of seronegative spondyloarthropathy is enthesitis (inflammation at the sites of insertion of tendons, ligaments or capsules on the bone).

The pathogenesis of SpA remains elusive, but it is possibly triggered by a microbe that enters the body when a physical barrier is breached (e.g. the skin in *psoriasis*, the gastrointestinal mucosa in *inflammatory bowel disease* or *diarrhoeal illnesses*, genitourinary mucosa in *sexually acquired infection*). A complex interplay between genetic factors (e.g. presence of *HLA B-27 gene*) and the microbe may then facilitate the T lymphocytes to target self-antigens, like entheses.

- Inflammation of the axial skeleton at sites of insertion of the ligaments connecting the vertebrae and sacroiliac joints causes *spondylitis* and *sacroiliitis* and manifests as inflammatory back pain and gluteal pain respectively.
- In the appendicular skeleton, manifestations include *synovitis*, *enthesitis* and *dactylitis*. Heel pain is a common presentation of enthesitis and occurs because of inflammation at the insertion sites of the Achilles tendon or plantar fascia. Enthesitis also causes dactylitis ('sausage-like' swelling of the whole finger or toe) because of extension of inflammation beyond the margins of the joint.
- At extra-skeletal sites, the autoimmune process may target those parts of the body where the connective tissue is 'loose', like iris, root of the aorta, conduction system of the heart and apex of the lung, manifesting as *iritis* (common), heart block, aortic regurgitation and apical lung fibrosis (rare).

Further questions to ask (*see Box 3.1*):

- Ask about *extra-articular symptoms*.

Features, such as psoriasis, inflammatory bowel disease and previous attacks of uveitis, would strengthen our suspicion of SpA.

- Ask about *diarrhoea, dysentery, dysuria or urethral discharge* prior to the onset of his joint symptoms.
- Obtain a *sexual history*.

Be tactful. You should start with '*I hope you won't mind if I ask you some sensitive questions*'.

- Obtain a *family history* of related illnesses.

This should not only include enquiry about arthritis and back problems but also inflammatory bowel disease and psoriasis.

- Ask what *medication* he takes for the pain and how the response has been.

Although non-specific, an excellent response to non-steroidal anti-inflammatory drugs would favour inflammatory arthritis or inflammatory back pain.

*He says that in the last two years, he has had two separate **episodes of pain and redness in his left eye**. On both occasions, he came to A and E, and the symptoms promptly responded to topical steroids. There is no history of psoriasis, inflammatory bowel disease or preceding diarrhoea, dysuria or urethral discharge. He has been in a steady relationship with his girlfriend for more than five years and not had any other sexual partner ever. His **father has psoriasis**, but not the arthritis.*

*He has been taking **diclofenac for the last two weeks and it has helped to ease the pain** in his joints and low back to some extent. He has never smoked and drinks one-to-two cans of beer during weekends. He works for a warehouse and his job is mostly manual. He is **struggling at work** because of the pain.*

The history of previous attacks of ocular inflammation, which is probably due to anterior uveitis, lends further support to seronegative SpA. The good response to diclofenac, although not specific, points to an inflammatory problem. The history of psoriasis in his father is also relevant.

WHAT SHOULD YOU LOOK FOR ON EXAMINATION?

You should

- Examine his *joints* to check for synovitis.
- Examine his *spinal movements*.
- Check for *psoriasis* (look at the nails, extensor aspect of the knees and elbows, trunk, scalp and gluteal fold).

Remember to ask for his permission before you look at the gluteal fold.

*There is evidence of **synovitis in his right ankle and left knee**, and **dactylitis in the left middle toe**. The rest of his joints are normal. His **lumbar movements are globally restricted**. His chest expansion is about 6 cm. Neck movements are full. There is no evidence of skin or nail psoriasis.*

Examination has confirmed the presence of synovitis and dactylitis. The global restriction of lumbar movements favours inflammatory back pain, especially in the context of his clinical presentation. Thus, his presentation is in keeping with axial as well as peripheral SpA (the term ankylosing spondylitis is now restricted to patients with axial SpA *and* plain radiographic changes in the sacroiliac joints or lumbar spine) (*see Figure 3.1*).

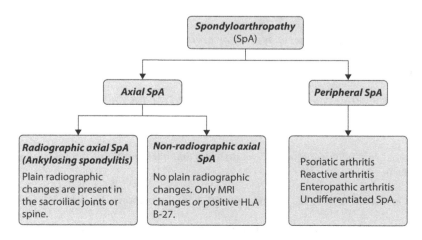

FIGURE 3.1   Classification of seronegative spondyloarthropathy.

HOW SHOULD THIS PATIENT BE INVESTIGATED FURTHER?

You should request

- *Blood tests*, including full blood count, erythrocyte sedimentation rate (ESR), liver function tests and serum creatinine.
- *Plain radiographs* of lumbar spine and sacroiliac (SI) joints.

Enthesitis may cause erosion of the underlying bone, followed by new bone formation. Thus, radiographic findings in the spine may include squaring of vertebrae (due to erosion of the corners of vertebral bones, where ligaments are attached), syndesmophytes (new bone that grows along the ligaments to eventually form a bridge between the bones) and bamboo spine appearance (due to the new bone causing fusion of vertebrae and facet joints, later on). In the sacroiliac joints, erosions are seen as widening of the joint space and new bone formation as sub-chondral sclerosis or fusion of sacroiliac joints.

- *Magnetic resonance imaging (MRI) scan of the SI joints*.

MRI is very sensitive in picking up bone marrow oedema, thus helping to make an earlier diagnosis, especially in patients with normal plain X-rays.

HLA-B27 is strongly associated with axial spondyloarthropathy. This gene is present in 10% of the healthy population, so its mere presence is not evidence of disease, and the test should not be requested unless there are supporting clinical features. It is most useful in patients with inflammatory back pain and normal imaging results.

WHAT SHOULD YOU TELL THE PATIENT?

You should tell him that

- His presentation is in keeping with inflammatory arthritis.

'Your joints are painful because they are inflamed. Inflammation causes fluid to collect in the joints and makes them stiff and swollen. This kind of inflammation occurs when the immune system mistakenly attacks the joints'.

- The back pain may be connected to the peripheral joint symptoms.

'I suspect your back pain is caused by inflammation of the ligaments, which are rope-like structures that connect the back bones together'.

- The history of uveitis is also probably related to the same problem.

'The pain and redness that you had in your eyes is also probably related to the same problem. In some people with this condition, the immune system not only attacks the joints and backbone, but also the eyes'.

- The family history of psoriasis in his father may be relevant.

'This kind of inflammation in the joints and backbone can occur in those with psoriasis. Although you do not have the skin rashes yourself, the fact that your father has psoriasis may be relevant'.

- You would refer him to a rheumatologist (*'joints specialist'*).
- You would arrange some blood tests and radiographs of the lumbar spine and sacroiliac joints in the meantime.

'I'll ask for some blood tests and X-rays of your backbone. The X-rays will tell us if your back pain is due to inflammation. The X-rays, however, may not show inflammation in the early stages. If the X-rays do not show inflammation, the specialist might ask for a scan of your backbone'.

- He could continue taking diclofenac.
- You will refer him to a physiotherapist, *'who will teach you some exercises for your back'*.
- You will update him when the results of the tests are back.

OUTCOME

*His full blood count, liver function tests and serum creatinine are normal. **ESR is 36 mm/hour**. Plain X-rays of the sacroiliac joints show evidence of **bilateral sacroiliitis**. HLA B-27 and MRI scan are not requested. He is advised to continue diclofenac, as he finds this helpful.*

He is referred to the rheumatologist, who commences him on sulphasalazine, as this is helpful for peripheral arthritis. He is also referred to a physiotherapist. He is told that it is important for him to follow an exercise routine to reduce the risk of ankylosis of the spine.

The 29-Year-Old Man with a Painful, Swollen Knee

Case 4

The orthopaedic registrar asks for your opinion on a 29-year-old man, who was admitted the night before with a two-day history of pain and swelling of his right knee.

The knee has been drained and the fluid sent for analysis, including crystals, Gram stain and culture. His blood test results show white cell count of 11.4 × 10⁹/L (normal 4–10) and C-reactive protein of 28 mg/L (normal <10). Rest of the blood counts, liver function tests and serum creatinine are normal. He has been commenced on diclofenac and cefazolin.

HOW SHOULD THIS PROBLEM BE APPROACHED?

After introducing yourself, you should first tell him why you have come to see him. Patients in hospital often wonder why they must keep repeating the story to multiple doctors!

'The orthopaedic doctor must have told you that your knee pain could possibly be due to infection. They have asked for my opinion to see if there are other possible reasons for the knee pain. I hope you won't mind if I asked you a few questions and briefly examined you. I'll then tell you what I think'.

Start with an open-ended question and ask if the pain has been better since coming to hospital.

*He tells you that the **pain started two days ago**. He was **struggling to walk because of the pain**. He feels much better since the knee was drained. The pink painkiller tablet also helps.*

You should

- Ask if he has **pain in the rest of his joints, neck or back** to establish if this is truly a monoarticular problem or part of a polyarticular problem.
- Ask about **preceding trauma or sporting activities** [if the pain is monoarticular], and constitutional symptoms like **fever**.

He has no pain in the rest of his joints, neck or low back. He denies preceding trauma or sporting activities. He was well apart from pain in the knee, and the nurse in A and E told him that his temperature was normal.

This patient presents with acute monoarticular pain, involving his right knee. In patients with monoarticular pain, it is important to first establish if the pain is **articular** (arising from the joint), **periarticular** (arising from structures outside the joint capsule, such as bursae, tendons or ligaments) or **referred** (pain referred

DOI: 10.1201/9781003430230-4

from an adjacent joint like hip). ***Bone pathology*** (e.g. osteonecrosis, stress fracture and tumour) can also present with acute monoarticular pain. In this patient, the pain is clearly articular, as he has already had his knee drained.

BOX 4.1   SOME UNDERLYING CAUSES OF ACUTE MONOARTICULAR PAIN AND SWELLING

- Trauma.
- Infective arthritis.
- Inflammation (e.g. crystal arthritis like gout or pseudogout, reactive arthritis and acute sarcoidosis).
- Haemarthrosis (bleeding into the joint cavity secondary to trauma *or* bleeding disorders).
- Degenerative (flare of osteoarthritis).

In the absence of preceding trauma, [a] septic arthritis, [b] gout and [c] reactive arthritis are the most likely diagnoses to consider in this patient (*see Box 4.1*). Of these, septic arthritis is the diagnosis not to miss, as delayed treatment could potentially lead to rapid joint destruction, spread of infection outside the joints *or* death.

Further questions should aim to explore the features suggestive of these diagnoses.

- Ask about other localising ***symptoms of infection***, like headache, cough, skin rash, diarrhoea, painful micturition and urethral discharge.
- Ask about symptoms of ***recent gastrointestinal or genitourinary infection*** (might suggest reactive arthritis).

Be tactful when you elicit the sexual history. Start with '*I hope you won't mind if I ask you some sensitive questions*'.

- Ask if he has had ***previous acute episodes of joint inflammation*** ('gout attacks').

Note: History of previous episodes of gout would not exclude septic arthritis.

- Complete the ***rest of the history***.

Ask about his other medical problems (particularly psoriasis and inflammatory bowel disease), medications taken, occupation, recent travel or infectious contacts, smoking history, alcohol consumption and family history of arthritis.

*After initial hesitation, he admits that when he went on a holiday to Bangkok three weeks ago, he **visited commercial sex workers** a couple of times. Although he used condoms, it slipped and fell during intercourse with one of them. A few days later, he felt a **burning sensation when he peed**, but no fever, urethral discharge, foul smelling urine or ulcers in his private parts. He did not see a doctor at the time, as his symptoms resolved in a few days. He has a girlfriend, but he has not had sexual intercourse with her since returning from Bangkok. He has no other sexual partners. He **asks if the information that he has shared with you could remain confidential**.*

Review of systems is unremarkable, with no localising symptoms of infection. His past medical history is blameless, and he takes no regular medication. He has never visited sex workers before or *been diagnosed with sexually acquired infection. There is no history of previous episodes of joint pain, psoriasis or inflammatory bowel disease. The relevant family history is unremarkable. He **smokes ten cigarettes/day** and **drinks a can of beer most evenings**. He manages a retail shop.*

Reactive arthritis due to sexually acquired infection is a possible differential diagnosis because of the recent history of dysuria soon after sexual intercourse with commercial sex workers (of which one was unprotected). The dysuria was possibly due to urethritis secondary to *Neisseria gonorrhoea or* Chlamydia trachomatis (also known as non-gonococcal urethritis). His presentation is not in keeping with gonococcal septic arthritis or disseminated gonococcal infection, as the arthritis occurs at the same time as the infection and not after three weeks. Although his dysuria has already resolved, his urine should be tested for Gonococcus and Chlamydia (*not* urethral swab, as he denies urethral discharge). If the urine polymerase chain reaction (PCR) is positive for Gonococcus and/or Chlamydia, he should receive appropriate antibiotics. He should also be tested for syphilis, hepatitis B and HIV (if he consents).

His reasons for requesting you to keep this information confidential are obvious.

- If there is no evidence of sexually acquired infection, we are not obliged to encourage him to tell the girlfriend.
- If he is found to have Gonococcus and/or Chlamydia and he is telling the truth, he may not have passed the infection to his girlfriend, and she need not be tested. He should be asked to abstain from intercourse with her (or indeed anyone else) until the infection is fully treated.
- If he turns out to be HIV positive, he should be strongly encouraged to tell his girlfriend.

If he refuses after repeated requests, confidentially would have to be breached (*after informing him*), to protect the health of his girlfriend.

WHAT SHOULD YOU LOOK FOR ON EXAMINATION?

You should

- Ask for his *vital signs*.
- Examine his *joints*, particularly the *right knee*.

If you had seen the patient before the knee was drained, you should have checked for redness, swelling, tenderness and restricted range of movements (*see Box 4.2* for features that help to differentiate articular from periarticular pathology).

- Offer to *examine his genitals*.
- Complete a *focussed general examination*.

Check for distant foci of infection, tophi and mucocutaneous lesions (e.g. erythema nodosum in sarcoidosis, conjunctivitis, circinate balanitis and keratoderma blenorrhagicum in reactive arthritis).

BOX 4.2   DIFFERENTIATING ARTICULAR FROM PERIARTICULAR PROBLEM

ARTICULAR PROBLEM	PERIARTICULAR PROBLEM
Global restriction of joint movements (e.g. global restriction of shoulder movements in gleno-humeral joint disease)	Restriction of movements in only a certain plane (e.g. restriction of abduction alone in supraspinatus tendinitis)
Active and passive movements are equally restricted[†]	Greater restriction of active range of movements
Swelling of the entire joint (e.g. filling of the parapatellar gutters and suprapatellar pouch with knee effusion)	Localised swelling (e.g. anterior swelling over the lower half of the patella in pre-patellar bursitis)

[†] Active range refers to movements performed by the patient (periarticular structures are used to move the joint), while passive range refers to movements performed by the examiner (periarticular structures are relaxed or not used). If the periarticular structures are diseased, the active range of movements would be expected to be more restricted compared to the passive range.

*His temperature is 36.2°C, pulse rate 76/minute, BP 116/74 mm Hg, respiratory rate 16/minute and oxygen saturation 96% on room air. **The right knee is bandaged.** The other joints are normal. Rest of the examination is unremarkable. There are no tophi or skin rashes. You are told that his genitals are normal, with no evidence of balanitis or ulcers.*

 Fever is not specific to septic arthritis. Patients with inflammatory arthritis due to any cause (e.g. crystal arthritis, reactive arthritis) may also develop fever. More importantly, the absence of fever would not exclude septic arthritis. The examination has not uncovered any distant sites of infection and there is no clinical evidence of tophaceous gout.

HOW SHOULD THIS PATIENT BE INVESTIGATED?

Investigations to request in patients with acute monoarthritis include:

- **Blood tests**, including full blood count, C-reactive protein (CRP), liver function tests, serum creatinine and uric acid.
- **Blood cultures** in those with suspected septic arthritis.
- **Synovial fluid analysis and culture**.

This is the crucial investigation in anyone presenting with acute monoarthritis. You should request [a] cell count, [b] Gram stain and culture and [c] polarising microscopy for crystals. In patients with suspected septic arthritis, joint aspiration should be performed *before* commencing antibiotics, whenever possible.

- There is no need to request *plain radiographs* of the knee (this is only indicated if there is a history of preceding trauma and in those with suspected pseudogout).

Ultrasound scan of the knee may be useful for guided aspiration in difficult cases.

In this patient, you should also request

- **Urine PCR for Gonococcus and Chlamydia**.
- **Tests for HIV** (if he consents), **syphilis and hepatitis B**.

WHAT SHOULD YOU TELL THE PATIENT AT THIS STAGE?

You should tell him that

- He should continue antibiotics until septic arthritis is excluded.

'We should continue the antibiotics until we know for sure that there is no infection in your knee. It could take a couple of days to get the results of your knee fluid'.

- He can continue taking diclofenac. If cultures are sterile and the knee is still painful, intra-articular steroid is an option.

'You can continue taking diclofenac, the "pink-coloured" tablet, for the pain. Once we rule out an infection, we can inject some steroid into the knee, if it is still painful. The steroid might be more effective than the painkiller'.

- His recent dysuria was most likely due to sexually acquired infection.

'I wonder if the burning sensation on peeing was due to an infection that you caught from one of the women in Thailand'.

- Another possible cause of the knee pain is sexually acquired reactive arthritis.

'Sometimes, the joints can get inflamed a few weeks after a sexually acquired infection. We call this reactive arthritis. If we do not find any infection in your knee, then reactive arthritis would be the most likely cause of your knee pain'.

- You would recommend a urine test to check for common sexually acquired infections.

'I would recommend testing your urine. If an infection is found, we can treat it with antibiotics'.

- You would also recommend an HIV test and tests for syphilis and hepatitis B.

'I'd also suggest testing for other sexually acquired infections, including HIV. I'll ask our nurse to talk to you about the HIV test in detail'.

- The information will remain confidential.

'We will treat this information as confidential. If we find an infection in the urine, you should abstain from sexual intercourse until the infection is treated fully. However, if your HIV result is positive, we would encourage you to tell your girlfriend so that she can be tested as well. The nurse will explain this further'.

- You will talk to him when his test results are back and seek the opinion of a rheumatologist (*'joints specialist'*) if needed.

OUTCOME

The following results are obtained:

- Synovial fluid shows normal white cell count and no crystals. Gram stain is normal. The cultures are sterile after two days.
- Urine PCR for Gonococcus and Chlamydia is negative.
- HIV test and tests for syphilis and hepatitis B are negative.

He is diagnosed with reactive arthritis. Cefazolin is discontinued after two days. Because the knee is still inflamed and painful, the rheumatologist injects steroid into his knee. He is referred to a physiotherapist, who teaches quadricep strengthening exercises. His symptoms completely resolve, and he is able to discontinue the diclofenac after two weeks.

The 68-Year-Old Woman with Pain in Her Right Knee and Hands

Case 5

A 68-year-old woman presents with a long history of pain in her right knee and hands.

HOW SHOULD THIS PROBLEM BE APPROACHED?

---

*She tells you that her **right knee has been painful** for the last three-to-four years. The pain was not too bad to begin with, and she was mostly able to cope. However, in the last six months, the pain has increased significantly. She was previously able to walk around the shopping mall without much problem, but now **struggles to walk** for even 15–20 minutes at a stretch because of the pain in her knee. She also gets **pain in her fingers**, but this is nowhere near as bad as the pain in her knee.*

You should

- Ask if she has **pain in the rest of her joints**, **neck or back**.
- Ask if the pain is **affecting her sleep**.
- Ask about inflammatory symptoms like **swelling**, and mechanical symptoms like **locking** and '**giving way**'.

*She has no pain in the rest of her joints, neck or back. The pain does not affect her sleep. She has not noticed any swelling in her joints, but the **knee becomes stiff if she sits for long periods** and it takes a few minutes to loosen up. Her **knee sometimes buckles**, but she has never experienced locking.*

Her presentation is in keeping with osteoarthritis (OA) as evidenced by (a) the long duration of her symptoms, with no recent change in the character of the pain, (b) absence of joint swelling and (c) aggravation of pain with activity (*see Box 5.1*). Patients with OA can develop an effusion in the knee because of cartilage breakdown products causing superimposed inflammation, but this is usually never as large as the effusions that occur in rheumatoid or psoriatic arthritis. The stiffness of the knee that she is experiencing after prolonged sitting, also known as *gelling*, is a common symptom of OA. The sensation of buckling or '*giving way*' suggests weakness of the quadriceps mechanism. *Locking* of the knee, which she denies, occurs because of cartilage fragments floating freely in the knee (loose bodies).

DOI: 10.1201/9781003430230-5

23

The effect on function and sleep is important to assess because surgical referral should be considered for those who *cannot walk*, *cannot work or cannot sleep*, especially if there is a poor response to conservative measures like pharmacological interventions and physiotherapy.

BOX 5.1   PATHOLOGY OF OSTEOARTHRITIS

Osteoarthritis is characterised by (a) degeneration of articular cartilage and (b) bone remodelling. The primary event in OA is breakdown of articular cartilage, which usually occurs at the central load-bearing portion of the joint. It is *not* due to preceding synovitis (unlike in rheumatoid arthritis, where the primary event is synovitis, and cartilage breakdown is a secondary event that occurs because of synovial hypertrophy and release of cytokines). The breakdown of cartilage can be visualised on plain radiographs as loss of joint space.

Bone remodelling leads to (a) thickening of sub-chondral bone (seen as sub-chondral sclerosis on plain radiographs), (b) formation of bone cysts and (c) growth of osteophytes at articular margins. The clinical effects of osteophytes depend on the site of formation. Osteophytes that form in hands usually do not cause symptoms, while those that form in the acromioclavicular joint could press on the rotator cuff and present with shoulder impingement, and those that form around the vertebrae could cause nerve root compression or spinal stenosis.

The breakdown products of cartilage may cause synovitis (as a secondary event) and expansion of the joint may stretch the surrounding ligaments, tendons or bursae, causing pain.

■ Explore her complaint of *pain in the hands*.

Ask about the duration, progression, presence of inflammatory features such as joint swelling and morning stiffness, and effect on function.

*Her **fingers have been painful** for the last two years. The pain has neither improved nor worsened during this time. It is a dull aching sensation, with no specific aggravating or relieving factors. Some of the **finger joints are swollen** (A quick inspection reveals Heberden's nodes over some of her distal interphalangeal joints) and they feel **stiff in the mornings for the first 10–15 minutes**. Her hand function is not affected.*

Her description of the pain in her hands also fits with OA. The presence of osteoarthritic changes in the joints would of course not rule out an inflammatory form of arthritis like rheumatoid, but the general pattern of evolution and absence of inflammatory joint swelling or prolonged early morning stiffness would make this less likely. Apart from hands and knees, other joints that are commonly affected by OA include weight-bearing joints (e.g. hips, knees and the first metatarsophalangeal joints) and those that are subject to excessive usage (e.g. carpo-metacarpal joints in thumbs and facet joints of cervical and lumbar spine).

■ Complete the *rest of the history*.

Ask about her other medical problems, regular medications, treatments tried for her joints so far, drug allergies, family history, occupation, smoking habit and alcohol consumption. Also, explore her *concerns and expectations*.

*Her medical problems include **hypertension**, **diabetes**, **hyperlipidaemia** and **stage 3 chronic kidney disease**. She takes amlodipine, atenolol, metformin, gliclazide and atorvastatin. She has tried paracetamol for the pain but only takes it about once every couple of days. It does take the edge off the pain. She has never seen* *a physiotherapist. Her **late mother had knobbly fingers**, but she was not formally diagnosed with arthritis. She has never smoked and drinks alcohol only socially. She is a retired secondary school teacher. She lives with her husband, who is well. She mostly spends her time at home and doesn't really exercise.*

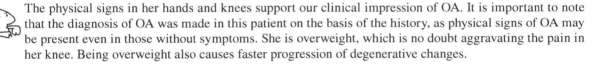 The multiple co-morbidities, especially hypertension and chronic kidney disease would preclude the use of some therapeutic options like non-steroidal anti-inflammatory drugs (NSAIDs). Our therapeutic strategies should be focussed on the knee, as this is her main concern and should aim to control her pain, improve her function and slow down the progression of disease.

WHAT SHOULD YOU LOOK FOR ON EXAMINATION?

You should

- Ask for her **body mass index**.
- Examine **her joints**, particularly the symptomatic knee and hands.

*She is **overweight**, with body mass index of 31.2. There is **bony enlargement** of the right knee with **loss of quadriceps bulk**. There is no varus or valgus deformity. There is no effusion in the knee. There is **restriction of knee movements** at the end of range. The left knee also looks enlarged with some crepitus, but there is a full range of movement. In the hands, there are **Heberden's** and **Bouchard's nodes**. There is no synovitis. The other joints are normal.*

The physical signs in her hands and knees support our clinical impression of OA. It is important to note that the diagnosis of OA was made in this patient on the basis of the history, as physical signs of OA may be present even in those without symptoms. She is overweight, which is no doubt aggravating the pain in her knee. Being overweight also causes faster progression of degenerative changes.

HOW SHOULD THIS PATIENT BE INVESTIGATED?

- Ask for **plain radiographs of her right knee** (weight-bearing anteroposterior, lateral and sky-line views). The sky-line view helps to look at the patellofemoral space.

Notes:

1. There is no need to request radiographs of her hands.
2. Joint space narrowing is best seen if radiographs are taken in the weight-bearing position.
3. There is no need to request radiographs for every patient with suspected osteoarthritis. In general, radiographs help to study the extent and severity of degenerative changes, although they may not correlate with symptoms. They also help to plan surgical management and look for other possible causes for the pain, such as osteonecrosis, stress fracture or tumour.

*Plain radiographs of her knee show evidence of **tricompartmental osteoarthritis**. Her lab tests (done three weeks ago) show **HbA$_1$c of 66 mmol/mol** (normal 20–42), **serum creatinine of 98 μmol/L and e-GFR of 54**.*

WHAT SHOULD YOU TELL THE PATIENT?

You should tell her that

- Her joint pain is due to OA.

'Your knee and hands are painful because of wear and tear in the joints. We call this osteoarthritis. We have this cushion or cartilage at the ends of our bones (draw a diagram and explain), *which ensures that the bones do not rub against each other, and movements of the joint are smooth. In osteoarthritis, the cartilage becomes worn out and thin'.*

- The X-rays *'show evidence of wear and tear in the knee'*.
- Most patients with OA *'do well and remain stable for many years'*, unlike those with an inflammatory form of arthritis.
- She should lose weight.

'Being overweight can place more strain on the knees and cause wear and tear changes to progress faster. You should therefore try to lose weight. You can go for short, gentle walks to begin with. You will not be causing more damage to your knees by exercising. Because your knees hurt when you walk, I would suggest that you take a painkiller about an hour before you start walking. You should also watch your diet and cut down the intake of sugars and fat. Exercise and healthy eating will help not only the knee problem, but also your diabetes'.

- You would refer her to a physiotherapist.

'Your muscles on the front part of your thigh appear to be weak and thin. This is the reason why your knee buckles when you walk. Strengthening this muscle can slow the progression of wear and tear changes in the knee and reduce pain. I'll refer you to a physiotherapist, who can help with this'.

- She should take paracetamol on a more regular basis. You would also prescribe a topical non-steroidal anti-inflammatory (NSAID) medication.

Explain to her that although oral NSAIDs may be more effective than paracetamol, this may not be ideal for her because *'they can affect the kidneys'*.

- If her response to the above measures is sub-optimal and she continues to struggle, you would refer her to an orthopaedic surgeon for an opinion.

Injecting some steroids into her knee is also an option.

- You would give her an information booklet on OA or suggest useful websites.

OUTCOME

*She tries regular **paracetamol**, **topical NSAID** plasters over her knee and a small dose of **tramadol** as and when necessary. The physiotherapist advises her on **quadriceps strengthening exercises** and suggests a **knee brace**. She starts with gentle exercises, but the pain stops her from walking for longer than ten minutes.*

*She follows a strict diet and manages to lose 3 kg over the next three months, but the pain continues to worsen. She is referred to the orthopaedic surgeon, who advises **total knee replacement**.*

The 72-Year-Old Man with Pain in All Four Limbs

Case 6

A 72-year-old man presents with a four-week history of pain in all his four limbs.

HOW SHOULD THIS PROBLEM BE APPROACHED?

Obtain a detailed history. Ask particularly about:

- The **distribution of pain**.
- **Inflammatory symptoms** like joint swelling and morning stiffness, and **constitutional symptoms** like fever and weight loss.
- **Duration of symptoms**, **onset** and **progression**.
- **Neurological symptoms**, like weakness and numbness.

*He tells you that his **arms and thighs have been painful** for the last four weeks. He has no pain in his neck and back, or below the elbows and knees. His joints are not swollen, but he **feels very stiff in the mornings for the first 2–3 hours**. He finds it difficult to wash his hair and put on his shirt in the mornings, but this improves as the day progresses. He feels **tired all the time** but denies fever or weight loss. Review of systems is unremarkable.*

His presentation is in keeping with polymyalgia rheumatica, as (a) he is over the age of 50, (b) the symptoms are confined to proximal limbs and (c) there is prolonged early morning stiffness. An excellent response to prednisolone would help to confirm the diagnosis.

His difficulty in washing hair and putting on his shirt in the mornings is most likely due to pain and stiffness rather than true neurological weakness, as the latter is unlikely to improve as the day progresses. Hence, we need not consider polymyositis, which is characterised by symmetrical, proximal limb *weakness* rather than pain.

The absence of prominent systemic symptoms, like fever or weight loss, reduces the likelihood of infection or malignancy, but these differentials should be revisited if his response to prednisolone is sub-optimal. There are no features of inflammatory arthritis at this stage, but there is a chance that he could develop this in the future. In most patients, rheumatoid arthritis begins in the small joints of the hands and feet and then spreads to larger joints, but in some elderly patients, pain begins in the girdle joints and then spreads to the smaller joints, usually when the dose of steroid is tapered ('*polymyalgic onset of rheumatoid arthritis*').

DOI: 10.1201/9781003430230-6

About 15–20% of patients with polymyalgia rheumatica develop giant cell arteritis (GCA) and it is important to ask about features that may suggest this diagnosis (use of the term 'temporal arteritis' is incorrect, as this condition can also affect other arteries).

- Ask about **headache, visual symptoms and jaw claudication** (most important questions to ask).

*He says he has had a **headache** for the last two weeks (and points to the right temple). He has never suffered from headaches before. His **scalp hurts when he combs his hair**. There is no pain on the left side of his head. He denies problems with his eyesight, double vision or pain in his jaw.*

The recent onset of headache, associated with scalp tenderness, is concerning. It is very likely that he has developed GCA. The most dreaded complication of GCA is **visual loss**, which may become irreversible, if not treated early. Visual loss occurs because of involvement of the central retinal artery and posterior ciliary arteries. Patients with GCA, without visual symptoms, should be commenced on 40–60 mg/day of prednisolone straightaway, even before the results of investigations are available and urgently referred to the rheumatologist. Those with visual symptoms should be commenced on a higher dose of oral prednisolone or intravenous pulse steroids and *referred to the ophthalmologist on the same calendar day.*

Patients with GCA may develop **double vision** or **jaw claudication** because of ischemia to the extraocular muscles and muscles of mastication, respectively. Rare complications of GCA include **stroke** (due to involvement of cerebral blood vessels) and **aortic aneurysm or dissection** (due to involvement of aorta).

- Complete the **rest of the history**.

Ask about his medical problems (particularly focusing on co-morbidities that would predispose him to adverse effects of corticosteroids), regular medications, smoking habit and alcohol consumption.

- Those who present with visual symptoms should **be asked if they drive** (very important).

*His medical history includes **type 2 diabetes, hyperlipidemia and benign prostate enlargement**. His regular medications are glipizide, metformin, linagliptin, atorvastatin and alfuzosin. His diabetic control has been poor, with the **most recent HbA₁c of 84 mmol/mol** (normal range 20–42), three months ago. He has never fractured a bone. He does not smoke. He drinks a glass of wine most evenings. He runs his own business and works three-to-four days a week. He drives a car. He lives with his wife.*

WHAT SHOULD YOU LOOK FOR ON EXAMINATION?

You should

- Ask for his **vital signs**.
- Palpate his **temporal arteries**, checking for thickening, tenderness and reduced pulsation.
- Record his **visual acuity** in both eyes separately, especially if there are visual complaints.

(Ask him to read something from a newspaper, magazine or booklet.)

- Examine his **hips and shoulders** to check the range of movements.

*His vital parameters are normal. Blood pressure is 122/82 mm Hg. His **right temporal artery is tender**, but pulsatile. The left temporal artery is pulsatile and non-tender. His visual acuity is normal. There is no restriction of shoulder or hip movements. The rest of the examination is unremarkable.*

HOW SHOULD THIS PATIENT BE INVESTIGATED?

You should request

- *Blood tests*, including full blood count, erythrocyte sedimentation rate (ESR) or C-reactive protein (CRP), liver function tests, serum creatinine, glucose, HbA_1c and vitamin D.
- *Temporal artery ultrasound* or *temporal artery biopsy* is the key investigation.

Where available, temporal artery ultrasound should be requested first. The characteristic ultrasound finding in GCA is a 'non-compressible halo' (caused by oedema around the vessel wall). If ultrasound service is not available, patients should be referred for temporal artery biopsy.

Note: If the pre-test probability is high and ultrasound is positive, GCA can be confirmed, and no further testing is necessary. If the pre-test probability is low and ultrasound is negative, GCA can be excluded. If the pre-test probability is high and the ultrasound is negative or *vice versa*, temporal artery biopsy should be requested.

WHAT SHOULD YOU TELL THE PATIENT?

You should tell him that

- His musculoskeletal symptoms are most likely due to polymyalgia rheumatica.

'I suspect you have developed a condition called polymyalgia. It affects people over the age of 50 and causes pain and stiffness of muscles around the shoulders and hips. We do not know what causes it'.

- The headache may be due to giant cell arteritis.

'I am concerned about your headache and wonder if this is due to inflammation of blood vessels in your scalp. This occurs in some people with polymyalgia'.

- You will arrange some blood tests and an urgent ultrasound scan of the temporal arteries.

'I'll ask for some blood tests and a scan of the blood vessels in your scalp. The scan will tell us if your headache is caused by inflammation of blood vessels'.

- You will speak to the rheumatologist (*'a specialist who deals with inflammation of blood vessels'*) and request an urgent appointment.
- He may need a temporal artery biopsy.

'Sometimes the scan may not show the inflammation clearly. In this case, the specialist might ask a surgeon to take a small piece of tissue from a blood vessel in your scalp to be examined under a microscope. This may not be needed if the scan clearly shows inflammation'.

- He should start treatment with steroids straightaway.

'I would suggest starting treatment with steroid pills straightaway. This inflammation could spread to blood vessels that supply the eye and potentially cause loss of sight. Steroid pills can rapidly control the inflammation and greatly reduce this risk'.

- Steroids can cause side effects.

'Steroids can affect the control of your blood sugar. It is therefore important that we closely monitor your blood sugar and adjust the treatment of your diabetes accordingly. Steroids can also raise your blood pressure, make you put on weight and cause thinning of the bones. The risk of developing these side effects depends on the dose of steroid and how long you take it for. The specialist might start you on other kinds of medications to get you off the steroid as soon as possible'.

- You will update him once you have seen the results of the scan and blood tests.

OUTCOME

The following results are obtained:

- Haemoglobin 122 g/L, white cell count 10×10^9/L and **platelets 598 $\times$ 10⁹/L**.
- **CRP 86 mg/L** and **ESR 76 mm/hour**.
- **HbA₁c 77 mmol/mol** (normal 20–42) and **plasma glucose 11.2 mmol/L**.
- Liver function tests show **alkaline phosphatase 187 IU/L**, GGT 57 IU/L. AST and ALT are normal.
- Serum creatinine 68 µmol/L.
- **Vitamin D 27 ng/mL** (normal >30).
- Ultrasound of the right temporal artery shows a **non-compressible halo**. Left temporal artery is normal.

 The ultrasound findings are in keeping with GCA. Given that the pre-test probability of GCA was high, there is no need to proceed with temporal artery biopsy. The elevated ESR and CRP, thrombocytosis and elevated alkaline phosphatase are in keeping with inflammation. There is evidence of poor diabetic control, which is likely to worsen further with corticosteroid treatment.

The rheumatologist finds no clinical evidence of involvement of extra-cranial arteries. All his peripheral pulses are normal, there are no bruits and blood pressure is the same in both arms. He starts him on 40 mg/day of prednisolone.

His headache and musculoskeletal symptoms resolved within two days. He suggests tocilizumab (monoclonal antibody that targets interleukin-6 receptor) so that he could rapidly taper the dose of prednisolone, given the risk of worsening diabetic control with prolonged steroid treatment. He starts him on a prophylactic dose of co-trimoxazole because of his increased risk of pneumocystis with a high-dose steroid, and 1000 units/day of vitamin D. He also arranges a bone density scan.

The 67-Year-Old Man with Back Pain **Case 7**

A 67-year-old man presents with a two-week history of back pain.

HOW SHOULD THIS PROBLEM BE APPROACHED?

Triaging is important to separate the vast majority of patients (about 93%) with ordinary or mechanical back pain from the few (about 7%) with a specific underlying problem (*see Box 7.1*).

BOX 7.1   SPECIFIC UNDERLYING CAUSES OF LOW BACK PAIN

- Cancer or infection.
- Axial spondyloarthropathy.
- Vertebral compression fracture.
- Prolapse of the intervertebral disc, cauda equina syndrome and spinal stenosis.

*He tells you that his back pain started two weeks ago. The pain is in the **middle part of his back*** (he points to the lower thoracic region). *Despite taking paracetamol and ibuprofen up to three times a day, **the pain is getting worse***. *He has never suffered from back pain before.*

Tell him that you are sorry to hear that he has been struggling with pain and explore his presenting complaint further.

- Ask about the *onset* and *progression* of the pain. Was there any *trauma to the back*?
- Is the pain localised to the back or *does it radiate down the leg(s)*?

If the pain radiates down the leg, ask about the character of the leg pain. Is the leg pain sharp and shooting and made worse by coughing or straining?

Note: Think of prolapsed intervertebral disc if the leg pain is sharp and shooting and made worse by coughing or straining. Mechanical back pain can also radiate to the legs, but this is usually a dull aching pain caused by muscle spasm.

- Are there any *neurological symptoms in the legs*, like weakness or numbness?

Note: Back pain with weak legs is a medical emergency. Spinal cord compression by tumour, abscess or tuberculosis are the usual causes.

DOI: 10.1201/9781003430230-7 31

- Any problems with control of his **bladder and bowels**?

Note: Urinary retention and faecal incontinence (from loss of anal tone) may be due to cauda equina syndrome (*see Box 7.2*). These patients should be referred to the neurosurgeon urgently, as permanent damage to sphincters can occur within a matter of hours.

BOX 7.2   FEATURES OF CAUDA EQUINA SYNDROME

- Retention of urine (the most consistent feature).
- Inability to feel the urine passing down the urethra.
- Loss of anal tone.
- Perineal anaesthesia ('*numb bum*').
- Bilateral leg pain.

- Are there any **exacerbating and relieving factors**?

Inflammatory back pain is typically worse with resting and better with activity, while mechanical pain is worse with certain postures and movements.

- Does he have **constitutional symptoms**, like fever, weight loss or fatigue?
- Is the pain affecting his **function or sleep**?

*He says the pain **began suddenly**. He is not sure what he was doing at the time. He is unable to recall any trauma or unusual physical activity prior to the onset of pain. The pain does not radiate down his legs, and there are no neurological symptoms. His bowel and bladder functions are intact. The **pain is more or less constant**, and there are no exacerbating or relieving factors. He has no pain elsewhere.*

*He has **lost about 7 kg** in the last three-to-four months. He always used to weigh around 70 kg but has now gone down to 63 kg. The weight loss is unintentional. He has **lost interest in food**. Of late, he has been **getting tired** very easily. He denies fever. He **struggles with his daily chores** and this **pain sometimes disturbs his sleep at night**.*

The story is quite concerning. There are several red flags (*see Box 7.3*), such as [a] older age (over 50 years), [b] the unintentional loss of about 10% of his body weight over a short span of time, [c] night pain and [d] progressively worsening pain that is unresponsive to analgesics. The tiredness is probably related to the underlying problem causing his back pain. Malignancy (e.g. metastatic deposits in the spine, multiple myeloma) or infection (e.g. tuberculosis) should be considered.

The sudden onset of pain suggests possible vertebral compression fracture. This is most likely a pathological fracture, as there is no history of preceding trauma. Cord compression seems unlikely because of the absence of neurological symptoms in the legs.

BOX 7.3   RED FLAG FEATURES IN PATIENTS WITH BACK PAIN[†]

- Age >50 years of age.
- History of malignancy.
- Unexplained weight loss.
- Unremitting or progressively worsening pain.
- Poor response to conservative measures.

[†] The likelihood of cancer is extremely low if none of these five features is present.

The next set of questions should explore the features that support a diagnosis of cancer or infection.

- A *review of systems* is essential.
- Obtain details of his *other medical problems*.

A previous diagnosis of cancer, history of fragility fractures or recurrent infection and tuberculosis contact history are particularly relevant.

Note: Fragility fractures and recurrent infection are features of multiple myeloma (*see Box 7.4*).

- Complete the *rest of the history*.

Ask about his regular medications, use of illicit drugs (increases risk of infection), smoking habit, alcohol consumption and occupation.

Note: Three important risk factors for osteoporosis to consider in men are alcohol, corticosteroids and hypogonadism.

Review of systems is unremarkable. There is no history of previous cancer, recurrent infection or fracture. He had a colonoscopy at the age of 55 and was told that it was 'clear'. He has not knowingly been in contact with anyone with tuberculosis.

*His past medical history is largely unremarkable except for **hypertension**, for which he takes 10 mg of amlodipine daily. He has never smoked and drinks alcohol only socially. He has never used illicit drugs. He is a retired immigration officer. He lives with his wife.*

WHAT SHOULD YOU LOOK FOR ON EXAMINATION?

- Examine his *spine* to check for tenderness, deformities and restriction of movements.
- Look for *signs that may suggest cancer* (e.g. finger clubbing, lymph node enlargement, hard liver, splenomegaly and abdominal mass).

Neurological examination of the legs is only indicated in those with radicular or neurological symptoms and could be abbreviated or omitted if the pain is confined to the back.

*He **looks tired** and **in some discomfort**. There is **tenderness at the level of the lower thoracic spine**, but there are no deformities. Spinal movements are not restricted. A brief neurological examination of the legs reveals normal power and sensation throughout. The rest of the examination is normal.*

HOW SHOULD THIS PATIENT BE EVALUATED FURTHER?

You should initially request

- *Plain radiographs of thoracic spine*.
- *Chest X-ray*.
- *Blood tests*, including full blood count, ESR, liver function tests, serum creatinine and electrolytes, calcium and phosphate, prostate-specific antigen and myeloma screen.

Depending on the results of the above tests, MRI scan of the thoracic spine *or* CT scan of the thorax, abdomen and pelvis should be considered.

WHAT SHOULD YOU TELL THE PATIENT?

You should tell him that

- You will prescribe stronger analgesia.

'I'll give you something stronger for the pain. It'll hopefully also help you get some sleep'.

- The back pain may be due to a fracture.

'I wonder whether you have broken a bone in your spine. I'll ask for an X-ray of your backbone to confirm this'.

- The back pain, weight loss and recent onset of tiredness may be due to an underlying medical problem.

'I am concerned that you have lost so much weight in the last few months. I'll ask for some blood tests first. I would like to get a scan of your backbone once I have seen the X-rays and blood test results. These tests will hopefully tell us why your back hurts and also why you have lost weight'.

- You would suggest admission to hospital.
- You will come back and talk to him once you have seen the results of the tests.

OUTCOME

- Plain X-ray of the thoracic spine shows a **vertebral compression fracture at T12**.
- **Haemoglobin 104 g/L**, MCV 85 fl, white cell count 4.2×10^9/L and platelet count 218×10^9/L.
- **ESR 86 mm/hour**.
- Liver enzymes normal. **Serum total protein 86 g/L** (normal 60–80) and **serum albumin 31 g/L** (normal 35–50).
- **Serum creatinine 168 μmol/L** (normal range 70–120).
- **Serum corrected serum calcium 2.94 mmol/L** (normal 2.2–2.7).
- Serum phosphate 1.22 mmol/L (normal 1.1–1.45).
- Prostate-specific antigen 1.6 ng/mL (normal <4).
- Myeloma screen pending.

 Plain X-ray of the thoracic spine has confirmed our suspicion of vertebral compression fracture. There are several abnormal results, including normocytic anaemia, elevated ESR, renal impairment, hypercalcemia, elevated total protein and low serum albumin. These results point to multiple myeloma (*see Box 7.4*). He should be referred to the haematologist urgently.

BOX 7.4   AN OVERVIEW OF MULTIPLE MYELOMA

Plasma cells produce immunoglobulins. There are five classes of immunoglobulin: IgG, IgM, IgD, IgA and IgE. Each immunoglobulin molecule consists of two heavy and two light chains. There are five types of heavy chains (γ, μ, δ, α and ε) and two types of light chains (κ and λ). Each individual plasma cell produces only one type of immunoglobulin, with any one of the five heavy chains and one of the two light chains.

In multiple myeloma, there is *monoclonal proliferation of plasma cells,* which results in excess production of one type of immunoglobulin, usually IgG, IgD or IgA. This is different from poly-clonal proliferation of plasma cells that occurs in infection or inflammation, where multiple clones of plasma cells produce different types of immunoglobulins.

The screening tests for myeloma (serum protein electrophoresis and serum-free light chains) essentially look for evidence of monoclonal proliferation of plasma cells.

■ *Serum protein electrophoresis* (SPEP)

The excess production of one type of immunoglobulin results in the appearance of a thick band on SPEP (known as the 'M' band, where 'M' stands for monoclonal). If the 'M' band is seen, the lab will proceed to do immunofixation to identify the type of immunoglobulin (the abnormal immu-noglobulin is known as paraprotein).

■ In some patients, myeloma cells only produce a part of the immunoglobulin molecule (either the heavy or light chain) *or* do not secrete any immunoglobulin at all.

Hence, *serum-free light chains* should also be measured. This is reported as kappa/lambda ratio (range 0.26–1.65). A kappa/lambda ratio >1.65 would suggest predominant production of kappa light chains, and a ratio <0.26 would suggest predominant production of lambda light chains. In inflam-mation, both kappa and lambda light chains are produced in excess, so the ratio would be normal.

Several other laboratory or radiographic abnormalities are also seen in myeloma:

■ *High ESR* because of elevated immunoglobulin.

(Immunoglobulins and fibrinogen cause sedimentation of erythrocytes.)

■ *Bone osteolysis* ('holes in the bones') because of osteoclast stimulation by myeloma cells.

A full skeletal survey (either plain X-rays or limited radiation CT scan of the long bones, skull, ribs and pelvis) should be requested to check for osteolysis.

■ *Hypercalcemia* because of stimulation of osteoclasts, which leads to release of calcium from the bones into blood.
■ *Renal impairment*, secondary to the direct toxic effect of light chains on renal tubules, hypercalcemia or hyperviscosity.
■ *Pancytopenia* because of myeloma cells taking up the bone marrow space and reducing the production of normal blood cells.

(CRAB is the acronym for high serum calcium, renal impairment, anaemia and bone osteolysis.)

■ *Immune paresis* occurs because the production of one type of immunoglobulin by myeloma cells suppresses the production of other types of immunoglobulin, thus increasing the risk of infection (e.g. suppression of IgA and IgM in patients with IgG myeloma).

In summary, myeloma is diagnosed based on (a) the 'M' band on SPEP and/or abnormal kappa/lambda ratio, (b) evidence of CRAB and (c) immune paresis. A ***bone marrow biopsy*** is necessary to confirm the diagnosis of myeloma. Serum ***β2 microglobulin*** level is useful for prognostication (higher levels are associated with poorer outcomes).

WHAT SHOULD YOU TELL THE PATIENT NOW?

You should tell him that

- The plain radiograph of the thoracic spine has confirmed the presence of fracture.

'The X-ray of your spine shows a fracture of one of the bones, as we suspected. This would explain your back pain'.

- The fracture may be pathological.

'Because you have broken this bone in the absence of any trauma to the back, I suspect your bones are weak'.

- The blood test results show anaemia, elevated ESR, renal impairment and hypercalcemia.

'I am still waiting for some more results, but the blood test results available so far show that your blood counts are low. The inflammation reading and calcium level are high. The kidneys are not working well'.

- You suspect that these abnormalities are due to a bone marrow problem.

'These results suggest that there could be a problem with the bone marrow, which is the inner part of the bone that produces blood cells. I suspect the bone marrow is producing some abnormal blood cells'.

- You would like to seek an urgent opinion from a haematologist (*'blood specialist'*).

*He is seen by the haematologist urgently. Myeloma screen shows **monoclonal production of IgG with elevated kappa/lambda ratio**. Further investigations, including serum immunoglobulin levels, skeletal survey and serum β2 microglobulin, are requested. The **bone marrow biopsy confirms the diagnosis of multiple myeloma**. The back pain gradually improves with narcotic analgesia. The haematologist plans to treat him with autologous stem cell transplant.*

The 38-Year-Old Woman with Widespread Pain and Tiredness

Case 8

A 38-year-old woman presents with a two-year history of widespread pain and tiredness.

HOW SHOULD THIS PROBLEM BE APPROACHED?

*She tells you that she is at the end of her tether. It **hurts all over** and no one seems to know what is wrong with her. She has **been suffering for the last two years** and during this time, she has consulted several doctors and they keep telling her that the test results are normal. She is frustrated that no one has been able to help her and says they probably don't believe her. She has tried painkillers and anti-inflammatory tablets, but they don't work.*

This is likely to be a difficult consultation because

- She is clearly very distressed and frustrated by her ongoing symptoms.
- The doctors who have seen her so far have not been able to provide a clear diagnosis.
- Analgesics and anti-inflammatories don't seem to be helping her pain.
- It may not be possible to explain her pain on the basis of a disease model.

The longer duration and widespread nature of symptoms reduce the likelihood of an underlying medical condition (*see Box 8.1*).

BOX 8.1   SOME ORGANIC CAUSES OF WIDESPREAD PAIN

- Inflammatory arthritis (e.g. rheumatoid arthritis, seronegative spondyloarthropathy).
- Osteoarthritis.
- Autoimmune connective tissue disease (e.g. systemic lupus erythematosus, Sjögren's syndrome).
- Osteomalacia.
- Thyroid dysfunction.
- Statin therapy.
- Malignancy.

DOI: 10.1201/9781003430230-8

After saying a few reassuring words, you should

- Establish the *extent of pain*.

Ask if she has pain in the joints as well as muscles. If the pain is widespread, ask if there are *specific troublesome areas* (that may be amenable to local corticosteroid injection or physiotherapy).

- If her joints are painful, check for *inflammatory features* like swelling and prolonged early morning stiffness.
- Ask about *features that may suggest seronegative spondyloarthropathy* (e.g. psoriasis, inflammatory bowel disease, uveitis and inflammatory back pain).
- Ask about *extra-articular symptoms that may suggest connective tissue disease* (e.g. skin rashes, recurrent oral ulcers, dry eyes and dry mouth, Raynaud's phenomenon, muscle weakness and breathlessness).
- Ask if she has *constitutional symptoms* like fever, sweats and loss of weight or appetite.

*She says **all her joints and muscles hurt**. They feel 'bruised'. There are no specific areas that are more painful than others. Her joints have never been swollen, but they **feel stiff all day**. Her **mouth is always dry** and her **hands sometimes get cold**, but she denies fever, sweats and other extra-articular symptoms that one would associate with an autoimmune connective tissue disease. She has **gained about 4–5 kg in the last two-to-three years**, which she thinks is because she has become sedentary.*

The history does not suggest inflammatory arthritis or autoimmune connective tissue disease (the dry mouth and cold hands are non-specific). Her description is more in keeping with medically unexplained chronic pain, which is sometimes labelled as fibromyalgia. The pathogenesis of fibromyalgia remains elusive.

Pain occurs in patients with injury or inflammation (e.g. appendicitis, fracture or synovitis) because of peripheral nociceptor stimulation. The pain is proportional to tissue injury or inflammation. Treating the underlying problem that stimulates the nociceptors abolishes pain in such patients (e.g. appendicectomy, fracture reduction or intra-articular steroids). Patients with fibromyalgia, on the other hand, experience pain because of *central pain sensitisation*, which simply means that peripheral sensory input is augmented in central pain pathways through complex mechanisms. The pain, instead of serving a protective function, becomes the 'disease'. Patients experience pain in the absence of tissue inflammation (pain that is out of proportion to injury or inflammation), hyperalgesia (pain amplification) and allodynia (light stimuli are perceived as painful).

Patients with fibromyalgia nearly always complain that they feel tired all the time. This is most likely because of *physical deconditioning* and *fragmentation of deep sleep*. A *chronic stress state* with resultant hyperadrenergic tone causes functional somatic manifestations, such as muscular discomfort due to increased muscle tension, disturbed bowel and bladder function, cold hands and dry mouth. Additionally, patients often develop *unhelpful thoughts and emotions*, such as anxiety, depression and fear. The chronic pain, poor sleep, psychological disturbance and physical deconditioning keep aggravating each other and set up a vicious cycle.

The next set of questions should explore the features of fibromyalgia.

- Ask about her *sleep*. Even if she says she sleeps well, ask if she wakes up feeling refreshed.

If her sleep is disturbed, it might be worth looking for other potential causes for the sleep disturbance, like obstructive sleep apnoea, restless legs syndrome or carpal tunnel syndrome.

- Ask about her *past medical history*, particularly if she was diagnosed with other functional somatic problems in the past.
- Obtain a full *medication history*.
- Ask about her *family* and obtain details of her *occupation* and *social history*.

*She only gets a few hours of sleep at night and always **wakes up feeling groggy and unrefreshed**. She used to be reasonably active before but has **become sedentary** in the last two years. She has been troubled with **alternating diarrhoea and constipation** for the last four-to-five years. She says this was investigated with a 'camera test' and the result was normal. The specialist diagnosed irritable bowel syndrome and suggested mebeverine, but that did not help at all. She also gets a **headache** from time to time and her **periods have always been painful**.*

*She is on regular codeine, ibuprofen and the occasional diazepam at night to help her sleep. She does not smoke or drink alcohol. She lives with her husband and two children, aged 14 and 12. She used to work part-time in an office but **hasn't been to work for more than a year**.*

- Enquire about **psychiatric problems** such as depression, preferably a little later during the consultation, after some rapport has been established. Be tactful.

It is important to be tactful because the patient is otherwise likely to feel that her symptoms are being dismissed as psychological (*'These symptoms must be getting you down'* is better than directly asking *'Do you feel depressed?'*).

*She **becomes tearful** and says she **feels low**. She once again mentions that she believes there is something seriously wrong with her. She is hoping that you will do some tests, find out what the problem is and give her the right pills to take the pain away.*

 There are several pointers suggestive of fibromyalgia in this story (*see Box 8.2*).

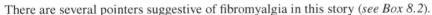

BOX 8.2   FEATURES OF FIBROMYALGIA

- The triad of chronic widespread pain, fatigue and non-restorative sleep.
- Other functional somatic symptoms, such as chronic headache, functional bowel disturbance and dysmenorrhoea.
- Psychological distress, and unhelpful thoughts, emotions and behaviours.
- Absence of clear evidence of an organic problem.

It is important to note that:

- Fibromyalgia is *not* a diagnosis of exclusion, so there is no need to not wait for other conditions that cause widespread pain or fatigue to be excluded before this diagnosis is considered.
- Fibromyalgia could co-exist with another rheumatic condition like rheumatoid arthritis (RA) or systemic lupus erythematosus (SLE), and complicate the presentation.

Thus, the presence of features suggestive of RA (e.g. synovitis, radiographic erosions, positive rheumatoid factor) would not exclude fibromyalgia. The pain in such patients would be expected to be out of proportion to any joint inflammation.

- The diagnosis of fibromyalgia generally becomes easier with longer duration of symptoms and presence of more suggestive features, but differentiating it from certain forms of rheumatic disease can be tricky.

For example, joint pain, tiredness, chest wall pain, cold hands, cognitive dysfunction, headaches and positive antinuclear antibody are common to both SLE and fibromyalgia.

WHAT IS THE ROLE OF PHYSICAL EXAMINATION?

You should

- Check for signs of ***inflammatory or degenerative joint disease*** and ***connective tissue disease***.

Note: The presence of Heberden's and Bouchard's nodes in the fingers or crepitus in the knees would not mean that all her symptoms are due to osteoarthritis. These findings may be incidental.

- Look for signs of ***regional pain problems*** in patients with specific troublesome areas (e.g. rotator cuff tendonitis or tenosynovitis).

Note: Allodynia (light stimuli being perceived as painful) and hyperalgesia (pain amplification) are features of central pain sensitisation.

*Examination is completely unremarkable except for **widespread non-specific muscular tenderness**. Even the slightest touch evokes a lot of grunting, sighing and moaning.*

WHAT INVESTIGATIONS SHOULD BE REQUESTED?

If not already done, a full blood count, erythrocyte sedimentation rate, thyroid function tests and vitamin D level could be requested.

Further investigations ('fishing expedition') should generally be avoided because it will only reinforce the patient's fear that *'something is seriously wrong and the doctor hasn't yet found out what the problem is'*. Indeed, none of the laboratory or imaging tests is specific for fibromyalgia.

WHAT SHOULD YOU TELL THE PATIENT?

Management of fibromyalgia is more of an art than science. The explanation should be tailored to the individual patient's expectations. In general, you should include the following points in your discussion and explain to her that:

- The pain is real. (Acknowledging this right at the beginning is important to get the patient on your side.)

'I don't want you to feel that we don't believe you just because the test results are normal. I can see that you are struggling, and I know you are not making up the pain'.

- Her presentation is not suggestive of some underlying medical condition.

'The pain is not due to a problem in your joints or muscles. This is the reason why painkillers and anti-inflammatory pills don't seem to work for you'.

- Her pain is due to central pain sensitisation.

'I believe that your pain is due to a problem with the way signals are carried in the nerves to the brain. We call this fibromyalgia. We do not know why exactly this happens. The headache, painful periods and diarrhoea could also be related to this'.

(Opinions may be divided on this, but despite the subjective nature of the illness, providing a diagnostic label might help the patient to get closure and equip herself with further knowledge through the internet or books. It would also help to stop the doctor from ordering unnecessary investigations or making further referrals.)

- Chronic pain differs from acute pain in that it is often accompanied by functional disturbance and psychological distress.

'When pain becomes long-standing, it affects your sleep and makes it hard for you to exercise. It makes you feel low and frustrated, which is only natural. But poor sleep, deconditioning and low mood can aggravate each other and make the pain worse. We should therefore try to not only reduce the pain, but also improve your sleep, fitness level and mood'.

- Further tests are not necessary.
- You would try a medication that targets the central pain pathways, but this alone will not help completely.

'Instead of giving you painkillers that work on the joints and muscles, I'd prefer to give you something that works on the nerves that carry pain signals to the brain. I'll prescribe a pill called amitriptyline, which you should take about 2–3 hours before you go to bed at night. This can also help to improve your sleep and make you feel fresh when you wake up. We can gradually increase the dose depending on how you respond, but pills alone are not enough to take the pain away'.

- She should start with some gentle exercises like walking and gradually build up her fitness. A physiotherapist can help with this.
- You would refer her to a psychologist for cognitive behavioural therapy.

'Our thoughts and beliefs can affect our emotions and behaviours in a positive or negative way. I can refer you to our psychologist. She can address some of the unhelpful thoughts and beliefs, which would help to alter the emotions and behaviours in a positive manner'.

- Improvement is certainly possible but will be a slow process. There is no quick-fix solution. Her active involvement is more important than any of the passive treatments that healthcare providers can offer.

OUTCOME

Her full blood count, ESR, thyroid function and vitamin D are normal. She is told that further investigations would not be helpful. She agrees to see a physiotherapist for a graded exercise program but declines a referral to the clinical psychologist.

She is prescribed 10 mg of amitriptyline to take at night. She is told that this could make her feel refreshed in the morning and improve her pain. Her GP is advised to gradually increase the dose of amitriptyline and add fluoxetine in the morning, in case of sub-optimal response. For pain relief, she is advised to wean herself off codeine and stop ibuprofen, and try tramadol instead, as this can help to reduce central pain transmission.

The 38-Year-Old Woman with Pain and Colour Changes in Her Fingers

Case 9

A 38-year-old woman presents with pain and colour changes in her fingers.

HOW SHOULD THIS PROBLEM BE APPROACHED?

- Ask **what exactly she means by 'colour changes'**.

*She tells you that her **fingers turn pale and become painful upon exposure to cold**. She must go indoors to warm her hands and the colour would then **turn red**, before slowly returning to normal after several minutes. If she is unable to get indoors in time, the fingers would become more painful and **turn blue or purple**. This has been occurring at least three to four times a week for the last three months. A few weeks ago, she developed an **ulcer on the tip of her right index finger**, but that is slowly healing.*

*She noticed **similar colour changes in her fingers during last winter as well**. She did not seek medical advice at the time, as the symptoms were not bad enough.*

 This patient is clearly describing symptoms that are consistent with Raynaud's phenomenon (RP). RP occurs because of spasm of digital arterioles. This is RP because

- Her symptoms are episodic.
- They are triggered by a drop in temperature.
- She is describing tri-phasic colour changes in her fingers.

The three colours represent [a] the reduction in blood flow because of vasospasm (white or pale) [b] stagnation of blood, resulting in accumulation of deoxygenated haemoglobin (blue or purple) and [c] hyperaemia, due to return of blood flow (red). Patients may not describe all three colours, but to diagnose RP, it would be useful if there is at least a bi-phasic colour change in the digits.

An additional helpful feature is the presence of a sharp line of demarcation separating the ischaemic and normal zones during an attack. Ask for **photographs taken during an attack**.

- Ask if her **symptoms are generalised or confined to only one limb**.

DOI: 10.1201/9781003430230-9

If colour changes only appear in one hand, especially in association with neurological symptoms, a local problem in the thoracic outlet should be excluded.

*Her symptoms occur in **both hands**. She has also noticed a bluish discoloration on the **tip of her nose and ear lobes**. She is not sure if similar colour changes have occurred in her feet.*

Having established that her symptoms are generalised, the next step is to decide whether this is **primary** (occurring on its own) or **secondary** (occurring in association with an underlying autoimmune connective tissue disease). Primary RP is a *functional* problem that only affects *thermoregulatory flow* (the flow that varies in response to a change in temperature), whereas secondary RP is a *structural* problem that also affects *nutritional* flow (the basic flow that is necessary to provide nutrition to tissues). Thus, digital tissue necrosis, ulcers and gangrene only occur in those with secondary RP. The commonest cause of secondary RP is systemic sclerosis (*see Figure 9.1*).

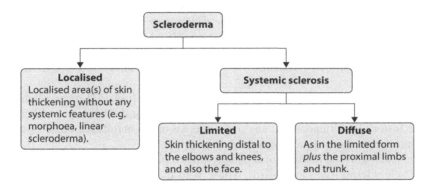

FIGURE 9.1   Classification of scleroderma.

Patients with systemic sclerosis may develop internal organ manifestations, such as [a] pulmonary hypertension, [b] interstitial lung disease, [c] renal crisis and [d] gastrointestinal tract involvement. These manifestations occur due to fibrosis and vasculopathy.

Further questions to ask:

■ Ask about **symptoms that may suggest an underlying connective tissue disease**, particularly scleroderma (*see Box 9.1*).
■ What **medications** does she take?

Drugs like β-blockers and ergot can cause vasoconstriction. Also ask if she takes the oral contraceptive pill or uses illicit drugs like cocaine.

■ Does she **smoke**?
■ What is her **occupation**?

Check if this involves the use of vibrating tools or exposure of hands to cold. The use of vibrating tools is associated with unilateral Raynaud's, usually on the dominant side.

■ Is there a **family history** of similar problems?

Up to half of those with primary RP may have a first-degree relative with a similar problem.

BOX 9.1   FEATURES THAT SHOULD RAISE THE SUSPICION OF AN AUTOIMMUNE CONNECTIVE TISSUE DISEASE

- Joint pain.
- Tightening of the skin (difficulty in making a fist or opening the mouth).
- Skin rashes (e.g. photosensitivity, telangiectasia).
- Dysphagia or symptoms of gastro-oesophageal reflux disease.
- Breathlessness (due to interstitial lung disease).
- Proximal muscle weakness.
- Sicca symptoms (dry eyes and mouth).

*Her **hands have been puffy** for the last six weeks. Her **joints generally hurt and feel stiff** but have not been swollen. She **finds it difficult to make a full fist** because of the puffiness. She is able to open her mouth fully. She has not noticed any skin rashes. She denies dysphagia, breathlessness, weakness in her limbs or sicca symptoms. She **smokes about 5–10 cigarettes/day**. She does not take any medication. She is not aware of anyone in her immediate family with autoimmune problems or similar symptoms. She works for a legal firm as an administrative assistant. She lives with her husband and two sons, aged 12 and 10.*

The [a] late onset of RP (primary RP usually begins much earlier in life), [b] history of ulcer in her index finger that is slow to heal and [c] puffiness of her hands suggest that the RP is most likely secondary to scleroderma. The history hasn't uncovered any overt internal organ manifestations of systemic sclerosis or other autoimmune connective tissue disease (*see Figure 9.2*).

Clinically, patients with the diffuse form usually present with RP, followed by development of the other features of scleroderma soon afterwards. Those with the limited form, on the other hand, often develop the features of systemic sclerosis, several years or even decades after the onset of RP. The limited form is also known as *CREST syndrome*, an acronym for *C*alcinosis, *R*aynaud's phenomenon, *E*sophageal dysmotility, *S*clerodactyly and *T*elangiectasia. The risk of interstitial lung disease and renal crisis is higher among patients with the diffuse form, whereas pulmonary hypertension is more common among those with the limited form. Occasionally, patients may present with internal organ manifestations alone, without skin thickening (*scleroderma sine scleroderma*).

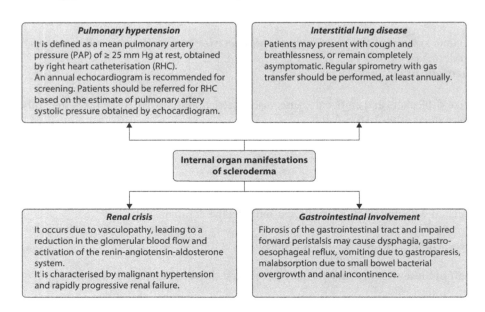

FIGURE 9.2   Internal organ manifestations of systemic sclerosis.

WHAT SHOULD YOU LOOK FOR ON EXAMINATION?

You should

- *Examine her hands* to look for evidence of sclerodactyly, telangiectasia and calcinosis.

In the early stages, the sclerodactyly is usually not evident and the hands may just be puffy, with a shiny appearance and loss of skin appendages.

- Check for signs of systemic sclerosis in her *face, trunk and legs*.

Facial features (usually seen in the later stages) include mask like facies, beaking of the nose, microstomia, peri-oral furrowing and telangiectasia.

- Check her *peripheral pulses*.
- Ask for her *blood pressure* (rising blood pressure should alert you to impending renal crisis).
- Listen to the *base of her lungs* for crackles and *heart sounds* for loud pulmonary component of the second sound.

Interstitial lung disease and pulmonary hypertension may be clinically silent, so it is important to request appropriate investigations to screen regularly.

*Both her **hands are puffy**, with a **shiny appearance** and **loss of skin appendages** over the dorsum. There is a tiny, healed **ulcer on the tip of her right index finger**, with no evidence of infection or gangrene. There is no synovitis, telangiectasia or calcinosis. All her peripheral pulses are felt. Facial features are normal, and there is no evidence of skin thickening in her trunk or legs. Her blood pressure is 116/72 mm Hg. Lungs are clear and heart sounds are normal.*

HOW SHOULD THIS PATIENT BE INVESTIGATED?

You should request

- *Blood tests*, including full blood count, liver function tests and serum creatinine.
- *Urinalysis*.

Note: Autoimmune conditions may cause anaemia, leucopenia and thrombocytopenia. In those with isolated RP, a full blood count may help to detect haematological conditions that cause hyperviscosity and sluggishness of the circulation (e.g. essential thrombocytosis, polycythaemia rubra vera). Urinalysis is important to screen for renal involvement, which may not be overt.

- *Anti-nuclear antibody* (ANA) and *antibodies to extractable nuclear antigens* (anti-ENA).

Note: A positive ANA result in a patient with isolated RP increases the likelihood of future development of scleroderma, while a negative result reduces the likelihood. The ANA result is irrelevant in this patient, as physical examination has revealed some early signs of scleroderma. Limited scleroderma is associated with anti-centromere antibody, and the diffuse form with anti-ScL-70 antibody.

■ *Pulmonary function tests* (with gas transfer) and *echocardiogram* to detect interstitial lung disease and pulmonary hypertension.

Note: A reduction in gas transfer may be secondary to interstitial lung disease or pulmonary hypertension.

WHAT SHOULD YOU TELL THE PATIENT?

You should tell her that

■ Her symptoms are due to Raynaud's phenomenon.

'I suspect the pain and colour changes in your fingers are due to reduced blood flow. This happens because of tightening of blood vessels when the outside temperature drops. We call this Raynaud's phenomenon'.

■ Her Raynaud's is most likely secondary.

'Raynaud's can occur on its own or it may be a sign of an underlying medical condition. Generally, the Raynaud's that occurs on its own starts at a very early age. The ulcer on the tip of your finger and puffiness of your hands suggest that your Raynaud's may be due to an underlying medical condition'.

■ The underlying medical condition is usually an autoimmune problem.

'Your immune system may be mistaking your own cells as foreign and attacking them'.

■ You would organise some blood and urine tests to look for evidence of an underlying medical condition.
■ She must stop smoking (very important.)

'I would strongly advise you to stop smoking because the harmful substances that are present in cigarettes could further reduce the blood flow to the fingers'.

■ She should try and avoid exposure to the cold.

'Make sure you wrap up warm when you are out in the cold. It might be a good idea to wear thermal gloves and socks. Do not handle frozen foods or anything cold with your bare hands'.

■ You would prescribe nifedipine to improve her symptoms.

'I'll prescribe a medication to improve the blood flow to the fingers. This medication may occasionally cause side effects like giddiness, constipation and swelling around the ankles'.

■ You would refer her to a rheumatologist (*'a specialist who deals with problems in the immune system'*).
■ You would give her an information booklet to read in the meantime.

'This booklet will explain more about Raynaud's and suggest a few tips on how to keep yourself warm'.

OUTCOME

The results of her investigations are as follows:

- Haemoglobin 128 g/L, white cell count 5.8×10^9/L and platelet count 276×10^9/L. ESR 26 mm/hour.
- Liver function tests and serum creatinine normal.
- Urinalysis normal, with no proteinuria, haematuria or casts.
- **ANA 1/160** and **anti-ScL-70 positive**.

She is seen by the rheumatologist urgently. He confirms the diagnosis of systemic sclerosis and explains this to the patient. Pulmonary function tests show FEV_1 82%, FVC 78% and DLCO 76%. 2D-echocardiogram is normal. She is advised to get a blood pressure machine and regularly check her blood pressure at home and also get a urine test on a monthly basis to detect renal involvement early. She is commenced on mycophenolate in the hope that this might slow down the progression of skin thickening, and omeprazole to reduce acid reflux. She is advised to continue taking nifedipine for her Raynaud's. The rheumatologist plans to monitor her closely.

The 65-Year-Old Man with a Painful Right Leg

Case 10

A 65-year-old man presents with a one-year history of pain in his right leg.

HOW SHOULD THIS PROBLEM BE APPROACHED?

---

*He tells you that his **right leg hurts when he walks**. It feels like a cramp. When his leg first **started hurting about a year ago**, he was able to walk for about 30 minutes before the pain forced him to stop. His **walking distance has since gradually reduced**, and he now gets pain after walking for just 10 minutes. The **pain abates if he stops for a few minutes**. He can then resume walking but has to stop again after walking another 10 minutes.*

 He gives a classical description of intermittent claudication (*Claudius* means limp in Latin). There are two types of claudication: vascular and neurogenic. Vascular claudication occurs because of narrowing of blood vessels supplying the legs, causing muscle ischaemia, while neurogenic claudication occurs because of narrowing of the spinal canal, causing pressure on spinal nerves. The spinal canal is spacious when the back is bent forward but becomes narrow when it is extended. Patients with spinal stenosis, therefore, report that pain is worse after prolonged standing (as the spine is extended) and better when they lean forward (e.g. while pushing a trolley in the supermarket or cycling). Typically, they relieve their pain by leaning forward.

Ask the following questions to ascertain if the leg pain is due to neurogenic claudication.

- Does he have **back pain**? Does the **leg feel weak or numb**
- Does he get **pain in his leg after standing for a long time**?
- What does he do when he gets pain? Does he tend to **lean forward**?

He denies back pain. His leg is not weak or numb. He only gets pain when he walks and not while resting or standing. He does not bend forward to relieve the pain.

 Although there are no features of spinal stenosis, this cannot be completely excluded at this stage. The other features of vascular claudication should be sought. Vascular claudication is most often caused by atherosclerosis. There are four key questions to ask in patients with suspected vascular claudication (*see Box 10.1*).

DOI: 10.1201/9781003430230-10

BOX 10.1   KEY QUESTIONS TO ASK PATIENTS WITH SUSPECTED VASCULAR CLAUDICATION

- What is the level of lesion (aortoiliac, femoropopliteal or distal)?
- What is the severity of disease?

This is based on the walking distance, rest pain and presence of leg ulcers or gangrene.

- Are there manifestations of atherosclerosis elsewhere (e.g. coronary, cerebral, renal, mesenteric)?
- What (modifiable) risk factors for vascular disease are present?

The extent of pain depends on the level of lesion. Aortoiliac disease presents with pain in the buttocks and thighs, and erectile impotence ('*Leriche syndrome*'), while femoropopliteal disease presents with pain in the whole of the calf, and distal disease with pain in the lower calves or foot (femoropopliteal occlusion only causes calf pain, as the thigh is supplied by the deep femoral artery).

As the vessels become progressively narrower, patients develop rest pain, leg ulcers and gangrene (*see Figure 10.1*). Patients with rest pain try to obtain relief by dangling the leg off the bed to improve circulation and their sleep is often disturbed at night because of this. Intermittent claudication, rest pain and gangrene could be equated to stable angina, unstable angina and myocardial infarction, respectively. Indeed, just like coronary artery disease, peripheral arterial disease (PAD) could be asymptomatic too.

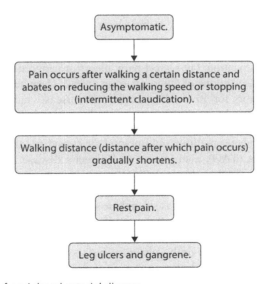

FIGURE 10.1 Progression of peripheral arterial disease.

Further questions to ask (*see Box 10.1*):

- Does he get ***pain in the left leg, thighs or buttocks***?
- Is he ***able to get an erection***? (Be tactful. Start with '*Would you mind if I ask you a sensitive question?*')
- Has he noticed any ***ulcers or blackish discolouration*** in the leg or foot?

Note: Arterial ulcers usually develop at the tips of the toes, heels or lateral aspect of the leg, as collaterals cannot compensate at these distal points. Venous ulcers, on the other hand, develop on the medial side of the leg, where venous pressure is higher.

- Does he get **chest pain on exertion** (angina) or **abdominal pain after eating** (due to mesenteric ischaemia)?
- Ask about **cardiovascular risk factors**, such as diabetes, hypertension, hyperlipidaemia, chronic kidney disease, smoking habit, and history of heart attack or stroke.

*He feels the **pain in the whole of his right calf**. He does not get pain in his left leg, thighs or bottom. His **erection hasn't been strong for many years**, but he put that down to his age and never sought medical advice. He has not noticed any ulcers or blackish discoloration in his leg or foot. He does not get chest pain on exertion or abdominal pain after eating.*

*He has been a **diabetic** since his late 40s. His most recent **HbA₁c was 66 mmol/mol** (normal 20–42), four months ago. He takes glipizide, metformin, atorvastatin and ramipril. He was told that his **kidneys were not working that well** and asked to take ramipril to reduce the protein in his urine. He goes for his eye checks every year and they have been fine so far. He has never had a heart attack or stroke. He has **smoked about 20 cigarettes/day** since the age of 20. He drinks a glass of wine once or twice a week. He used to work as a supervisor in a garments factory until three years ago. He lives with his wife.*

In summary,

- His symptoms are suggestive of vascular claudication.
- The lesion is likely to be at the femoropopliteal level (superficial femoral and popliteal arteries), as the whole of his calf is painful.

The problem with erection is probably due to his age or atherosclerosis and may not be due to lesion at the aortoiliac level, especially as there is no gluteal or thigh pain.

- He has intermittent claudication, but no rest pain, ulcers or gangrene.
- There are no *overt* manifestations of atherosclerotic disease elsewhere.
- He has several risk factors for atherosclerotic vascular disease, including older age, diabetes mellitus, hyperlipidaemia, chronic kidney disease and smoking habit.

Of these, advancing age, diabetes mellitus and smoking are considered the 'big 3' risk factors for PAD. Thromboangiitis obliterans (TAO), also known as Buerger's disease, is a differential diagnosis in patients presenting with chronic limb ischaemia. TAO causes segmental inflammation and thrombosis of small- and medium-sized arteries and veins, superficial thrombophlebitis and Raynaud's phenomenon, usually in the distal extremities of the limbs. It is strongly associated with use of tobacco products (including chewing tobacco). Patients are typically young men (<45 years), *without* risk factors for atherosclerosis. TAO is unlikely in this patient, as he is older and has risk factors for atherosclerosis. Embolic occlusion is the diagnosis not to miss in patients with limb ischaemia, but these patients present acutely with the 5Ps (pain, pallor, paralysis, paraesthesia and pulselessness) and not with long-standing intermittent claudication.

WHAT SHOULD YOU LOOK FOR ON EXAMINATION?

You should expose his legs adequately and carefully inspect the front and back of the legs and feet (including soles and web spaces between toes).

- Look for **ischaemic changes**, like pallor (especially when the limb is elevated), loss of hair, nail dystrophy, reduced capillary refill (>2 seconds is abnormal), coldness, ulcers and gangrene.

In patients with gangrene, you should note if it is dry (well demarcated and black) or wet (moist, swollen and blistering). Patients with wet gangrene should be referred to a vascular surgeon urgently.

- *Palpate the peripheral pulses*, including femoral, popliteal, dorsalis pedis, posterior tibial, radial, brachial and carotids.
- Check for *irregular pulse* (atrial fibrillation), and auscultate over the femoral and popliteal arteries for *bruits*.
- Ask for his *blood pressure*.
- Listen to the *heart for murmurs*.
- Test the *sensation and power* in the distal legs.

*He is **overweight**, with **body mass index of 31**. There is **tar staining** in the fingers. There is **loss of hair** and some **nail dystrophy** in the right leg. There are no ulcers or gangrene. Capillary refill is <2 seconds on both sides. There is no temperature difference between the two sides.*

*His **right popliteal, posterior tibial and dorsalis pedis pulses are barely palpable**. The rest of the pulses are normal. Rhythm is regular. There are no bruits. His **blood pressure is 138/88 mm Hg** in the right upper limb. Heart sounds are normal. There is normal sensation and power in the distal legs.*

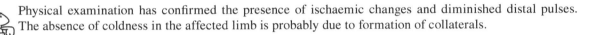

Physical examination has confirmed the presence of ischaemic changes and diminished distal pulses. The absence of coldness in the affected limb is probably due to formation of collaterals.

HOW SHOULD HE BE EVALUATED?

You should ask for

- *Blood tests*, including blood counts, renal function, glucose and HbA_1c.
- *Ankle-brachial pressure index* (ABPI).

ABPI compares the systolic pressure at the ankle (posterior tibial or dorsalis pedis artery) and the higher of the two systolic pressures in the arms (brachial artery). The blood pressure cuff is tied around the arm and leg, and the Doppler probe is placed over the artery. An ABPI of ≤0.9 is suggestive of PAD (*see Box 10.2*).

BOX 10.2   INTERPRETATION OF ABPI

≥1.4	Arterial wall stiffening due to calcification.
1–1.39	Normal.
0.91–0.99	Equivocal.
0.41–0.9	Mild-to-moderate peripheral arterial disease.
≤0.4	Severe peripheral arterial disease.

In patients with ABPI of ≥1.4 (indicates arterial wall stiffening due to calcification, in patients with advanced age, diabetes or chronic kidney disease), the *toe-brachial pressure index* (TBPI) should be measured, as toe vessels are less susceptible to developing stiffness. A TBPI below 0.7 is considered abnormal.

■ *Duplex arterial scan*.

It is called a Duplex scan, as it combines traditional ultrasound scan with Doppler. Doppler helps to see how well the blood is flowing along arteries. It is an excellent modality for screening and diagnosis of PAD. Duplex is not ideal for aortoiliac disease, as the gas in intestine is not a good conductor of sound.

Digital subtraction CT-angiography (DSA) provides high-resolution three-dimensional images and is considered the gold standard. Radio-opaque structures like bones are excluded (or subtracted) digitally from the image, thus allowing for an accurate depiction of blood vessels. It is generally reserved for patients who need endovascular intervention and those with suspected aortoiliac disease.

WHAT SHOULD YOU TELL THE PATIENT?

You should tell him that

- His leg pain is due to atherosclerotic narrowing of blood vessels.

'I suspect the blood vessels in your legs have become narrow because of fat deposition on their inner lining. Your leg hurts because when you walk, your calf muscles need extra blood, but the narrowed blood vessels are unable to provide this'.

- You would arrange a few investigations to assess the leg circulation.

'I'll arrange a few tests to confirm this. In one of these tests, we'll measure the blood pressure in your arms and legs. If the blood vessels are healthy, the pressure should be the same in the arm and leg. But if the blood vessels are narrow, the pressure in your leg will be lower. The pressure test will only broadly tell us if your blood vessels are narrowed. So once you have had the pressure test, I'll ask for a scan of your legs to find out which blood vessels are blocked'.

- He must stop smoking (most important advice).
- You would recommend low-dose aspirin (*'blood thinning medication'*).

Warn him about the risks of aspirin, particularly peptic ulcer and risk of bleeding.

- Cessation of smoking, better diabetic control and low-dose aspirin would help to reduce the risk of further progression and development of complications.

'If the blood vessels continue to narrow, your leg will start to hurt even when you are resting. In due course, this may lead to the formation of sores or ulcers in the leg. If the blood supply is completely cut off, the foot could turn black. You can greatly reduce the risk of developing these problems if you stop smoking. It is also important to control your diabetes better and take the blood thinning medication'.

- You would refer him to the physiotherapist.

'The physiotherapist will teach you some exercises, which will hopefully help to increase your walking distance'.

- You would refer him to the vascular surgeon.

'I'll refer you to a blood vessel specialist. If your pain continues to worsen, he might suggest an operation to improve the blood flow to the leg'.

OUTCOME

- His full blood count is normal, **e-GFR is 46** and **HbA$_1$c is 68 mmol/mol** (normal 20–42).
- The **ABPI is 0.7 in the right leg** and **0.9 in the left leg**. The **TBPI is 0.55 in the right leg**.
- Duplex scan confirms **narrowing of the superficial femoral, popliteal, posterior tibial and dorsalis pedis arteries in the right leg**.

He manages to quit smoking. He is referred to a diabetologist, who increases the dosages of his anti-diabetic medications and refers him to a dietician. He is also referred to a physiotherapist for supervised exercise program. The vascular surgeon adds pentoxifylline to low-dose aspirin. He decides to follow him in his clinic and offer surgery if symptoms continue to worsen.

The ABPI and TBPI readings and results of Duplex scan have confirmed PAD in the right leg at the femoropopliteal level. Management of PAD should include (a) cessation of smoking, (b) control of vascular risk factors, particularly diabetes, and (c) anti-platelet therapy. Single anti-platelet therapy (aspirin or clopidogrel) should be considered in all patients with symptomatic PAD, while dual anti-platelet therapy is reserved for those who undergo revascularisation. Pentoxifylline and cilostazol (phosphodiesterase inhibitor), which promote vasodilatation and improve blood flow, are useful in patients with symptomatic PAD. For patients who are unable to quit smoking, varenicline or bupropion can help to reduce cravings and symptoms of nicotine withdrawal.

A supervised exercise program can help to improve walking distance, hence the referral to the physiotherapist. Surgical options include angioplasty for short-segment occlusion, surgical bypass *or* amputation (in patients with gangrene).

The 24-Year-Old Woman with a Painful and Swollen Leg

Case 11

A 24-year-old woman presents to the acute medical unit with a two-day history of pain and swelling in her right leg.

HOW SHOULD THIS PROBLEM BE APPROACHED?

---

*She tells you that her **leg suddenly became painful and swollen two days ago**.*

Deep vein thrombosis (DVT) is the most important diagnosis to exclude in anyone presenting with unilateral painful and swollen leg. The main concern in patients with DVT is the risk of pulmonary embolism (PE). You should therefore first ensure that

- Her ***vital signs*** are satisfactory.
- There are no ***symptoms suggestive of pulmonary embolism***, like breathlessness, pleuritic chest pain or haemoptysis.

Her oxygen saturation is 98% on room air, pulse rate 68/minute, respiratory rate 16/minute, blood pressure 124/76 mm Hg and temperature 36.8°C. She denies breathlessness, chest pain or haemoptysis.

 Having ensured that her vital signs are satisfactory and there are no clinical symptoms of PE, the aim of clinical assessment is to stratify into high or low probability for DVT based on the presence of [a] risk factors for thrombosis and [b] features suggestive of other conditions that can present similarly (*see Figure 11.1*).

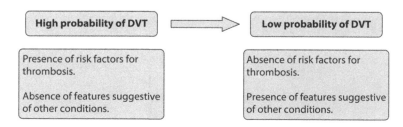

FIGURE 11.1 Assessing the probability of deep vein thrombosis.

DOI: 10.1201/9781003430230-11

- Check if there are *risk factors for venous thrombosis*, such as recent prolonged immobilisation, high oestrogen state or active malignancy (*see Box 11.1*).

BOX 11.1   RISK FACTORS FOR DEEP VEIN THROMBOSIS

- Recent prolonged immobilisation (e.g. major surgery, hospitalisation or confinement to bed for >3 days, long distance travel).
- High oestrogen state (e.g. pregnancy, combined oral contraceptive pill, hormone replacement therapy).
- Active malignancy, congestive heart failure and inflammatory bowel disease.
- Obesity (body mass index >30).
- Smoking habit.

- Look for *features that may suggest an alternative condition*, like fever (both cellulitis and DVT can present with fever), redness of the skin (cellulitis), knee swelling (ruptured Baker's cyst) and history of trauma to the leg.
- Ask if she has *previously been diagnosed with thrombosis* ('*blood clots*').
- Ask if there is *anyone in her immediate family with history of thrombosis*.

Note: A tendency to develop thrombosis because of hypercoagulable state is called thrombophilia. It may be inherited or acquired. Thrombophilia should be suspected if (a) thrombosis is unprovoked (i.e. it occurs in the absence of risk factors), (b) it is recurrent, (c) it occurs in an unusual site or (d) there is a positive family history (unprovoked thrombosis in a first-degree relative <50 years of age).

- Complete the *rest of the history*.

Ask about her past medical and surgical problems, regular medications, occupation, social, obstetric and menstrual history.

Note: The *obstetric history* is particularly important in women with unprovoked or recurrent thrombosis. In women with thrombophilia, there may be a history of recurrent pregnancy loss, premature delivery, intrauterine growth retardation or pre-eclampsia (due to placental insufficiency).

She denies fever, redness of the skin, preceding trauma to the leg or knee swelling. She works as a healthcare assistant in a private hospital and is normally very active. She did not travel anywhere recently. She started taking the combined oral contraceptive pill four months ago, just before she got married. She does not take any other medication. She has never been pregnant.

Her past medical history is blameless. She has not been diagnosed with blood clots before. There is no one in her immediate family with blood clotting problem, as far as she is aware. She does not smoke or drink. She lives with her husband.

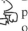

DVT is the most likely diagnosis. The recent initiation of oral contraceptive pill is relevant, as it may have provoked the thrombosis. It is possible that the contraceptive pill was the 'second hit' on a background of thrombophilia. There are no features to suggest an alternative diagnosis like trauma, ruptured Baker's cyst or cellulitis.

WHAT SHOULD YOU LOOK FOR ON EXAMINATION?

You should *examine the swollen leg* and check for

■ The extent of swelling and presence of pitting.

Her calf circumference should be measured at identical points on both sides, about 10 cm below the tibial tuberosity. A difference of more than 3 cm between the two sides is significant.

■ Redness, warmth and tenderness of the affected leg.
■ Presence of superficial collateral veins.
■ Signs of knee effusion (swelling and restricted range of motion).

Inspection of the right leg reveals **swelling of the whole leg**, *extending up to the level of mid-thigh. There is a* **difference of 4.5 cm between the two sides**. *There is no redness or warmth, but the* **leg is tender**. *There are no superficial collateral veins. Examination of the knee is normal. The left leg is normal. Rest of the examination is unremarkable.*

Based on the examination findings, the diagnosis must be presumed to be proximal DVT until proven otherwise. The pre-test probability of DVT can be estimated with the help of 'Well's criteria'. She would score 3 points ('DVT likely') because [a] the whole leg is swollen, [b] there is pitting oedema confined to the symptomatic leg and [c] there is a difference of >3 cm between the two sides (one point for each, adding up to a total of 3 points).

HOW SHOULD THIS PATIENT BE INVESTIGATED?

You should request

■ *Blood tests*, including full blood count, liver function tests, serum creatinine, prothrombin time (PT) and activated partial thromboplastin time (APTT).
■ *Urine pregnancy test*.
■ *D-dimer*.
■ *Venous ultrasonography* (DVT scan).

Both D-dimer and venous ultrasound are useful for risk stratification (*see Figure 11.2*).

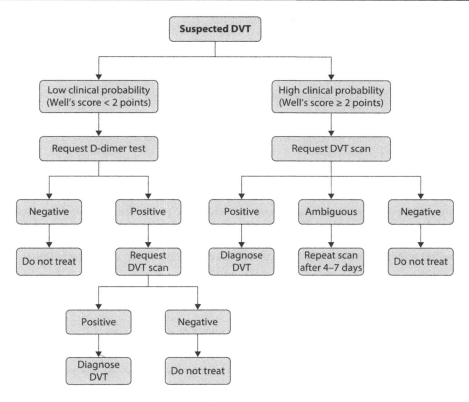

FIGURE 11.2   Simple algorithm for diagnostic approach to suspected DVT.

Notes:
1 A negative D-dimer would nearly exclude DVT because of its high negative predictive value. A positive result should however be followed by a DVT scan, as there are several causes for high D-dimer.
2 Venous ultrasound is >95% sensitive and 95% specific for diagnosis of proximal DVT.

WHAT SHOULD YOU TELL THE PATIENT?

You should tell her that

- Her leg pain is most likely due to DVT.

'I am keen to rule out a blood clot in your leg. A blood clot is a common reason for pain and swelling of the leg'.

- You would be requesting some blood tests and a DVT scan.

'I'll arrange for a scan of your leg. This will tell us if there is a blood clot. I'll also ask for a few blood tests'.

- You will start her on anticoagulant treatment if the scan confirms the thrombosis.

'If the scan confirms the blood clot, I would recommend a blood thinning tablet to take for at least three months'.

(If there is a delay in getting scan, she should be commenced on low molecular weight heparin straightaway, pending the results of the scan).

■ Anticoagulant treatment can reduce the risk of PE.

'There is a chance that the blood clot in the leg could break and travel to the lungs. The blood thinning medication can greatly help to reduce this risk'.

■ (She asks about the risks of anticoagulant treatment.)

'It can make you bleed more than normal, as your blood will not clot as easily. Your periods, for example, may become heavy or you may bleed for longer than usual if you cut yourself. I'll discuss this further once you have had the scan'.

■ She should discontinue the oral contraceptive pill.

'The contraceptive pill can make the blood sticky and increase the risk of blood clots. If the scan confirms the blood clot, I would advise you to stop taking it'.

■ You would refer her to a gynaecologist to discuss alternative forms of contraception.

'I'll then discuss alternative forms of contraception and refer you to a gynae doctor, if needed. This is particularly important because you should not get pregnant while you are on the blood thinning tablet'.

■ You will come back and talk to her once she has had the scan.

OUTCOME

■ Her haemoglobin is 132 g/L, white cell count 9.4×10^9/L and **platelet count 84×10^9/L**.
■ Liver function tests and serum creatinine normal.
■ PT normal. **APTT is prolonged at 62 seconds**.
■ Urine pregnancy test negative.
■ Venous ultrasound scan of right leg confirms the presence of **proximal DVT**.

Although her thrombosis was most likely provoked by the oral contraceptive pill, the low platelet count and prolonged APTT point to anti-phospholipid syndrome (APS), which is a form of acquired thrombophilia (*see Figure 11.3* and *Boxes 11.2* and *11.3*).

Inherited thrombophilia is less likely in the absence of a positive family history. There is no suggestion of malignancy or myeloproliferative disorder in the history or initial blood test results.

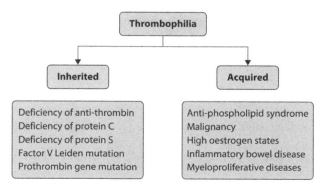

FIGURE 11.3   Classification of thrombophilia.

BOX 11.2   INHERITED THROMBOPHILIA

There are natural pro-coagulants and anticoagulants.

■ *Anti-thrombin* (AT) is a natural anticoagulant that prevents thrombin from needlessly converting fibrinogen to fibrin.

Hence, a deficiency of AT would lead to excess fibrin formation and hypercoagulable state.

■ *Factor V Leiden* (FVL) converts prothrombin to thrombin, while *protein C* and *protein S* keep breaking down the FVL.

In the presence of FVL mutation *or* deficiency of protein C or protein S, prothrombin gets converted to excess thrombin, leading to hypercoagulable state.

■ A *prothrombin gene mutation* (PGM) also has the same effect as FVL mutation, causing prothrombin to get converted to thrombin.

BOX 11.3   ANTI-PHOSPHOLIPID SYNDROME

Anti-phospholipid syndrome (APS) is characterised by (a) recurrent arterial or venous thrombosis, or pregnancy morbidity *and* (b) the presence of one or more of the anti-phospholipid antibodies. Arterial events usually occur in the cerebral territory, manifesting as strokes or transient isch-aemic attacks, while venous events commonly manifest as DVT or PE. Other manifestations of APS include thrombocytopenia, cardiac valvular vegetations and livedo reticularis. APS may be *primary*, when it occurs on its own, or *secondary*, when it occurs in association with systemic lupus erythematosus.

The anti-phospholipid antibodies (aPL) include the following:

■ *Anti-cardiolipin antibody* (aCL) IgM and IgG.

The aCL is an antibody that is either directed against a co-factor called $\beta2$ glycoprotein I ($\beta2$ GPI) that is bound to cardiolipin (cardiolipin is a phospholipid) *or* just cardiolipin alone. It is more specific when it is directed against both $\beta2$ GPI and cardiolipin.

■ *Lupus anticoagulant* (LAC).

The antibody with 'lupus anticoagulant activity' is directed against prothrombin plus phos-pholipid *or* $\beta2$ GPI plus phospholipid. The presence of lupus anticoagulant prolongs phospholipid-dependent coagulation assays like APTT.

■ *$\beta2$ glycoprotein I antibody* IgM and IgG.

The $\beta2$ GPI that is not bound to anti-cardiolipin can be detected by separately testing for $\beta2$ GPI (the anti-cardiolipin antibody test only detects the $\beta2$ GPI that is bound to cardiolipin).

The aPL should be persistently positive (at least twice ≥12 weeks apart) for the result to be con-sidered significant, as some infections and drugs may cause these antibodies to appear transiently.

*Her **aCL IgG and β2 GPI IgG are reported to be significantly positive**. The LAC is negative. The haematologist plans to repeat the aPL tests three months later to check if they are persistently positive.*

She reports no symptoms suggestive of systemic lupus erythematosus, and her ANA and anti-DNA are both negative, so if her aPL antibodies were to remain persistently positive after three months, she would be labelled as primary APS and given advice to continue the anticoagulant therapy long term. The anticoagulant of choice would be warfarin, as there is no evidence (as yet) for the benefit of novel oral anticoagulants in APS.

The 56-Year-Old Woman with Microcytic Anaemia

Case 12

A 56-year-old woman, who was previously in good health, presents with a three-month history of tiredness.

Her blood tests (done two weeks ago) show Hb 94 g/L with mean corpuscular volume 74 fl (normal 80–100). Her white cell and platelet count, liver, renal and thyroid function are normal. Her Hb was 131 g/L when it was last checked five years ago.

HOW SHOULD THIS PROBLEM BE APPROACHED?

*She tells you that she has been **feeling very tired** for the last three to four months. The tiredness is making it **difficult for her to manage the daily chores**. She works for a private bank and she has been **struggling at work** too.*

There are several causes for tiredness, such as chronic inflammation or infection, cancer, anaemia, thyroid disease, poor sleep, depression and deconditioning. Of these, it appears that her tiredness is most likely due to anaemia. Her anaemia is microcytic, as the mean corpuscular volume (MCV) is low. The red cells become smaller when there is a problem with production of haem or globin (*see Figure 12.1*).

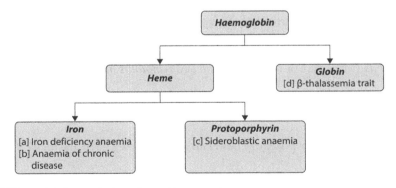

FIGURE 12.1   Differential diagnosis for microcytic anaemia.

Notes:
1 In patients with iron deficiency, the total amount of body iron is *reduced*.
2 In anaemia of chronic disease (e.g. rheumatoid arthritis, inflammatory bowel disease), increased production of hepcidin prevents the release of iron from storage sites to developing red cells. Here, the total body iron is *not reduced*.
3 Sideroblastic anaemia is caused by a biochemical block that prevents iron from combining with protoporphyrin (e.g. pyridoxine deficiency).

DOI: 10.1201/9781003430230-12

In this patient, β-thalassemia trait can be ruled out, as her haemoglobin was normal five years ago. Anaemia of chronic disease is unlikely, as she was previously healthy. Sideroblastic anaemia is very rare. Thus, her anaemia is most likely secondary to iron deficiency. Iron deficiency may result from reduced dietary intake of iron, reduced gastrointestinal absorption or increased loss (*see Box 12.1*).

BOX 12.1   CAUSES OF IRON DEFICIENCY ANAEMIA

■ *Increased loss.*

This is most commonly due to (a) gastrointestinal blood loss in men and post-menopausal women, or (b) menorrhagia in pre-menopausal women. Other possible sources of blood loss are hae-maturia (e.g. renal cell carcinoma), chronic epistaxis (e.g. hereditary haemorrhagic telangiectasia) and regular blood donation.

■ *Reduced dietary intake* (e.g. red meat, green leafy vegetables).
■ *Reduced absorption* (e.g. coeliac disease, Crohn's disease).

■ Ask about *other symptoms of anaemia*, such as dizziness or light headedness, palpitations, shortness of breath and ankle swelling.

Breathlessness, orthopnea and ankle swelling might point to cardiac failure secondary to anaemia.

Further questions should explore the features of possible underlying causes of iron deficiency. Ask about

■ *Symptoms that may suggest a gastrointestinal source of blood loss* (*see Box 12.2*), such as dysphagia, dyspepsia, weight loss, recent change in bowel habits, and melena or rectal bleeding.

Patients over the age of 50 should also be asked if they have been screened for colon cancer.

■ *Her regular medications* (particularly aspirin and non-steroidal anti-inflammatory drugs).
■ *Other sources of blood loss*, like epistaxis, vaginal bleeding, haematuria and regular blood donation.
■ *Dietary habits* (vegetarian or non-vegetarian) and *symptoms of malabsorption*.

Features of malabsorption include diarrhoea, bloating and wind (carbohydrates), oedema (protein), steatorrhea (fat), osteoporosis, peripheral neuropathy and weight loss.

■ *Previous surgeries*, *family history of bowel disease*, *smoking* habit and *alcohol* consumption.

Gastrectomy increases the risk of iron deficiency anaemia (hydrochloric acid in the stomach aids absorption of iron by converting the unabsorbable ferric form in the diet to absorbable ferrous form). Smoking increases the risk of peptic ulcer, while both smoking and alcohol increase the risk of oesophageal and gastric cancer.

BOX 12.2   GASTROINTESTINAL SOURCES OF BLOOD LOSS†

- Ingestion of aspirin or non-steroidal anti-inflammatory drug (NSAID).
- Oesophagitis or oesophageal carcinoma.
- Peptic ulcer disease.
- Gastric cancer.
- Coeliac disease.
- Colon cancer.
- Haemorrhoids.
- Angiodysplasia.

† NSAIDs are the commonest cause of iron deficiency anaemia. Gastric cancer, colon cancer and coeliac disease are the three diagnoses not to miss.

*She **feels lightheaded at times** but denies palpitations, shortness of breath or ankle swelling. She also denies dysphagia, dyspepsia, weight loss, change in bowel habit, steatorrhea, melena and rectal bleeding. She has **been taking diclofenac** about three to four times a week for the last one year to relieve her knee pain, which was diagnosed as osteoarthritis by a GP. She does not take gastro-protective agents. She denies epistaxis, vaginal bleeding and haematuria. She has never donated blood.*

She eats meat and green leafy vegetables. There is no one in her immediate family with bowel problems. She has never had a colonoscopy. She has not had any surgeries. She does not smoke or drink. She lives with her husband.

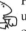

Her regular consumption of diclofenac for the knee pain is relevant. NSAIDs increase the risk of peptic ulcer and small bowel mucosal injury. The other causes of iron deficiency anaemia, particularly colon cancer, cannot be excluded at this stage on the basis of the history of NSAID ingestion, especially in someone of her age. There don't seem to be any pointers to suggest malabsorption or reduced dietary intake of iron.

WHAT SHOULD YOU LOOK FOR ON EXAMINATION?

There may be pallor of the palmar creases and mucous membranes, but the goal of examination in this patient is really to look for clues that may suggest an underlying cause of iron deficiency anaemia. You should

- Perform a **general examination**.

Look for telangiectasias in the nose and mouth (hereditary haemorrhagic telangiectasia), oral ulcers (Crohn's disease), buccal pigmentation (Peutz-Jeghers syndrome) and dermatitis herpetiformis over the extensor aspect of the elbows (coeliac disease). All these signs are rare.

- ***Examine her abdomen***.

Check for tenderness (e.g. peptic ulcer), mass (e.g. stomach or colon cancer) and organomegaly (e.g. palpable liver due to metastases).

- Examine the ***cardiovascular system***.

Signs of severe anaemia include tachycardia, ankle oedema and flow murmurs.

*Physical examination is unremarkable except for **conjunctival pallor**. Her abdomen is soft and non-tender, with no palpable mass or organomegaly. Cardiovascular examination is normal.*

HOW SHOULD THIS PATIENT BE EVALUATED FURTHER?

You should ask for

- ***Iron studies***, including serum iron, total iron-binding capacity, ferritin and transferrin saturation (*see Box 12.3*), ***serum vitamin B_{12}*** and ***folate***.

BOX 12.3   SERUM IRON, FERRITIN, TOTAL IRON-BINDING CAPACITY AND TRANSFERRIN SATURATION

Iron that is absorbed from the gastrointestinal tract is transported in the blood by *transferrin*. Two-thirds of iron is transported to the bone marrow for haemopoieses, and the remaining one-third to storage sites, where it binds to *ferritin*.

- ***Serum iron*** is low in both iron deficiency anaemia (IDA) and anaemia of chronic disease (ACD).

In IDA, total body iron is reduced, while in ACD, iron is sequestered inside cells.

- ***Serum ferritin*** is (a) low in IDA, as the total body iron stores are reduced, and (b) increased in ACD, as it is an acute phase reactant protein.
- ***Total iron-binding capacity*** (TIBC) is an indirect measure of transferrin.

Ferritin and transferrin have an inverse relationship, which means when ferritin is low, the liver produces more transferrin in an attempt to bind more iron and *vice versa*. Hence, TIBC is high in IDA and low in ACD.

- ***Transferrin saturation*** refers to the proportion of transferrin that is saturated with iron (serum iron/TIBC × 100).

Although the liver produces more transferrin in IDA, there is not enough iron, so the transferrin saturation is low. In ACD, the liver produces less transferrin, so transferrin saturation is normal.

If the patient is found to be iron deficient, you should

- Refer to the gastroenterologist for further evaluation, including ***upper and lower gastrointestinal (GI) endoscopies***.

Note: How far to investigate someone with iron deficiency anaemia depends on the age, sex and socio-economic background. Endoscopies may be appropriate for this patient, but not for a young girl from a deprived background living in a third-world country, in whom the anaemia is likely to be secondary to poor dietary intake of iron or hookworm infection.

- Request ***screening test for coeliac disease***, either tissue transglutaminase antibody *or* anti-endomysial antibody (especially if the iron deficiency anaemia is unexplained).

Ask for serum IgA at the same time, as coeliac antibodies are IgA, and those with IgA deficiency may have a falsely negative coeliac screen.

■ Test her *urine for red blood cells (RBCs)* (to screen for renal cell carcinoma).

Haemoglobin electrophoresis is the investigation of choice to diagnose β-thalassemia trait. A normal haemoglobin molecule consists of two α and two β chains (α2 β2). In β-thalassemia trait, there is absence of β chains, which leads to increased production of HbA$_2$ (α2 δ2) and foetal haemoglobin (α2 ϒ2). Hb electrophoresis helps to detect the increased HbA$_2$ and HbF.

The RBC count and red cell distribution width (RDW) are also useful to differentiate iron deficiency anaemia and β-thalassemia trait.

■ In iron deficiency, fewer red cells are produced because of lack of iron, but in β-thalassemia trait, the red cell count is usually normal.

■ RDW refers to variation in the size and shape of RBCs (higher the RDW, more the variation). In iron deficiency, RDW is high because successive batches of new red cells become progressively smaller in size as the limited supply of iron gets used up. In β-thalassemia trait, RDW is normal, as the red cells are uniform in size.

WHAT SHOULD YOU TELL THE PATIENT?

You should tell her that

■ Her tiredness is most likely due to anaemia.

'The blood tests that you had two weeks ago show that you are anaemic. This is probably the reason why you feel so tired. Anaemia simply means that your haemoglobin level is low. Haemoglobin is the blood protein that helps to carry oxygen around'.

■ Her anaemia is most likely due to iron deficiency.

'I suspect you are anaemic because of a lack of iron. I'll ask for a few blood tests to confirm this'.

■ The iron deficiency is possibly due to gastrointestinal blood loss.

'When you bleed, you lose iron from the body. It is possible that you are bleeding from your stomach or bowel. If there is only a tiny amount of oozing, you may not notice blood in the stool, but if this bleeding continues for a long time, a large amount of iron can be lost, leading to anaemia'.

■ She should stop taking diclofenac (this is a key advice) and try simple painkillers like paracetamol and/or a topical anti-inflammatory agent for the knee pain instead.

'Diclofenac can cause ulcers in the stomach, and these ulcers can bleed. I would suggest that you stop taking the diclofenac straightaway. For your knee pain, I'll prescribe paracetamol tablets and an anti-inflammatory plaster to apply over the knee'.

■ Other causes of iron deficiency are still possible, and it would be advisable for her to undergo further evaluation.

'I'll refer you to a bowel specialist because it is important to check if there are other possible reasons for your anaemia. He might suggest passing a camera through the upper and lower ends to look inside your stomach and bowel'.

- You would prescribe iron pills to improve her iron levels in the meantime, but this alone is not sufficient.

'I'll prescribe iron pills to take in the meantime, while we try and find out why you are losing iron'.

- Warn her about the side effects of iron therapy.

'Your stools may turn black when you start taking iron. It may cause tummy discomfort and constipation, but most people do not experience any side effects'.

OUTCOME

---

*Her **serum iron is 37 µg/dL** (normal range 50–170), **total iron-binding capacity 460 µg/dL** (normal range 250–370), **serum ferritin 6 ng/mL** (normal range 12–150) and **transferrin saturation 8%** (normal 15–50) in keeping with iron deficiency anaemia. Serum B$_{12}$ and folate are normal.*

*Urinalysis is normal, with no RBCs. She discontinues diclofenac and tries paracetamol and topical ketoprofen for her knee pain. She is prescribed ferrous sulphate and referred to the gastroenterologist. Upper GI endoscopy shows **gastric erosions**. The CLO test is positive for **Helicobacter pylori**, so she is treated with triple therapy. Colonoscopy is normal.*

The 38-Year-Old Woman with Macrocytic Anaemia

Case 13

A 38-year-old woman presents with a four-week history of tiredness.

Her haemoglobin is 46 g/L, mean corpuscular volume 118 fl (normal 75–96), white cell count 8.1×10^9/L and platelet count 368×10^9/L. Her liver and renal function, serum ferritin, vitamin B_{12}, folate and thyroid stimulating hormone are normal. Previous blood test results are unavailable.

HOW SHOULD THIS PROBLEM BE APPROACHED?

---

*She tells you that she has been feeling **very tired** and **lightheaded** for the last four to five weeks. She denies shortness of breath, palpitations, chest pain or ankle swelling.*

Her vital parameters are satisfactory, with pulse rate 84/minute, blood pressure 118/74 mm Hg, respiratory rate 16/minute, oxygen saturation 98% on room air and temperature 35.9°C.

Her tiredness and light headedness are most likely due to severe anaemia. Severe anaemia is generally due to bone marrow failure, blood loss or haemolysis (*see Figure 13.1*).

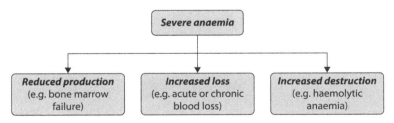

FIGURE 13.1 Classification of the causes of severe anaemia.

The differential diagnosis can be narrowed based on the high mean corpuscular volume (*see Box 13.1*).

Vitamin B_{12} and folate deficiency can be excluded on the basis of her blood test results. Acute blood loss need not be considered, as her symptoms began more than a month ago. Although chronic blood loss may co-exist with another cause of anaemia, the normal serum ferritin would make this less likely. A bone marrow problem is also unlikely, as her white cell and platelet counts are normal. Haemolytic anaemia, therefore, seems the most likely diagnosis.

DOI: 10.1201/9781003430230-13

BOX 13.1   CAUSES OF HIGH MCV†

- Vitamin B_{12} and folate deficiency.
- Haemolytic anaemia.
- Aplastic anaemia or myelodysplasia.
- Alcohol.
- Hypothyroidism.

† Vitamin B_{12} and folate are essential for synthesis of DNA, so their deficiency leads to delayed nuclear maturation in the haematopoietic precursor cells. Cytoplasmic maturation proceeds normally, as protein synthesis is unaffected. The asynchrony between nuclear and cytoplasmic maturation allows the cell to grow larger, as cell division cannot happen until nuclear maturation is complete.

† In haemolytic anaemia, the high MCV is due to the presence of large-sized red cell precursors like reticulocytes in the peripheral blood. There are more reticulocytes because of increased bone marrow erythropoiesis in response to premature destruction of red blood cells.

† Red cells become larger in conditions that cause 'sluggishness of the bone marrow' (e.g. aplastic anaemia, myelodysplasia, alcohol-induced bone marrow suppression or hypothyroidism).

- Ask if she has noticed *yellowing of the skin or eyes*.

Note: Jaundice occurs in haemolytic anaemia because of increased unconjugated bilirubin, but not all patients may report this (*see Figure 13.2*). The jaundice is usually a light lemon-yellow tinge.

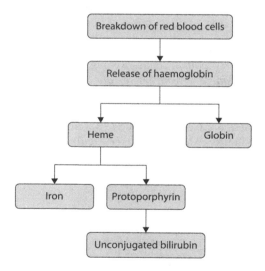

FIGURE 13.2   Jaundice in patients with haemolysis.

*She says her friends and husband have recently been telling that her **eyes look yellow**. There is no change in the colour of her urine or stools.*

The yellowing of sclera points to haemolytic anaemia, especially as her liver function tests are normal. Congenital haemolytic anaemias (e.g. thalassemia, hereditary spherocytosis) are unlikely, as they would not present for the first time at the age of 38. Her haemolytic anaemia is most likely due to immune or acquired non-immune cause (*see Figure 13.3*). A thorough review of systems is essential in order to look for a possible underlying cause of haemolytic anaemia (e.g. drugs, infection, haematological malignancy and autoimmune disease).

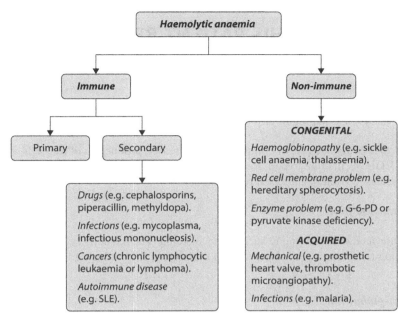

FIGURE 13.3   Overview of the causes of haemolytic anaemia.

Review of systems is unremarkable. In particular, she denies fever, sweats, recent illnesses, weight loss, swelling in her neck, armpits and groins, joint pain and skin rashes.

Her medical history is unremarkable. She does not take any medication. She has never had any surgeries. She has not travelled anywhere recently. The relevant family history is unremarkable. She has never been pregnant. Her menses are regular. She does not smoke or drink. She lives with her husband and works as a librarian.

WHAT SHOULD YOU LOOK FOR ON EXAMINATION?

You should perform a general examination and particularly check for:

- Evidence of *icterus* in the sclerae.
- *Lymphadenopathy, hepatomegaly and splenomegaly.*
- *Signs of autoimmune disease* (e.g. synovitis, skin rashes).

*There is evidence of **conjunctival pallor** and **lemon-yellow tinge in her sclerae**. The **spleen is palpable** about three fingerbreadths below the left costal margin. There is no hepatomegaly or lymphadenopathy. Rest of the examination is unremarkable.*

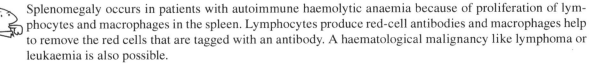

Splenomegaly occurs in patients with autoimmune haemolytic anaemia because of proliferation of lymphocytes and macrophages in the spleen. Lymphocytes produce red-cell antibodies and macrophages help to remove the red cells that are tagged with an antibody. A haematological malignancy like lymphoma or leukaemia is also possible.

HOW SHOULD THIS PATIENT BE INVESTIGATED?

You should request

- ■ *Tests to look for evidence of haemolysis*, including reticulocyte count, bilirubin, lactate dehydrogenase (LDH) and haptoglobin.

Note: Reticulocytosis occurs because of compensatory increased production of red cells by the bone marrow. Elevation of LDH occurs due to cell breakdown. Haptoglobin becomes depleted because it binds to the haemoglobin released from haemolysed red cells.

- ■ *Peripheral blood film*.

Spherocytes are seen in autoimmune haemolytic anaemia. The red cells become spherical because of the immune reaction removing a part of the red cell membrane, thus reducing the red cell surface area to volume ratio.

- ■ *Direct anti-globulin test*.

The direct anti-globulin test detects *autoantibodies* that are bound to red cell antigens *on the surface of the red cell*. Red cell agglutination occurs when the patient's serum (which contains red cells, with autoantibodies on their surface) is mixed with Coomb's reagent (which contains anti-human globulin).

- ■ *Anti-nuclear antibody* (screening test for SLE.)
- ■ *Group and save* (in anticipation of the need for blood transfusion.)
- ■ *CT scan of the neck, thorax, abdomen and pelvis* to check for evidence of haematological malignancy (e.g. cervical, intra-thoracic or intra-abdominal lymphadenopathy, splenomegaly and hepatomegaly).

WHAT SHOULD YOU TELL THE PATIENT?

You should tell her that

- ■ She is tired because of anaemia.

'Your blood tests show that you are anaemic. This is probably the reason why you feel so tired. Anaemia simply means that haemoglobin level is low. Haemoglobin is the protein in blood cells that helps to carry oxygen around'.

- ■ Her anaemia could be secondary to haemolysis.

'I suspect your blood cells are getting destroyed prematurely. This may be due to the immune system mistakenly attacking your blood cells. Your eyes look yellow because of a pigment that is released from blood cells when they get destroyed'.

- ■ Further investigations are necessary.

'I would like to ask for a few more blood tests. These tests will tell us if your blood cells are getting destroyed prematurely. I'll also arrange a scan of your chest and tummy to look for medical conditions that can cause premature destruction of the blood cells'.

■ She needs admission to hospital for blood transfusion.

'I would recommend blood transfusion to temporarily increase your haemoglobin and make you feel better'.

■ You will discuss the next steps once the blood test results are back.
■ You would refer her to a haematologist. Treatment of her anaemia depends on the cause.

'I'll ask a blood specialist to see you once the results of the tests are available. The specialist will start you on appropriate treatments depending on the results of these tests'.

OUTCOME

The results of her investigations are as follows:

■ **Reticulocytes 14.8%** (normal range 0.5–1.5%).
■ **Bilirubin 46 μmol/L** (normal <17). Liver enzymes normal.
■ **Haptoglobin <0.08 g/L** (normal range 0.35–2.50).
■ **LDH 544 U/L** (normal range 125–220).
■ Peripheral blood film shows **macrocytic red cells, spherocytes** and **reticulocytes**. The white blood cells and platelets are normal.
■ **Direct anti-globulin test positive**.
■ ANA negative.
■ Urine pregnancy test negative.
■ CT scan of the neck, thorax, abdomen and pelvis shows **moderate splenomegaly** but is otherwise unremarkable.

The reticulocytosis, hyperbilirubinemia, low haptoglobin and elevated LDH are in keeping with haemolysis. The presence of spherocytes and positive direct anti-globulin test point to an autoimmune process. The negative ANA makes it extremely unlikely that her haemolytic anaemia is due to SLE. An underlying leukaemia or lymphoma is unlikely, as CT scan of the neck, thorax, abdomen and pelvis is normal and there are no abnormal cells on the peripheral blood film. From the history, we have already ruled out medication-induced haemolysis and there are no clues to a possible infectious aetiology. Her autoimmune haemolytic anaemia is therefore most likely idiopathic.

The haematologist commences high-dose prednisolone, folic acid (to support the haemopoiesis), vitamin D and co-trimoxazole (as prophylaxis against pneumocystis). The patient initially declines blood transfusion but agrees to this, two days later, when the haemoglobin drops further to 39 g/L. Her bone density scan shows T scores of 0 and +0.2 in her lumbar spine and left femoral neck, respectively. Her fasting glucose is 5.2 mmol/L.

Her haemoglobin gradually improves to 112 g/L over the next few days. The haematologist arranges to follow her in the clinic and gradually taper the dose of her prednisolone.

The 27-Year-Old Woman with Thrombocytopenia

Case 14

A 27-year-old woman presents to the emergency department with menorrhagia.

Her blood tests show haemoglobin 122 g/L, white cell count 8.4×10^9/L and platelet count 26×10^9/L. Liver function tests, serum creatinine and peripheral blood film are normal. No previous blood test results are available for comparison.

HOW SHOULD THIS PROBLEM BE APPROACHED?

*She tells you that her **menses is heavy** and hasn't stopped even after seven days. She **feels exhausted**. Her menses usually lasts only four days at the most and it has never been so heavy.*

After introducing yourself, explain to her that her platelet count is low (the focus of this consultation is the low platelet count, *not* the menorrhagia): *'The blood tests done just now show that your platelets are reduced in number. Platelet is a type of blood cell that helps the blood to clot, so not having enough platelets can make you bleed more easily. I hope you won't mind if I ask you a few questions and quickly examine you. I'll then try and explain why your platelet count might be low and what we can do about it'.*

- First ensure that (a) her ***vital parameters*** are satisfactory and (b) she is not ***bleeding from any other site***.

Ask about epistaxis, bleeding from gums, haemoptysis, hematemesis, rectal bleeding and haematuria. Although major bleeding (e.g. intra-cranial or intra-abdominal) is uncommon, it would be prudent to screen for neurological and abdominal symptoms.

Note: Although thrombocytopenia is defined as platelet count below 150×10^9/L, patients seldom bleed spontaneously unless the platelet count drops below $10–20 \times 10^9$/L.

Her vital signs are satisfactory. She is alert and oriented. She denies epistaxis, bleeding from gums, haemoptysis, haematemesis, rectal bleeding, haematuria, neurological symptoms or abdominal pain.

 Although no previous blood test results are available for comparison, the short history of menorrhagia suggests that her platelet count might have dropped recently.

In some patients, thrombocytopenia may be artefactual. This occurs when the platelet count is checked with an ethylene diamine tetra acetic acid (EDTA) sample. The apparent lowering of platelet

DOI: 10.1201/9781003430230-14

count is due to *in vitro* platelet clumping, which prevents all the platelets from being counted. If this is suspected, the full blood count should be repeated with a citrate sample. The thrombocytopenia in this patient is unlikely to be artefactual, as she has presented with bleeding.

Having ensured that she is stable and there is no major bleeding, the next step is to try and ascertain the underlying cause of thrombocytopenia. This can be done with the help of the history and results of some laboratory tests. From a practical perspective, there are five important causes to consider (*see Figure 14.1* and *Box 14.1*).

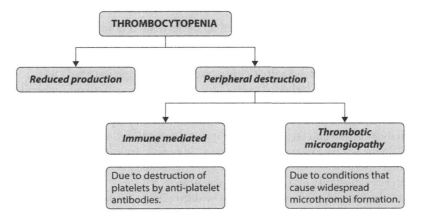

FIGURE 14.1   Mechanisms of thrombocytopenia.

BOX 14.1   UNDERLYING CAUSES OF THROMBOCYTOPENIA

■ Thrombotic microangiopathy.
■ Bone marrow failure.
■ Infections[†].
■ Drugs[†].
■ Immune-mediated thrombocytopenia.

[†] Infections and drugs cause thrombocytopenia by reducing the production of platelets and/or increasing the destruction.

Of these, immune-mediated thrombocytopenia, drugs and infections are the most likely causes to consider in this patient. Bone marrow failure is unlikely, as the other cell lines are not affected. Thrombotic microangiopathy (TMA) is also unlikely, as her haemoglobin is normal, and there are no features of haemolysis *or* fragmented red cells in her peripheral blood film (*see Box 14.2* and *Figure 14.2*).

BOX 14.2   THROMBOTIC MICROANGIOPATHY

Thrombotic microangiopathy (TMA) is characterised by widespread formation of microthrombi in the circulation. It is the *diagnosis not to miss* in someone presenting with thrombocytopenia.

The endothelium produces von Willebrand factor (vWF), which helps to clump platelets during the formation of a primary haemostatic plug. A small amount of vWF is continuously secreted in the basal state (i.e. even when there is no need to form a haemostatic plug) in the form of ultra-large multimers, but inappropriate platelet aggregation is prevented because the protease enzyme ADAMTS-13 keeps breaking these multimers into smaller units. Thus, deficiency of ADAMTS-13 *or* increased production of ultra-large multimers of vWF can lead to formation of *platelet thrombi.* Platelet thrombi occur in ***thrombotic thrombocytopenic purpura*** (TTP) due to deficiency of ADAMTS-13, and in ***haemolytic uraemia syndrome*** (HUS) due to increased production of vWF. In both TTP and HUS, clotting factors and fibrinogen are not used, as the coagulation cascade is not activated. Hence, prothrombin time (PT), activated partial thromboplastin time (APTT), thrombin time (TT) and fibrinogen level are normal.

Features of TMA are as follows:

1. ***Thrombocytopenia***, as platelets are used up for formation of microthrombi.
2. ***Microangiopathic haemolytic anaemia*** (MAHA), as red cells get severed when they try to get past the microthrombi.
3. ***Fragmented or severed red cells*** (schistocytes) in the peripheral blood film.
4. ***Elevated serum lactate dehydrogenase*** (due to haemolysis and tissue ischaemia).

The classical pentad of TTP includes [a] thrombocytopenia, [b] MAHA, [c] fever, [d] central nervous system dysfunction and [e] acute kidney injury. In practice, the presence of thrombocytopenia and MAHA in the absence of an alternative cause is considered sufficient for a diagnosis of TTP because of its high mortality (>90%) and the need to commence plasma exchange urgently. Plasma exchange reduces the mortality of TTP to less than 10%.

The increased release of vWF in HUS could be due to Shiga toxin produced by *E. coli* 0157:H7 (typical or diarrhoea (+) HUS), a dysregulated complement system (atypical or diarrhoea (−) HUS), activation of renin-angiotensin-aldosterone system (malignant hypertension) or release of bioactive substances from an oxidatively stressed placenta (pre-eclamptic toxaemia).

TMA also occurs in ***disseminated intravascular coagulation*** (DIC). In DIC, the coagulation cascade is activated by release of tissue factor by various insults such as infection, trauma, burns, snake venom, dead foetus or amniotic fluid embolism, resulting in the formation of a *fibrin blood clot.* Because clotting factors and fibrinogen are used up in the process, laboratory findings of DIC include prolongation of PT, APTT and TT, with low fibrinogen and elevated D-dimers (D-dimers, also known as fibrin degradation products, are elevated because of lysis of the fibrin clot by plasmin).

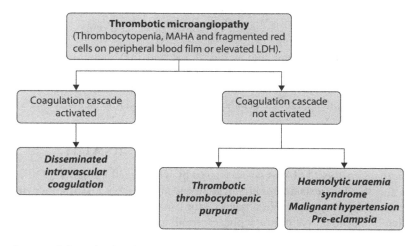

FIGURE 14.2   Causes of thrombotic microangiopathy.

The next set of questions should elicit the features that may suggest an underlying cause for her thrombocytopenia. You should

- Check for *clues that may suggest an underlying infection* (e.g. fever, history of recent travel or residence in an endemic area, infectious contacts, high-risk sexual behaviour).

Note: Several infections like malaria, dengue, human immunodeficiency virus, hepatitis C, infectious mononucleosis, cytomegalovirus infection and leptospirosis can cause thrombocytopenia.

- Obtain a detailed *drug history*, including 'over-the-counter' preparations and illicit drugs. Also ask about her *alcohol intake*.

Note: Several drugs are known to cause thrombocytopenia (e.g. co-trimoxazole, antibiotics, heparin, quinine, statins, rifampicin, angiotensin-converting enzyme inhibitors).

- Ask about *features of autoimmune connective tissue disease* (e.g. joint pain, skin rashes, muscle weakness, dry eyes and mouth, Raynaud's phenomenon, previous thrombosis or pregnancy loss).

Note: Immune thrombocytopenic purpura (ITP) is mediated by anti-platelet antibodies. It can occur on its own (primary ITP) or with other features of systemic lupus erythematosus (SLE-associated ITP).

She denies fever, joint pain or skin rashes. Review of systems is unremarkable, with no symptoms of infection or autoimmune disease. There is no history of recent travel, previous residence in tropical countries or infectious contacts. Her past medical history is blameless. She takes no regular medications, 'over-the-counter' preparations or illicit drugs. She does not smoke and seldom drinks alcohol. She is an optometrist and lives with her husband. She has never been pregnant.

WHAT SHOULD YOU LOOK FOR ON EXAMINATION?

Apart from checking her *vital signs*, you should

- Perform a *general examination* to look for signs of autoimmune connective tissue disease (e.g. synovitis, skin rashes).
- Check for *purpura or petechiae*.
- Examine the abdomen to check for *splenomegaly*.

Note: In patients with thrombocytopenia, splenomegaly may be caused by infections like malaria, haematological malignancy (e.g. leukaemia or lymphoma) or myelofibrosis (due to extra-medullary haemopoiesis). Massive splenomegaly due to any cause may lead to thrombocytopenia by causing platelet sequestration.

Physical examination is completely unremarkable. There are no signs of autoimmune connective tissue disease. Her spleen is not palpable.

WHAT FURTHER INVESTIGATIONS SHOULD BE REQUESTED?

You should request

- *Coagulation profile* (prothrombin time [PT] and activated partial thromboplastin time [APTT]).
- *Anti-nuclear antibody* (ANA).

In patients with positive ANA, you should request double-stranded DNA antibody, complement levels and urinalysis (to screen for renal involvement).

- *Chest X-ray*, *blood glucose* and *screening tests for hepatitis B and C* (in anticipation of commencing steroid therapy).

Other investigations that may be requested in selected patients (depending on clinical presentation) include

- Lactate dehydrogenase, disseminated intravascular coagulation (DIC) screen (TT, fibrinogen, D-dimers), stool cultures or serology for *E. coli* 0157: H7 and ADAMTS-13 activity (in patients with suspected TMA).
- Screening tests for malaria, dengue, Epstein-Barr virus, cytomegalovirus, HIV and hepatitis C [in patients with suspected infection-related thrombocytopenia].
- Bone marrow biopsy, vitamin B_{12} and folate (in patients with suspected bone marrow failure).

WHAT SHOULD YOU TELL THE PATIENT?

You should explain to her that

- Her menorrhagia is due to the low platelet count.

'I feel that the low platelet count is the reason for your heavy menses. As I mentioned earlier, not having enough platelets can make you bleed more easily'.

- Her low platelet count is immune mediated.

'I suspect your immune system is mistakenly attacking the platelets. We do not know why the immune system makes this mistake in some people'.

- You would like to ask for further tests to ascertain the cause of her thrombocytopenia.

'I hope you won't mind if I ask for a few more blood tests. These tests will help to find out why your platelet count is low'.

- You would like to admit her to the hospital and monitor closely.

'Your platelet count could drop further, so I'd like to admit and monitor you closely'.

- You would ask a haematologist (*'blood specialist'*) to see her urgently.
- She should follow some general precautions to prevent bleeding.

'You should take some precautions to reduce the chance of bleeding. You should not brush your teeth hard or blow your nose forcefully. I'll give you a laxative so that you don't strain while having a bowel movement'.

- The haematologist will discuss the treatment options depending on the results of the tests.
- You would update her when the results of the tests are available.

OUTCOME

Her blood test results are as follows:

- PT and APTT normal.
- **ANA positive 1/320**.
- Anti-double-stranded DNA and complement levels normal.
- Urinalysis normal.
- Chest X-ray normal.
- Blood glucose normal.
- Hepatitis B and C screen negative.

The positive ANA result points to immune-mediated thrombocytopenia. As there are no other features of lupus such as joint pain, skin rashes, cytopenia (other than thrombocytopenia) or abnormal urinalysis, we have to label this as primary-ITP.

She is referred to the haematologist, who commences treatment with high-dose oral prednisolone. She is also given tranexamic acid (it reduces bleeding by inhibiting fibrinolysis). A gynaecologist is also consulted. Her platelet count gradually picks up over the next two weeks. The haematologist plans to follow her in the clinic and gradually taper the dose of prednisolone.

The 33-Year-Old Man with Eosinophilia

Case 15

A 33-year-old man presents with painful joints.

His blood results show haemoglobin 128 g/L, white cell count 14.8 × 10⁹/L, eosinophils 9.36 × 10⁹/L (normal <0.35 × 10⁹/L) and platelets 316 × 10⁹/L. Liver function tests and serum creatinine are normal. Erythrocyte sedimentation rate (ESR) is 68 mm/hour.

HOW SHOULD THIS PROBLEM BE APPROACHED?

Explore his presenting complaint first.

- Ask about his ***joint pain*** and determine the extent and distribution, presence of inflammatory features, duration, mode of onset and progression.

*He tells you that his **ankles, wrists and elbows have been painful and stiff** for the last two weeks. He has not noticed any swelling. The pain started in all these joints at the same time. It has since neither improved nor worsened. He has never suffered with joint pain in the past.*

 The most striking laboratory abnormality (apart from the high ESR) is the severe eosinophilia (*see Figure 15.1*).

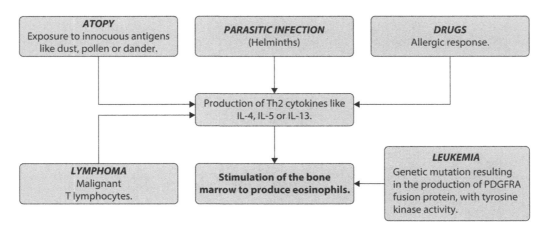

FIGURE 15.1 Pathogenesis of eosinophilia.

DOI: 10.1201/9781003430230-15

When healthy individuals are exposed to innocuous antigens like dust, pollen, dander or feather, they mount a Th1 (Th = helper T cell) cytokine response that helps to induce the production of IgG by plasma cells. The IgG combines with antigens and efficiently clears them, without causing an inflammatory response. Thus, most of us do not suffer any ill effects when we are exposed to innocuous antigens.

In those with an atopic tendency, on the other hand, Th2 cytokines like IL-4, IL-5 and IL-13 are produced instead. These cytokines, IL-5 in particular, stimulate the (a) plasma cells to produce IgE instead of IgG and (b) bone marrow to produce eosinophils. The IgE, upon exposure to the antigen, causes the release of inflammatory mediators like histamine from mast cells. These inflammatory mediators cause vasodilatation, increased vascular permeability (nasal stuffiness, urticaria and in extreme cases, hypotension and shock) and bronchospasm (breathlessness and wheezing).

The antigen that induces an allergic response could be a medication, like a prescription drug or an 'over-the-counter' preparation. Eosinophils are also released in response to tissue helminthic infections, as cationic proteins produced by eosinophils are an important line of defence against such parasites (e.g. Filariasis, Strongyloides, Schistosomiasis, Toxocara and Trichinella). Thus, [a] *atopy*, [b] *allergic drug reaction* and [c] *helminthic infection* are the three most common causes of eosinophilia. The fungus *Aspergillus*, to which most of us are frequently exposed, may cause a similar aberrant response in susceptible individuals, leading to bronchospasm (*allergic bronchopulmonary aspergillosis*).

Less common, but sinister causes include *lymphoma* (the malignant lymphocytes produce excess amounts of IL-5, resulting in eosinophilia) and *eosinophilic leukaemia* (a genetic mutation leads to the production of a fusion protein called FIP 1L1 PDGFRA, with tyrosine kinase activity). In the absence of reactive or clonal causes, the eosinophilia is labelled as *idiopathic*.

In some patients, the 'allergen' that induces eosinophilia may target the blood vessel wall and cause vasculitis (*eosinophilic granulomatosis with polyangiitis*, EGPA). EGPA may manifest with systemic symptoms, inflammatory arthritis, vasculitic skin rashes, mononeuritis multiplex, glomerulonephritis and gastrointestinal involvement (e.g. abdominal pain, rectal bleeding).

In patients with eosinophil count of $>1.5 \times 10^9$/L, it is important to check if the hypereosinophilia is causing any tissue damage, particularly in the heart. Eosinophilic infiltration and release of cytotoxic products may lead to myocarditis, endomyocardial fibrosis and formation of intra-cardiac thrombi, manifesting as heart failure and rhythm or conduction disturbance.

In this patient, the eosinophilia, joint pain and elevated ESR are possibly due to an underlying systemic condition (e.g. vasculitis, infection, lymphoma).

Further questions to ask:

- Ask about *features suggestive of atopy*, such as bronchial asthma, rhinitis or nasal polyps, eczema and family history of atopic diseases.
- Check for clues that may suggest helminthic infection.

Ask about *travel* to tropical countries (including residence in such countries, even if it was decades earlier), *pets at home* (e.g. Toxoplasma infection may be spread by handling cats) and *dietary habits* (e.g. trichinella infection may be acquired by eating pork).

- Obtain a *detailed medication history*. This should include not only prescription drugs, but also 'over-the-counter' preparations and nutritional supplements.
- Ask about *symptoms suggestive of cardiac involvement*, such as shortness of breath, orthopnoea and ankle swelling.
- Complete a *review of systems* to check for features of EGPA and lymphoma.

Ask particularly about swollen lymph glands, fever, weight loss, skin rashes, neurological symptoms like weakness and numbness, and gastrointestinal symptoms like abdominal pain and rectal bleeding.

*He was in good health until six months ago, when he was **diagnosed with asthma**. He was admitted to hospital at the time with chest tightness and wheezing and treated with oral steroid and nebulisers. He subsequently had some breathing tests and the diagnosis of asthma was confirmed by a lung specialist. Although he was prescribed inhalers, he did not use them, as he felt well.*

*He did not suffer with asthma during his childhood. He has never suffered with nasal stuffiness or eczema, and there is no one in his family with atopic diseases. He denies shortness of breath, orthopnoea or ankle swelling. He says he has **lost about 3–4 kg in weight** in the last two months without trying and his **appetite has not been great**. He also **feels increasingly tired**. Review of systems is otherwise unremarkable, with no lymph gland swelling, fever, sweats, neurological or gastrointestinal symptoms.*

He has never travelled to a tropical country. He does not keep any pets at home. He is non-vegetarian but does not eat beef or pork. He does not take any regular medication. He has never smoked and seldom drinks alcohol. He is a software programmer. He lives with his wife and a five-year-old son.

From the history, we can exclude medication or toxin-induced eosinophilia. Helminthic infection is less likely, as he has never travelled to a tropical country. Also, his overall presentation does not support this diagnosis. The late onset of asthma at the age of 33 is significant, which, when taken together with the inflammatory joint symptoms, unintentional weight loss, tiredness, eosinophilia and elevated ESR, points to systemic vasculitis. The history does not suggest involvement of any of the major organs from vasculitis, but he should be screened for renal involvement, as it may be occult. The absence of lymph node swelling would not exclude lymphoma, but the late-onset asthma seems to be more in keeping with vasculitis. Although he denies breathlessness, an echocardiogram should be requested to screen for cardiac involvement.

WHAT SHOULD YOU LOOK FOR ON EXAMINATION?

You should

- Ask for his *vital signs*.
- Perform a *general examination*.

Particularly look for synovitis, cutaneous lesions that may suggest vasculitis (e.g. purpura, infarcts, ulcers or gangrene) and lymphadenopathy (may suggest lymphoma).

- Examine the ***abdomen*** to check for enlarged liver and spleen (may suggest lymphoma or leukaemia).
- Listen to the ***heart and lungs***.

*His vital parameters are satisfactory. Blood pressure is 124/78 mm Hg. His **wrists and ankles are tender**, but there is no swelling or restriction in range of movements. There are no cutaneous lesions. There is no organomegaly. Heart and lung sounds are normal. Rest of the examination is unremarkable.*

HOW SHOULD THIS PATIENT BE EVALUATED FURTHER?

You should ask for

- *Urinalysis* to screen for renal involvement in vasculitis.
- *Anti-neutrophil cytoplasmic antibody* (ANCA).

Note: A negative ANCA result would not exclude ANCA-associated vasculitis, and a positive result would not confirm the diagnosis. The result should always be interpreted in the context of the whole clinical picture.

- **Chest X-ray**.
- **2D echocardiogram** (in all patients with eosinophil count >1.5 × 10^9/L).

Further tests to request in selected patients, depending on the clinical presentation or results of the initial tests, include:

- Screening tests for hepatitis B and C, glucose and vitamin D (if steroid therapy is contemplated).
- Renal biopsy in patients with abnormal urinalysis.
- FIP1L1-PDGFRA mutation (for eosinophilic leukaemia).
- CT scan of the thorax, abdomen and pelvis, lymph node or bone marrow biopsy (in patients with suspected lymphoma or leukaemia).

WHAT SHOULD YOU TELL THE PATIENT?

You should explain to him that

- His presentation is most likely due to vasculitis.

'I suspect you have developed a condition called vasculitis. Vasculitis means inflammation of blood vessels. Vasculitis can cause joint pain and make you feel tired and lose weight'.

- The late onset of asthma is related to the vasculitis.

'Inflammation generally occurs when our immune system attacks harmful proteins that are present in bacteria or viruses. In some people, inflammation occurs even when the immune system tries to clear harmless proteins like pollen or dust. We call this allergy. The asthma that you developed six months ago is a form of allergy. The allergic tendency usually develops at a very early age and often runs in families, but in some people, this can begin during adulthood. Those who develop the allergic tendency during adulthood can sometimes develop inflammation of blood vessels. We do not exactly know why this happens'.

- His blood test results show eosinophilia and elevated ESR.

'Your blood test results show that you have a higher number of a certain type of white blood cell called eosinophil. Your inflammation reading is also high. This fits in with my suspicion of vasculitis'.

- You would refer him to a rheumatologist (*'specialist who deals with inflammation of blood vessels'*).
- You would arrange further investigations to support the diagnosis of vasculitis and an echocardiogram.

'I'll ask for a few blood and urine tests, and an X-ray of your chest in the meantime. These tests will give us more information about the vasculitis and tell us if any of your internal organs are affected. Sometimes, eosinophils can cause inflammation of the heart muscle, so I'll arrange for a scan of your heart as well'.

- The specialist will discuss the treatment options.
- You would update him when the results of the tests are available.

OUTCOME

His results show

- Urinalysis shows **2+ protein, 2+ blood, 54 red blood cells and 5 white blood cells**, but no casts.
- **Proteinuria estimated by urine protein/creatinine ratio is 1.2 grams/day.**
- Chest X-ray normal.
- 2D Echocardiogram normal, with ejection fraction of 65%.
- **Myeloperoxidase-ANCA positive at 164 IU/mL** (normal <5). Proteinase 3-ANCA negative.
- Hepatitis B and C screen negative.
- Blood glucose normal.
- **Vitamin D 18 ng/mL** (normal >30).

*Renal biopsy is arranged by the rheumatologist and this is reported as showing **focal segmental crescentic glomerulonephritis**. He is diagnosed with EGPA and treated with pulse methylprednisolone, followed by high-dose oral prednisolone along with rituximab (anti-CD20 monoclonal antibody, which depletes B cells). He is also given co-trimoxazole as prophylaxis against pneumocystis infection, and vitamin D replacement. The rheumatologist arranges to follow him in clinic and gradually taper the dose of prednisolone.*

The 64-Year-Old Woman with an Enlarged Cervical Lymph Node

Case 16

A previously healthy 64-year-old woman presents with a three-week history of swelling over the right side of her neck.

HOW SHOULD THIS PROBLEM BE APPROACHED?

---

*On quick examination, the swelling appears to be an **enlarged lymph node** in the right jugulodigastric region.*

The two most common causes of lymphadenopathy are [a] infection and [b] malignancy (secondary deposits from cancer in the drainage area *or* haematological malignancy like lymphoma or leukaemia). The history should aim to differentiate these two entities.

Initial questions to ask:

- Is the swelling *painful or painless*?
- Is it *increasing or decreasing in size*?

Note: A painful lymph node that is decreasing in size is usually due to reactive lymphadenitis secondary to an infection in the drainage area, while a painless lymph node that is increasing in size is suspicious of a sinister cause like lymphoma.

- Is there *similar swelling elsewhere*?

Ask particularly about swelling on the other side of the neck, axillae and groins, as the neck swelling could be part of a generalised lymphadenopathy (*see Box 16.1*).

- Are there any '*B symptoms*'?

Lymphoma may be associated with 'B symptoms', which include [a] fever >38°C, [b] drenching night sweats and [c] weight loss of >10% over the previous six months.

- (If the swelling is localised to one region) Are there are any *symptoms suggestive of infection or malignancy* in the area(s) drained by the lymph node(s)?

DOI: 10.1201/9781003430230-16

BOX 16.1   UNDERLYING CAUSES OF GENERALISED LYMPHADENOPATHY

- *Infections* (e.g. infectious mononucleosis, cytomegalovirus infection, tuberculosis, HIV infection, hepatitis B and C, secondary syphilis, toxoplasmosis).
- *Malignancy* (e.g. Hodgkin's disease, NHL, leukaemia).
- *Inflammatory conditions* (e.g. systemic lupus erythematosus, sarcoidosis).
- *Drugs* (e.g. serum sickness).

---

*She says she first noticed the swelling about three to four weeks ago. The swelling is gradually **increasing in size**, but it is **not painful**. There is a **small lump in her right groin** as well, but none on the left side of the neck, armpits or left groin. She denies fever, weight loss or night sweats. Her GP recently prescribed a week's course of **co-amoxiclav**, but it **did not help to reduce the size of the swelling**.*

- Complete the *rest of the history*.

Ask about her other medical problems, regular medications, recent travel, occupation, pets at home, hobbies and contact with tuberculosis (think of the causes listed in *Box 16.1*).

Note: Do not obtain a sexual history, unless you think it is absolutely necessary.

Her past medical history is blameless. She denies joint pain or skin rashes. Review of systems is unremarkable. She has never knowingly been in contact with anyone with tuberculosis. She hasn't travelled anywhere for more than three years. She does not keep any pets at home. She does not take any medication. She has never smoked and seldom drinks alcohol. The relevant family history is unremarkable. She is a retired secondary school teacher. She lives with her husband.

Although she says she only noticed the swelling three to four weeks ago, she might have had it for longer. The [a] absence of pain, [b] increasing size of the swelling and [c] absence of response to the antibiotic are concerning. A haematological malignancy like lymphoma should be considered, especially as there are no features suggestive of any of the infections that are known to cause generalised lymph node enlargement. The lymph node in her groin may or may not be related to the same disease process. It is quite common for inguinal nodes to be slightly enlarged, so they are not considered significant unless they are >1.5 cm in diameter.

WHAT SHOULD YOU LOOK FOR ON EXAMINATION?

Ask for her *vital signs* and examine the following areas in particular:

- The *swelling in the neck*, noting the size, consistency, mobility and presence of tenderness.

Note: A tender lymph node is usually due to infection, while hard and fixed lymph nodes would suggest malignancy. In lymphoma, the lymph nodes are usually firm and rubbery.

- The *other lymph node regions*, like the other side of her neck, axillae and inguinal region.

Certain lymph nodes may offer specific clues (e.g. enlarged left supraclavicular node due to intra-abdominal or testicular malignancy, enlarged right supraclavicular node due to intra-thoracic malignancy, enlarged epitrochlear node due to syphilis).

- The abdomen, to check for **enlarged liver and spleen**.
- The **drainage areas**, to look for evidence of cancer or infection (e.g. the breasts in patients with axillary lymphadenopathy, ENT examination in those with cervical lymphadenopathy).

*Her vital parameters are normal. There is a **solitary swelling in the right jugulodigastric region**. The swelling is firm, rubbery and non-tender. It measures 3 cm across. The **swelling in the left inguinal region** is also firm, rubbery and non-tender, and it measures 2.5 cm across. Rest of the examination is unremarkable. There are no other palpable lymph nodes and examination of the abdomen reveals no organomegaly.*

HOW SHOULD THIS PATIENT BE INVESTIGATED?

You should request

- **Full blood count, liver function tests and serum creatinine**.
- **Peripheral blood film**, to look for evidence of leukaemia.
- **Erythrocyte sedimentation rate** (ESR).
- **Lactate dehydrogenase** (LDH).

Note: LDH may be elevated in patients with lymphoma, but this is non-specific. Other causes of LDH elevation include conditions that cause cell death (e.g. myocardial infarction, liver disease, haemolysis).

- A **chest X-ray**, to look for evidence of mediastinal lymphadenopathy.
- **Tests to look for supportive evidence of** infection, like Epstein-Barr virus IgM, cytomegalovirus IgM, hepatitis screen, HIV test, toxoplasma IgM and syphilis screen.

These tests (apart from HIV test, *see below*) are probably not necessary for this patient.

- She should be referred for an **excision biopsy of the cervical lymph node**, as lymphoma is a strong possibility.

Note: A fine needle aspiration for cytology (FNAC) is adequate to diagnose tuberculosis, but not lymphoma, as the nodal architecture should be studied.

WHAT SHOULD YOU TELL THE PATIENT?

You should tell her that

- The swelling in the neck and inguinal region are lymph nodes.

'The swelling in your neck and groin are lymph glands. Lymph glands are present throughout the body. Lymph glands can get bigger for a variety of reasons, the most common of which would be an infection'.

- Further evaluation is recommended, as her lymph nodes are painless and increasing in size.

'When lymph glands get bigger because of an infection, they tend to be painful. As your lymph glands are not painful and they are increasing in size even after the course of antibiotics, I would recommend further tests to check for other possible reasons for enlargement of your lymph glands. I'll first ask for some blood tests and an X-ray of your chest'.

■ You plan to refer to the surgeon.

'Once the results of these tests are back, I'll refer you to a surgeon so that the lymph gland in the neck can be removed and examined under the microscope. We call this a biopsy. It is a minor procedure that can be performed after numbing the skin. The results of the biopsy will tell us why your lymph glands are enlarged'.

■ You will get in touch with her once the results of her blood tests are available.

OUTCOME

The results of the initial investigations are as follows:

■ Haemoglobin 134 g/L, white cell count 7.8×10^9/L and platelet count 248×10^9/L.
■ Peripheral blood film shows no evidence of leukaemia.
■ Liver function tests normal.
■ Serum creatinine normal.
■ **ESR 36 mm/hour.**
■ **LDH 624 U/L** (normal 240–480).
■ Chest X-ray normal.

The normal blood counts suggest that her bone marrow is functioning normally. The elevated ESR is non-specific and could be secondary to infection, inflammation or malignancy. The elevation of LDH is probably due to lymphoma in the context of her clinical presentation.

*She is referred to a surgeon, who performs an excision biopsy of the cervical lymph node. After a couple of days, the preliminary biopsy result is reported as showing features of **non-Hodgkin's lymphoma** (NHL) (see Boxes 16.2 and 16.3).*

She is urgently referred to the haematologist. HIV test is requested, as it is a risk factor for NHL. She arranges a positron emission tomography (PET)-CT scan in order to stage the disease.

BOX 16.2 OVERVIEW OF LYMPHOMA

Lymphomas are caused by *neoplastic proliferation* of the *lymphocytes* in *lymphoid tissues*. Broadly, they are classified into (a) Hodgkin's disease and (b) non-Hodgkin's lymphoma (NHL). NHL is far more common, accounting for more than 90% of the cases of lymphoma.

The cell of origin in Hodgkin's disease is not known, but the characteristic histopathological finding is the presence of Reed-Sternberg cells. There are four pathological types, including [a] nodular sclerosis, [b] lymphocyte predominant (best prognosis), [c] lymphocyte depleted (worst prognosis) and [d] mixed cellularity.

NHL is classified based on

■ *The cell of origin* (B cells [80%] or T cells [20%]).
■ *Site of origin* (nodal or extra-nodal).

Examples of extra-nodal sites are mucosa-associated lymphoid tissues and salivary glands.

■ *Grade* (high grade or low grade).

The grading is based on the predicted rate of progression. High-grade lymphomas are fast-growing and aggressive (they respond better to chemotherapy), while low-grade lymphomas are slow growing and indolent.

BOX 16.3   THE ANN ARBOR STAGING OF LYMPHOMA

Stage I: Involvement of one single lymph node region.
Stage II: Involvement of two or more regions, but on the same side of the diaphragm (either above or below the diaphragm).
Stage III: Involvement of lymph nodes above and below the diaphragm.
Stage IV: Diffuse involvement of extra-nodal sites (e.g. bone marrow, liver), **with or without** involvement of nodes.

Note: Each of the above stages is sub-staged into A (B symptoms absent) or B (B symptoms present).

*The final biopsy result is reported as **diffuse large B cell** NHL, which is a form of high-grade lymphoma. PET-CT scan shows **involvement of the para-aortic nodes in addition to the cervical and inguinal nodes**. Her lymphoma is staged as IIIA. HIV test is negative. The haemato-oncologist decides to treat with chemotherapy.*

The 64-Year-Old Man with Abdominal Discomfort

Case 17

A 64-year-old man presents with a two-month history of left-sided abdominal discomfort.

HOW SHOULD THIS PROBLEM BE APPROACHED?

Start with an open-ended question and **explore his main complaint**.

- Ask about the site of discomfort and whether it radiates, character, onset and progression, and aggravating and relieving factors.
- Ask about **associated symptoms** (respiratory, gastrointestinal and urinary).

*He tells you that he feels a **discomfort on the left side of his tummy** (he points to the left hypochondrium). It is **dull ache**. The pain does not radiate anywhere and there is no back pain. This **started about two months ago** and it has since neither improved nor worsened. The **discomfort is there most of the time**, with no specific aggravating or relieving factors.*

*He used to be very active until three months ago, but does not have that energy now. He **gets tired very easily**. He has **lost interest in food** and thinks he has **lost about 3–4 kg over the last three months** without trying. He denies chest pain, cough, breathlessness, dysphagia, nausea, vomiting, change in bowel habit, rectal bleeding or urinary symptoms.*

The dull nature of the discomfort suggests that it is arising from a solid rather than tubular organ like intestine, as the latter is more likely to cause colicky pain. The solid organ in the left hypochondrium is the spleen, so it is possible that his discomfort is caused by a gradually enlarging spleen. Problems in the base of the left lung, left kidney or spine can present with left hypochondrial pain, but they seem less likely because of the absence of associated cough, breathlessness, urinary symptoms and back pain.

There are some concerning features in the history, such as (a) the unintentional weight loss, (b) loss of appetite and (c) the recent onset of fatigue. The differential diagnosis includes malignancy (e.g. lymphoma or leukaemia), chronic inflammation and infection. You should

- Complete a **full review of the systems**.
- Complete the **rest of the history** and particularly ask about his other medical problems, regular medications, smoking habit and alcohol intake, occupation, hobbies and details of recent travel.

DOI: 10.1201/9781003430230-17

*He denies fever, sweats, joint pain and muscle aches. His medical history is largely unremarkable except for **hyperlipidaemia and gout**. He takes atorvastatin and allopurinol. He has **smoked about 20 cigarettes a day since the age of 20**, but seldom drinks alcohol, as it triggers an attack of gout. He is a retired civil servant. He has no hobbies. He has not travelled abroad for more than four years. He lives with his wife.*

WHAT SHOULD YOU LOOK FOR ON EXAMINATION?

You should

- Ask for his ***vital parameters*** and perform a ***general examination***.
- ***Examine the abdomen***.

*His vital parameters are normal. He is moderately built and comfortable at rest. He is not pale or jaundiced, and there is no finger clubbing or oedema. His **spleen is palpable** and extends about four fingerbreadths below the left costal margin. It is not possible to get above the swelling and there is no notch. It is not bimanually palpable or ballotable. It is dull to percussion. There is no hepatomegaly or free fluid in the abdomen.*

The mass in the left hypochondrium is most likely the spleen and not the left kidney because (a) it is not possible to get above the swelling, (b) it is not bimanually palpable or ballotable and (c) it is dull to percussion. See *Box 17.1* for some common causes of splenomegaly.

BOX 17.1   SOME COMMON CAUSES OF SPLENOMEGALY

- ***Portal hypertension***.
- ***Haemolytic anaemia*** (e.g. hereditary spherocytosis, thalassemia).
- ***Blood borne infections*** (e.g. malaria, leishmaniasis, typhoid, infective endocarditis).
- ***Haematological malignancy*** (e.g. leukaemia, lymphoma).

Notes:
1 Rare causes of splenomegaly include Felty's syndrome, amyloidosis, sarcoidosis and glycogen or lipid storage disorders.
2 Splenomegaly occurs because of (a) a larger volume of blood being held in the venous sinuses (portal hypertension), (b) proliferation of splenic macrophages to phagocytose the red cells that are pre-maturely destroyed or extra-medullary haemopoiesis (haemolytic anaemia), (c) reactive proliferation of white cells (infection) *or* (d) clonal proliferation of white cells (leukaemia or lymphoma).

A further history should be obtained and focussed examination performed, bearing in mind the underlying causes of splenomegaly (*see Box 17.1*).

He confirms that he has never been a heavy drinker. He has not been diagnosed with liver or blood problems. He has never been tested for hepatitis B or C. There is no family history of liver disease. He has lived in the UK all his life and it is more than four years since he travelled abroad.
   There are no markers of chronic liver disease or enlarged lymph nodes in the neck, axillae and groins.

Although hyperlipidaemia may be associated with non-alcoholic fatty liver disease, portal hypertension seems less likely because of the absence of markers of chronic liver disease. A chronic infection like malaria or leishmaniasis is also unlikely in a man who has never lived outside the UK. Haemolytic anaemias, like hereditary spherocytosis and thalassemia, or storage disorders would not present for the first time at the age of 64. Felty's syndrome can be ruled out because of the absence of a background diagnosis of rheumatoid arthritis. Secondary amyloidosis is also unlikely in the absence of chronic inflammatory disease. A haematological malignancy like lymphoma or leukaemia is possible, so the results of the blood counts are crucial.

HOW SHOULD THIS PATIENT BE EVALUATED FURTHER?

As the most important concern is haematological malignancy, you should request

- *Blood tests*, including full blood count, peripheral blood film, liver function tests and serum creatinine.
- *Ultrasound scan of the abdomen*.

If available, a bedside ultrasound may be performed to quickly confirm splenomegaly. Further investigations can be decided based on the results of these tests.

WHAT SHOULD YOU TELL THE PATIENT?

You should tell him that

- His spleen is enlarged, which is probably the cause of his abdominal discomfort.

'We have an organ here on the left side called spleen. It stores our blood cells and helps us to fight infections. I can feel a lump here. I suspect it is your spleen, which has become bigger. This is probably the reason why your tummy hurts'.

- The cause of his splenomegaly is not clear.

'I am not sure why your spleen has become bigger. The usual causes are infection, or a problem in the liver or blood cells'.

- His tiredness and weight loss could be due to the same problem causing the splenomegaly.
- Further investigations are necessary.

'I'll first ask for some blood tests and a scan of your tummy. You may need further tests depending on the results of these blood tests'.

- You will update him as soon as the results of the blood tests are available. The results should be available in less than a couple of hours.

OUTCOME

A little later, the lab technician phones you to inform the results of his blood tests.

- **Haemoglobin 112 g/L**.
- **Total white cell count 68×10^9/L**. Predominant increase in neutrophils (82%) and basophils (10%).
- **Platelet count 524×10^9/L**.

- **Peripheral blood film shows myelocytes, promyelocytes, metamyelocytes and mature neutrophils. There are occasional myeloblasts**. Red cells are normocytic and normochromic. Platelets look normal.
- Liver function tests and serum creatinine normal.
- Ultrasound scan is reported as showing an **enlarged spleen**, which extends about 9 cm below the left costal margin. There is no free fluid in the abdomen.

 The elevated white cell count and the peripheral blood film findings are very concerning and in keeping with chronic myeloid leukaemia (CML) (*see Box 17.2*). There is also evidence of normocytic normochromic anaemia and thrombocytosis. He should be referred to the haematologist urgently.

WHAT SHOULD YOU TELL THE PATIENT NOW?

You should tell him that

- The blood counts and peripheral blood film show some abnormalities.

'We have different kinds of cells in the blood, like red blood cells, white blood cells and platelets. These blood cells are produced by the bone marrow, which is the inner part of our bones. Your results show that you have a much higher number of white blood cells in your blood. An infection is the most common reason for a high white blood cell count, but your results seem to suggest that there may be a problem with the bone marrow'.

- You would refer him to a haematologist.

'I'll ask a blood specialist to see you urgently. He might arrange further tests to find out why the white blood cell numbers are so high'.

BOX 17.2   OVERVIEW OF LEUKAEMIA

The pluripotent stem cells in bone marrow differentiate into myeloid or lymphoid stem cells. Lymphoid stem cells develop into lymphocytes, while myeloid stem cells develop into red cells, platelets, granulocytes (neutrophils, eosinophils and basophils) and monocytes.

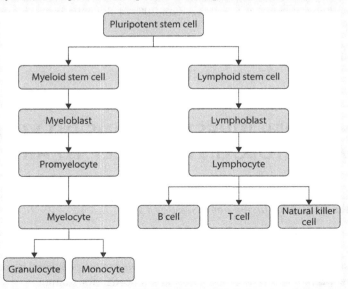

Leukaemia occurs because of maturation arrest along the developmental cycle, leading to *clonal proliferation* of *haematopoietic precursor cells* in the *bone marrow*. They are broadly classified into acute and chronic.

In *acute leukaemia*,

- The maturation arrest occurs at an early phase of the developmental cycle, leading to clonal proliferation of *more immature cells*, like blasts. The immature cells retain the ability to multiply but lose the ability to differentiate.

Normally, less than 5% of the cells in the bone marrow are blast cells, but in acute leukaemia, this increases to more than 20% (anything between 5 and 20% is known as myelodysplasia). Blast cells may also be seen in the peripheral blood film. The type of blast cell depends on the cell line of origin (lymphoblast in acute lymphoblastic leukaemia or myeloblast in acute myeloblastic leukaemia).

- The blast cells *proliferate rapidly* and take up the normal bone marrow space, causing anaemia (fatigue), leukopenia (infection) and thrombocytopenia (bleeding).

The rapidly multiplying blasts may infiltrate other tissues like skin, gums (causing gum hypertrophy), meninges, liver, spleen, lymph nodes and testis.

In *chronic leukaemia*,

- The maturation arrest occurs during a later phase of the development cycle, leading to clonal proliferation of more *mature haematopoietic precursor cells*.

The type of mature cell(s) seen in the peripheral blood film depends on the cell line of origin (mature lymphocytes in chronic lymphocytic leukaemia (CLL) *or* a variety of cells such as myelocytes, promyelocytes, metamyelocytes and mature granulocytes in CML).

- The proliferation *occurs at a slower pace*. Thus, patients usually do not manifest symptoms of bone marrow failure at the time of presentation.

The slowly multiplying cells initially infiltrate the spleen (in CML) or lymph nodes (in CLL). Bone marrow failure may occur only in the later stages when there is increasing multiplication of cancer cells in the bone marrow. When more than 20% of the cells in the bone marrow become blasts, we call it blast transformation.

Thus, acute leukaemia is characterised by *rapid proliferation of more immature elements*, while chronic leukaemia is characterised by *slower proliferation of more mature elements*.

WHAT FURTHER INVESTIGATIONS DO YOU THINK THE HAEMATOLOGIST IS LIKELY TO ARRANGE?

- Fluorescence in situ hybridisation (FISH) or polymerase chain reaction (PCR) to check for evidence of the *BCR-ABL fusion gene* (*see Box 17.3*).

A peripheral blood sample should be sufficient for both FISH and PCR.

- Cytogenetic studies to look for *Philadelphia chromosome* in the peripheral blood or bone marrow.
- *Bone marrow studies* will provide the information needed for staging.

There are different stages in CML: chronic phase, accelerated phase and blast phase. Progression to blast phase is marked by increasing number of blast cells.

BOX 17.3   PHILADELPHIA CHROMOSOME AND BCR/ABL FUSION GENE

Translocation is the process where a part of one chromosome breaks off and attaches to another chromosome. In CML, there is reciprocal translocation between chromosomes 9 and 22, which means a part of chromosome 9 attaches to chromosome 22, and vice versa.

The Abelson (ABL) gene on chromosome 9 is translocated to the breakpoint cluster region (BCR) of chromosome 22, resulting in the formation of the BCR-ABL fusion gene in the latter. Chromosome 22 becomes shorter because of this translocation because it loses a longer piece to chromosome 9 and only gains a smaller piece in return. This shorter *chromosome 22 with the BCR-ABL fusion gene* is known as Philadelphia chromosome (or Ph chromosome in short).

The BCR-ABL fusion gene codes for BCR-ABL protein, which has tyrosine kinase activity. Tyrosine kinase is an enzyme that phosphorylates certain proteins to aid the transmission of signals into cells (transduction). The abnormal tyrosine kinase activity leads to the wrong signals being sent into myeloid cells of the bone marrow *'asking them to keep multiplying'*, thus leading to uncontrolled myeloid proliferation. Drugs like imatinib that are used to treat CML act by blocking tyrosine kinase activity.

Fluorescence in situ hybridisation (FISH) uses fluorescent probes to light up ABL and BCR genes with different colours. Thus, it helps to detect the presence of BCR-ABL fusion gene by showing two different colours in the same location on chromosome 22. The *polymerase chain reaction* (PCR) is another method to look at the BCR-ABL gene. The DNA segments of interest are amplified to see whether a specific m-RNA molecule is being produced by this gene.

Cytogenetic analysis is the process of studying the number and structure of the chromosomes. Cytogenetic analysis can help to identify the short chromosome 22 (Ph chromosome) in bone marrow or peripheral blood sample and confirm the diagnosis of CML.

*The haematologist sees him urgently and arranges further tests. The FISH test done with the peripheral blood sample shows that he is **BCR-ABL positive**. His bone marrow studies confirm that he is in the **chronic phase of CML**, with less than 10% blast cells. He is commenced on imatinib.*

The 52-Year-Old Man with Headache

Case 18

A 52-year-old man presents with a six-month history of gradually worsening headache.

HOW SHOULD THIS PROBLEM BE APPROACHED?

---

*When you greet him, you note **acromegalic features on his face**.* (The key is to recognise acromegaly from the facial features and ask the right questions.)

- ***Explore his presenting complaint*** and ask about the site of headache, character, duration of symptoms, and aggravating and relieving factors.

Is the headache worse with coughing or straining? Does it wake him from sleep?

- Ask if his ***hat, glove, ring or shoe size has increased recently***.
- Ask if he has got any ***old photographs***.
- Ask about ***visual symptoms***.

Even if he says that he can 'see normally', ask if he is ***bumping into objects*** on his sides.

- If he reports visual symptoms, ask if he ***drives a car*** (an important question to ask in all patients with visual symptoms).

*He tells you that he has been troubled with this **headache** for the last six months. It feels like a dull ache over the forehead. There are no specific aggravating or relieving factors. It is not worse with coughing or straining, and his sleep is not disturbed because of headache.*

*His **shoe size has gradually increased** from size 9 to size 12 in the last four to five years. He doesn't wear a hat, ring or gloves. He is not in possession of any old photographs at the time of this consultation. He says his eyesight is good but admits that he has been **bumping into objects on his sides**. He is an estate agent and **drives to work every day**.*

The gradual increase in his shoe size strengthens the suspicion of acromegaly (*acral* = peripheral parts, *megaly* = enlargement). The most common cause of acromegaly is increased secretion of growth hormone (GH) by a benign pituitary tumour. Very rarely, acromegaly may be caused by excessive production of GH-releasing hormone by the hypothalamus or an ectopic tumour.

DOI: 10.1201/9781003430230-18

Enlargement only occurs in the peripheral parts, as GH hypersecretion begins *after* puberty, when the epiphyses would have already fused (GH hypersecretion that starts *before* epiphyseal fusion causes longitudinal growth of the long bones and leads to gigantism and tall stature). He is bumping into objects on his sides, most likely because of bitemporal hemianopia. The hemianopia occurs because of compression of decussating nasal fibres in the optic chiasma by a pituitary tumour. He is still driving in the presence of a possible visual field defect, which is concerning.

Further questions to ask:

- Check for possible **complications of acromegaly** (*see Box 18.1*).

BOX 18.1   COMPLICATIONS OF ACROMEGALY

- Hypertension.
- Diabetes mellitus.
- Proximal myopathy.
- Carpal tunnel syndrome.
- Congestive cardiac failure.
- Obstructive sleep apnoea.
- Osteoarthritis.
- Colon cancer.

The excess GH facilitates the growth of colonic polyps, which could potentially turn cancerous.

- Ask if he **sweats a lot**.

Note: Excessive sweating is a feature of active acromegaly.

- Ask about **sexual dysfunction** ('*Have you had problems with your erection recently?*'.) Be tactful. In women, you should ask about amenorrhoea and galactorrhoea.

Note: Patients may develop sexual dysfunction because of increased prolactin. There are two possible mechanisms for increased prolactin in patients with acromegaly: (a) Co-secretion of prolactin by the pituitary tumour (both GH and prolactin are secreted by the same cell type) or (b) compression of the pituitary stalk (the part that connects the hypothalamus and pituitary) by the tumour, thus preventing dopamine from the hypothalamus reaching the pituitary (dopamine secreted by the hypothalamus inhibits the release of prolactin from anterior pituitary).

- Complete the **rest of the history**.

Ask about his other medical problems, regular medications, occupation, smoking habit and alcohol intake.

*He says his **blood pressure was noted to be around 150/100** on a few occasions. His GP suggested a medication to lower his blood pressure, but he was not keen. When he last had his blood sugar tested, which was just over a year ago, the result was normal. He denies weakness, numbness, breathlessness or joint pain. He is not sure if he snores at night. There is no recent change in his bowel habit, rectal bleeding or weight loss. He has not been screened for colon cancer before.*

*He has been **sweating a lot** for quite some time now. He has no problems with getting an erection. His past medical history is unremarkable, and he does not take any regular medication. His family* *history is unremarkable too. He does not smoke. He drinks a can of beer about three to four times a week. He has been living alone since getting divorced more than ten years ago.*

WHAT SHOULD YOU LOOK FOR ON EXAMINATION?

- Look for *features of acromegaly*.

You should (a) inspect the face from the front and sides, (b) look at the hands and feet, (c) ask the patient to show you his teeth (hypertrophy of gingival tissues will increase the space between teeth), (d) look at the tongue for evidence of macroglossia and (e) check for evidence of thick, greasy skin.
Once the features of acromegaly have been identified,

- Ask for his *blood pressure*.
- Examine his *visual fields* to check for evidence of bitemporal hemianopia (very important).
- Check for evidence of *proximal myopathy*.
- Check for *signs of carpal tunnel syndrome*.

This is *not necessary* if the patient denies tingling or weakness in his hands.

- Look around the *axillae for skin tags* and *acanthosis nigricans*.
- *Palpate the abdomen* for a mass (because of increased risk of colorectal cancer).

*Examination reveals **acromegalic features**, including prominent supra-orbital ridges, mandibular prognathism, enlargement of lips and nose, increased inter-dental cleft space, macroglossia and spade-like hands and feet. There is evidence of **bitemporal hemianopia**. Blood pressure is **162/98 mm Hg**. His power is grade 5/5 in the proximal upper and lower limbs. The axillae look normal, with no evidence of skin tags or acanthosis nigricans. Examination of the abdomen is normal.*

Physical examination has confirmed the presence of acromegalic features and bitemporal hemianopia. (In the early stages, the pituitary tumour only causes bitemporal superior quadrantanopia, as the inferior fibres in optic chiasma are compressed first.) He should be referred to an optometrist for a more detailed assessment of his visual fields.

HOW SHOULD THIS PATIENT BE INVESTIGATED?

- *Insulin-like growth factor-1* (IGF-1) is a good screening test for acromegaly (GH mediates its action through IGF-1).

If IGF-1 level is equivocal, an *oral glucose tolerance test* (OGTT) should be requested. OGTT is preferred because glucose normally suppresses the production of GH. The GH level fluctuates widely throughout the day; hence, measuring random levels is unhelpful.

- *MRI scan of the pituitary* is the investigation of choice to look for evidence of a pituitary tumour.
- *Fasting blood glucose*, *serum calcium* (ask for serum parathyroid hormone, if serum calcium is high) and *serum prolactin* (as ~30% of patients with acromegaly co-secrete prolactin).

Note: Think of multiple endocrine neoplasia (MEN) if hyperparathyroidism is present in a patient with a pituitary tumour.

Once the diagnosis of acromegaly is confirmed,

- ***Pituitary function*** should be fully assessed, as large tumours may compress the normal pituitary gland and reduce the secretion of other pituitary hormones.

This includes checking the pituitary-thyroid, pituitary-adrenal and pituitary-gonadal axes (thyroid-stimulating hormone, thyroxine, adrenocorticotrophic hormone, cortisol, prolactin, follicle-stimulating hormone, luteinising hormone, testosterone or oestradiol).

- All patients with acromegaly should be referred to a gastroenterologist for ***colonoscopy***.

WHAT SHOULD YOU TELL THE PATIENT?

You should tell him that

- The headache is caused by a pituitary tumour.

'We have a tiny gland below the brain called pituitary. I suspect your headache is caused by a growth in this gland'.

- The pituitary tumour is making too much GH.

'This gland makes a few hormones, including one called growth hormone that helps us to grow when we are young. If this gland makes too much growth hormone, the hands and feet can become larger. We call this acromegaly. This is probably the reason why your shoe size has gone up to 12'.

- The pituitary tumour is causing bitemporal hemianopia. He should therefore stop driving (very important to tell him).

'I suspect this growth is pressing on a nerve that connects the eyes to the brain. This is the reason why you are not able to see clearly on your sides. It is not safe for you to continue driving. You may be able to resume driving once the problem is treated and if your vision improves, but I am unable to say anything more at this stage'.

- You would refer him to an endocrinologist (*'hormone specialist'*).
- You would arrange some blood tests and a scan of the pituitary gland.

'I'll discuss with the specialist and ask for some blood tests to check the hormones that are produced by this gland. I'll also ask for a scan of the pituitary gland. It will help to confirm the presence of a growth and also tell us how big it is. The specialist will discuss the treatment options with you after you have had these tests'.

- You would refer him to an optometrist for a more detailed assessment of his visual fields.

'I'll refer you to the eye clinic for a more detailed examination of your eyes'.

- You would recommend colonoscopy.

'Bowel cancer is more common among those with acromegaly. It may not cause any symptoms in the early stages, so I would recommend having a bowel examination. I can refer you to a bowel specialist, who will explain this to you'.

■ You would suggest a medication for his high blood pressure.

'I would suggest taking a medication to lower your blood pressure. It is important to control the blood pressure, as it may increase the risk of heart attack and stroke'.

■ You will update him when the test results are available.

OUTCOME

*His **serum IGF-1 is elevated**. The MRI scan is reported as showing **macroadenoma of the pituitary gland**. His serum prolactin, TSH, thyroxine, ACTH, cortisol and testosterone levels are normal. Blood counts, renal function, fasting glucose and serum calcium are normal. His colonoscopy is normal. He is referred to an endocrine surgeon, who performs a trans-sphenoidal resection of the pituitary tumour.*

 Radiotherapy and medical therapy are options for patients in whom surgery is not successful or contraindicated. Medications used for acromegaly include [a] octreotide (somatostatin receptor agonist), [b] cabergoline or bromocriptine (dopamine agonists) and [c] pegvisomant (GH receptor antagonist).

The 28-Year-Old Woman Who Is Losing Weight

Case 19

A 28-year-old woman presents with a six-month history of weight loss.

HOW SHOULD THIS PROBLEM BE APPROACHED?

*When you greet her, you note **proptosis in both eyes**.*

- Explore her principal complaint of **weight loss**.

How much weight has she lost? How is her **appetite**?

- Ask relevant questions to assess her **thyroid status** (*see Box 19.1*).

BOX 19.1   QUESTIONS TO ASK TO ASSESS THE THYROID STATUS[†]

- Weight and appetite.
- Bowel habits.
- Preference for heat or cold.
- Menstruation.
- Sleep.
- Tremors.
- Palpitations.[††]

[†] Weight gain despite eating less, constipation, cold intolerance, menorrhagia or oligomenorrhoea, hypersomnolence, tiredness and lack of energy are features of hypothyroidism, while weight loss despite eating more, diarrhoea, heat intolerance, oligomenorrhoea, reduced sleep, anxiety, tremors and palpitations are features of hyperthyroidism.

[††] If the patient reports palpitations, ask about the frequency, rate, rhythm (regular or irregular) and associated symptoms like breathlessness, dizziness or syncope.

- Ask if she has any difficulty in raising her arms or rising from a seated position (***proximal myopathy***).
- Ask about her ***eyes***. Is there any pain, swelling or redness in her eyes? Is she able to close her eyes fully? Is she able to see normally? Is she seeing double?
- Ask if she has noticed ***swelling over the front of her neck*** (goitre).

DOI: 10.1201/9781003430230-19

If she reports swelling, ask about **pressure symptoms** like dysphagia, stridor and change in voice (due to compression of the left recurrent laryngeal nerve).

*She tells you that she has **lost about 6–7 kg** in the last six months. She is quite pleased about this, as she has managed to lose weight **despite eating more**! She moves her bowels about three to four times a day, and her **stools are watery**. Until three to four months ago, she was moving her bowels once daily, passing solid stools. She has not noticed blood in her stools. She has been **sweating a lot** recently and her **periods have become scanty**. She **hasn't been able to sleep for more than 4–5 hours** at night but still feels refreshed. She denies tremors, palpitations or limb weakness.*

*Her **eyes seem to be bulging**, but they are not painful or red. She can close her eyes fully and see normally. She is not seeing double. She thinks the **front of her neck is swollen**. She has no problem with swallowing or breathing, and there is no change in her voice.*

There are several features in keeping with hyperthyroidism, including [a] the unintentional weight loss despite an increase in appetite, [b] diarrhoea, [c] heat intolerance ('feeling sweaty'), [d] oligomenorrhoea, [e] poor sleep, [f] change in appearance of the eyes and [g] swelling over the front of her neck. The proptosis suggests that hyperthyroidism is due to Graves' disease (as it is caused by autoimmune mediated inflammation of retro-orbital tissues).

Some further questions to ask (depending on the presentation)

- **Pain** over the front of the neck. (This question is not relevant in this patient, as her presentation is in keeping with Graves' disease.)

De Quervain's thyroiditis may cause fever, pain and tenderness over the thyroid, but this is *not* hyperthyroidism. The hormones that are stored in the thyroid are simply released into the circulation.

- Ask about her **other medical problems**, particularly if she has asthma.

Non-selective ß-blockers, which are useful to control the symptoms of thyrotoxicosis, are contraindicated in patients with asthma.

- Ask what **medications** she is taking.

Amiodarone, lithium and very rarely thyroxine ingestion ('factitious hyperthyroidism') can all cause hyperthyroidism (not relevant in her case.)

- Is she **pregnant** or planning to get pregnant soon? Has she **just delivered**?

Note: Radioiodine and carbimazole should be avoided during pregnancy; think of post-partum thyroiditis in patients who have just delivered.

- Ask if she **smokes** (thyroid eye disease is worse among smokers).

*Her past medical history is blameless. She does not take any medication. She is not pregnant or planning to get pregnant anytime soon. She is single and not sexually active. She **smokes about 10 cigarettes/day** and drinks alcohol when she goes out with friends. She works in the immigration office.*

WHAT SHOULD YOU LOOK FOR ON EXAMINATION?

You should

- Assess the **thyroid status**.

[a] Ask the patient to stretch the hands and look for tremors (placing a piece of paper on the outstretched hands would make it obvious), [b] check for sweaty palms and palmar erythema and [c] count the pulse rate and check for irregular rhythm (atrial fibrillation).

■ Examine her *eyes* (*see Box 19.2*).

BOX 19.2   EXAMINATION OF THE EYES IN PATIENTS WITH GRAVES' DISEASE

■ Go behind the patient and look at the eyes from above and the sides to check for *proptosis*.
■ Check for *lid retraction*.

Lid retraction is present if you are able to see the sclera above the upper margin of iris.

■ Test for *lid lag*.

Lid lag simply means that movement of the eyelid lags behind that of the eyeball. To test this, move the finger in a vertical plane and ask the patient to follow your finger.

■ Ask the patient to *close the eyes fully*.

Inability to close the eyes fully increases the risk of corneal ulceration.

■ Check her *visual acuity* (ask her to read something from a book or magazine).

Reduced visual acuity may be due to optic nerve compression by retro-orbital swelling.

■ Check her *eye movements* to detect evidence of ophthalmoplegia.

■ Examine the *swelling in her neck*. Ask her to drink some water and see if the swelling moves with deglutition. Stand behind the patient and feel the swelling.

What is the consistency of the swelling? Are you able to get below the swelling? Are there any enlarged lymph nodes? Do you hear a bruit over the thyroid?

■ *Inspect the shins* for evidence of pretibial myxoedema.
■ *Test the power in proximal limbs* (myopathy).

A full neurological examination is not necessary. The deep tendon reflexes may be brisk in hyperthyroidism, but there is no need to test this.

*There is a **fine tremor** in her hands. Her hands are not warm or sweaty. The **pulse rate is 100/minute** and regular. There is **bilateral proptosis**, with **lid retraction** and **lid lag**. She is able to close her eyes fully. Near visual acuity is normal and eye movements are full. There is a diffuse, firm and non-tender **swelling over the anterior neck** that moves with deglutition. It does not extend retrosternally. There is no bruit over the thyroid. There is no evidence of pretibial myxoedema, and power is grade 5/5 in her proximal upper and lower limbs.*

The fine tremor and tachycardia further support our impression of hyperthyroidism. The normal visual acuity, unrestricted eye movements and her ability to close the eyes fully are all reassuring. Examination has confirmed the presence of goitre.

HOW SHOULD SHE BE EVALUATED FURTHER?

You should ask for

- Full blood count, liver function tests and serum creatinine.
- *Thyroid panel* including [a] serum free thyroxine (T4) and [b] thyroid-stimulating hormone (TSH).

Check serum triiodothyronine (T3) only if T4 is normal and TSH is low.

- *Thyroid antibodies*.

TSH receptor and thyroid peroxidase (TPO) antibodies may be present in patients with Graves' disease.

- *Ultrasound scan* of the thyroid (helps to distinguish solid from cystic swelling).
- *Radioactive iodine (RAI) scan*.

The cause of hyperthyroidism can be deduced from the pattern of uptake (diffuse increased uptake in Graves' disease, single area of focal uptake in focal nodular goitre and multiple areas of increased focal uptake in multi-nodular goitre). RAI scan is also useful to detect retrosternal extension of the goitre.

- *CT or MRI of the orbits* is useful to further assess the eye disease.

WHAT SHOULD YOU TELL THE PATIENT?

You should tell her that

- You suspect her symptoms are due to hyperthyroidism.

'The swelling at the front of your neck is an enlarged thyroid gland. The thyroid produces a hormone that controls the workings of various organs. I suspect you are losing weight because your thyroid is overactive and producing too much of this hormone. This is also the reason for your loose bowels, scanty periods, poor sleep and excessive sweating'.

- The hyperthyroidism is most likely due to Graves' disease.

'This can happen when the immune system mistakenly attacks the thyroid gland. We call this Graves' disease'.

- The proptosis is also due to thyroid disease.

'The bulging of your eyes is also because of the thyroid problem. This occurs because of swelling behind the eyes'.

- You would organise some blood tests and a scan of her thyroid gland.

'I'll ask for some blood tests to measure your thyroid hormones and check if the immune system is attacking your thyroid. I'll also ask for a scan of your thyroid gland'.

- She should stop smoking, as it *'could worsen the eye problem'* (very important.)
- You would refer her to an endocrinologist.

'I'll refer you to a thyroid specialist. She will discuss the treatment options based on the test results and your preferences'.

- You would refer her to an ophthalmologist for assessment of her proptosis.

'I'll also refer you to the eye clinic, where they'll check your eyes thoroughly. The bulging can make it difficult to fully close the eyes, and the swelling behind the eyes can affect your eyesight or cause double vision. It is therefore important that you are monitored closely in the eye clinic'.

OUTCOME

Her results are as follows:

- Full blood count, liver function tests and serum creatinine normal.
- **Serum free thyroxine 7.16 ng/dL** (normal range 0.9–2.3).
- **TSH 0.08 miu/L** (normal range 0.35–5.50).
- **TSH receptor antibody and anti-TPO positive**.
- **Ultrasound of the neck shows diffuse enlargement of the thyroid**.

The endocrinologist commences carbimazole after discussing the treatment options. She is also commenced on propranolol to improve her symptoms. She is advised not to get pregnant while on carbimazole and to get her blood counts monitored regularly.

Baseline assessment in the eye clinic reveals normal eyesight and no ophthalmoplegia. She is advised to use moisturisers and sunglasses and sleep propped up to reduce the peri-orbital oedema. She is followed up by the endocrinologist and ophthalmologist.

The 54-Year-Old Woman with Weight Gain

Case 20

You are asked to see a 54-year-old woman who complains of weight gain. She has gained over 20 kg in the last two years.

HOW SHOULD THIS PROBLEM BE APPROACHED?

*When you greet her, you note that **she looks Cushingoid**, with truncal obesity and moon facies.*

- Start by exploring her presenting complaint of **weight gain**.

*She tells you that she used to weigh around 68–70 kg until two years ago but weighs nearly 90 kg now. She feels **hungry all the time** and **keeps craving sugary foods**. Of late, she has been feeling very **tired and weak** as well.*

- Ask what exactly she means by **weakness**.

Is the weakness particularly affecting tasks that require the use of her proximal limb muscles (**proximal myopathy**)?

*She finds it **difficult to raise her arms above the level of her shoulders or rise from a seated position**. She denies distal limb weakness or numbness.*

In a vast majority, weight gain is caused by imbalance between calorie consumption and expenditure. In this patient, the weakness, which is most likely due to proximal myopathy, suggests that her weight gain is due to an underlying medical condition. Even if you did not make a spot diagnosis earlier, the combination of weight gain and proximal weakness should alert you to either Cushing's syndrome or hypothyroidism. Of the two, the former is more likely, as she reports increased appetite.

Further questions should explore possible complications or other features of Cushing's syndrome (*see Box 20.1*).

DOI: 10.1201/9781003430230-20

BOX 20.1   FEATURES OF CUSHING'S SYNDROME[†]

- Hypertension.
- Diabetes mellitus.[††]
- Proximal myopathy.
- Osteopenia or osteoporosis, leading to an increased risk of low-trauma fractures.
- Avascular necrosis of the bone.
- Redistribution of fat to the upper half of the body and face ('*moon facies*') and accumulation of fat in the supraclavicular and dorsocervical regions ('*buffalo hump*').
- Thinning of skin (e.g. abdominal striae, easy bruising, poor wound healing).
- Acne and hirsutism.
- Cataract and glaucoma.
- Insomnia, depression or mood swings.
- Menstrual irregularities.

[†] The four most important complications not to miss in the history are hypertension, diabetes, osteoporosis and proximal myopathy.
[††] If she says she is not a diabetic, ask if she has been tested for it recently.

*She has not been tested for diabetes or had her blood pressure measured anytime recently. She has never fractured a bone or had scans to check her bone density. She says some **stretch marks have appeared over her tummy**. She has not had acne since her teenage years, and there is no abnormal hair growth over her face or elsewhere. She uses reading glasses, but her vision is otherwise normal. She has always been a **poor sleeper**. She denies feeling 'low' or having mood swings. She went through her menopause at the age of 50.*

- Screen for ***hypothyroidism***.

Ask about change in her bowel habit, cold intolerance and neck swelling.

Her bowel movements are regular, with no recent change. She denies intolerance to cold. There is no neck swelling.

The next set of questions should aim to determine the underlying cause of glucocorticoid excess (*see Box 20.2*).

BOX 20.2   UNDERLYING CAUSES OF GLUCOCORTICOID EXCESS

- Glucocorticoid therapy (by far, the most common cause).
- Increased cortisol production by an adrenal tumour.
- Increased adrenocorticotrophic hormone (ACTH) production by a pituitary tumour (the commonest cause of endogenous hypercortisolism).
- Ectopic ACTH production (usually due to small cell lung cancer).

- Ask if she takes ***glucocorticoids*** (including steroid inhalers or topical preparations) or ***traditional preparations***.

Note: Some traditional Chinese medications, which are popular in some Asian countries, contain steroids.

- Ask if she has ***headache*** or ***visual disturbance***.

Even if she denies visual disturbance, ask if she **bumps into objects on her sides** (due to bitemporal hemianopia secondary to compression of optic chiasma by a pituitary tumour).

■ Ask about respiratory symptoms, like **cough and haemoptysis** (might suggest lung cancer).

She takes prednisolone tablets every day. She saw a private doctor for pain and stiffness around her shoulders and hips about three years ago and he prescribed prednisolone. She was told that her pain was caused by polymyalgia. She was initially given 20 mg of prednisolone to take every day and her pain resolved within a few days. She has been taking at least 10 mg/day since then but often increases the dose to 15–20 mg. She tried to lower the dose below 10 mg on a couple of occasions, but her muscles became painful. She denies headache, visual disturbance, cough or haemoptysis.

*Her past medical history is otherwise unremarkable and she takes no other medication. She works in an office, doing a desk-bound job. She **smokes about ten cigarettes/day** and drinks a glass of wine about once or twice a week. She lives with her husband.*

 The long-term use of corticosteroids for possible polymyalgia is the most likely cause of her Cushing's syndrome. Apart from possible myopathy, there are no overt complications of Cushing's, but her blood pressure should be measured and she should be screened for diabetes mellitus, hyperlipidaemia and osteoporosis.

WHAT SHOULD YOU LOOK FOR ON EXAMINATION?

Having already spotted the truncal obesity and moon facies, you should now

■ Test the **power in her limbs** to confirm that she is weak.

There is no need for a full neurological examination.

■ Ask for her **blood pressure**.
■ Look at the **abdominal wall for striae**.
■ **Examine her joints** to quickly check for synovitis or joint deformities.

Note: Her visual fields need not be examined routinely, as there is a clear underlying cause for her Cushing's syndrome, and she denies headache or visual symptoms.

*The power is **grade 4/5 in her proximal upper and lower limbs**. Distal power is normal. Her **blood pressure is 158/94 mm Hg**. There are **striae on her abdominal wall**. The joints look normal.*

HOW SHOULD SHE BE EVALUATED FURTHER?

You should request the following tests:

■ **Fasting blood glucose** and **HbA₁c** to screen for diabetes.
■ **Lipid panel**.
■ **Serum vitamin D level**.
■ **Bone density scan** to check for osteopenia or osteoporosis.

The evaluation of patients with suspected Cushing's syndrome that is not caused by exogenous steroids is outlined in *Figure 20.1*. These patients should be discussed with the endocrinologist.

WHAT SHOULD YOU TELL THE PATIENT?

You should tell her that

- Her weight gain is due to prednisolone.

'I suspect the steroid pills have made you put on weight'.

- Her muscle weakness and striae are also due to prednisolone.

'Steroid pills can affect the muscles and make them weak. This is the reason why you find it so difficult to stand up from the seated position or raise your arms. Steroid pills can also make the skin thinner. This would explain the stretch marks on your tummy'.

- You would suggest gradually tapering the dose of prednisolone. Prednisolone should not be stopped abruptly.

'We should try and gradually taper the dose of your steroid pill. It should not be stopped suddenly. Our body produces a small amount of steroid, which helps us cope with stressful states like illnesses. If steroid pills are taken for a long time, our body stops making this natural steroid. If you abruptly stop taking the steroid pills, it can take a while, sometimes even several months, for the body to resume the production of steroid and you may be left with no steroid during that time. If we gradually lower the dose of your steroid, the body will slowly increase its production of steroid'.

- You would refer her to a rheumatologist for an opinion regarding her polymyalgia.

'I appreciate your concern that your pain may return if you come off the steroid pills. I'll ask a specialist to see you. He might suggest other kinds of medications to treat your problem'.

- Corticosteroids increase the risk of diabetes, hypertension and osteoporosis.

'Steroid pills can increase the risk of developing diabetes, high blood pressure and thinning of bones. Your blood pressure reading was in fact high when we checked it just now'.

- You will arrange blood tests to screen for diabetes and hyperlipidaemia (*'high cholesterol'*), and also a bone density scan (*'a scan to check for thinning of the bones'*).
- If the blood pressure is persistently high, you would recommend *'starting a pill to lower the blood pressure'*.
- She should stop smoking, eat healthily (*'cut down sugars and fats'*) and start some gentle exercises like walking.
- You will update her once the test results are available.

OUTCOME

Her results are as follows:

- Full blood count, serum creatinine, thyroid function and creatine kinase normal.
- Erythrocyte sedimentation rate 16 mm/hour.
- **Fasting glucose 6.4 mmol/L and HbA$_1$c 49 mmol/mol** (normal 20–42).

- **Low-density lipoprotein 4.8** (target <2.7), **triglycerides 3.6 mmol/L** (target <1.7) and high-density lipoprotein 1.1 mmol/L (target >1.0).
- **Vitamin D 22 ng/mL** (normal >30).
- Bone density scan shows **T scores of −1.8 in her lumbar spine and −2.3 in her femoral neck**.

She is commenced on alendronate and vitamin D to reduce the risk of fragility fracture, atorvastatin for hyperlipidaemia and amlodipine for hypertension (as her blood pressure is persistently above 160/ 90 mm Hg). An oral glucose tolerance test shows impaired glucose tolerance. She is advised to quit smoking and follow healthy lifestyle measures. She is referred to a rheumatologist, who plans to gradually taper the dose of prednisolone and closely monitor her progress.

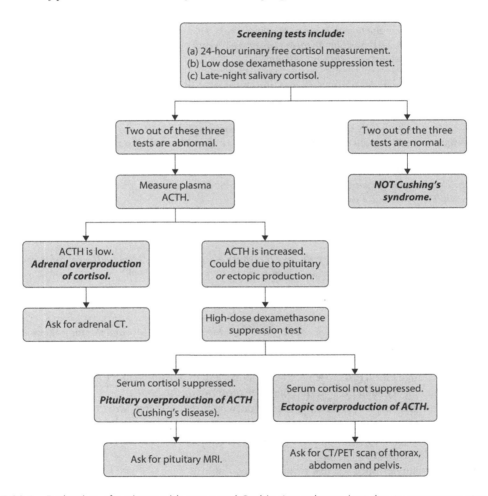

FIGURE 20.1   Evaluation of patients with suspected Cushing's syndrome (not due to exogenous steroid).

Notes:

1 The screening tests reflect different physiological abnormalities: increased cortisol production (24-hour urinary free cortisol), loss of the bedtime cortisol nadir (salivary cortisol) and impaired response to glucocorticoid negative feedback (dexamethasone suppression test).

2 The use of more than one test is recommended for screening.

3 If biochemical and anatomical investigations are inconclusive, inferior petrosal sinus sampling is useful to distinguish between pituitary and ectopic overproduction of ACTH.

The 45-Year-Old Man with Giddiness

Case 21

A 45-year-old man presents to the medical admissions unit with giddiness.

His blood test results show normal full blood count, blood glucose 5.1 mmol/L, serum urea 4.3 mmol/L (normal 2–7), creatinine 74 μmol/L (normal 70–120), sodium 126 mmol/L (normal 135–145) and potassium 5.2 mmol/L (normal 3–5).

HOW SHOULD THIS PROBLEM BE APPROACHED?

- Explore his main complaint of giddiness.

Is it **vertiginous or non-vertiginous**? Is it **related to posture**? Are there any **cardiac or neurological symptoms**?

*He tells you that he has been feeling giddy for the last few weeks. The room doesn't spin around him. He just **feels light headed**. This occurs **whenever he tries to stand up from a lying or seated position**. The giddiness usually improves after a short while.*

He denies cardiac symptoms like chest pain, shortness of breath or palpitations, and neurological symptoms like headache, weakness or numbness.

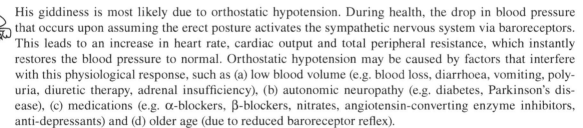

His giddiness is most likely due to orthostatic hypotension. During health, the drop in blood pressure that occurs upon assuming the erect posture activates the sympathetic nervous system via baroreceptors. This leads to an increase in heart rate, cardiac output and total peripheral resistance, which instantly restores the blood pressure to normal. Orthostatic hypotension may be caused by factors that interfere with this physiological response, such as (a) low blood volume (e.g. blood loss, diarrhoea, vomiting, polyuria, diuretic therapy, adrenal insufficiency), (b) autonomic neuropathy (e.g. diabetes, Parkinson's disease), (c) medications (e.g. α-blockers, β-blockers, nitrates, angiotensin-converting enzyme inhibitors, anti-depressants) and (d) older age (due to reduced baroreceptor reflex).

Based on the hyponatremia, the differential diagnosis can be narrowed down to diarrhoea, vomiting, medications such as diuretics and anti-depressants, and primary adrenal insufficiency (Addison's disease) (*see Box 21.1*). Of these, Addison's disease seems more likely, as his serum potassium is elevated (diarrhoea, vomiting and diuretic therapy would be expected to cause hypokalaemia). In Addison's disease, hyponatremia and hyperkalaemia occur because of mineralocorticoid (aldosterone) deficiency. Secondary adrenal insufficiency does not cause hyponatremia or hyperkalaemia because aldosterone production is unaffected (*see Figure 21.1*).

DOI: 10.1201/9781003430230-21

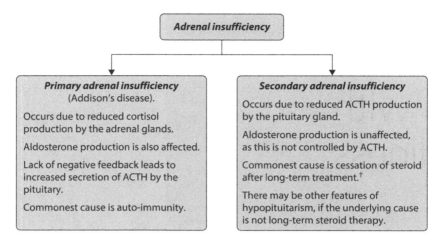

FIGURE 21.1   Primary and secondary adrenal insufficiency. ACTH = adrenocorticotrophic hormone.

† Long-term steroid therapy causes suppression of the hypothalamo-pituitary-adrenal (HPA) axis. Sudden cessation of steroid therapy leads to adrenal insufficiency, as it may take a while for the HPA axis to resume the production of steroid.

- Ask if he recently had ***diarrhoea or vomiting***.
- Obtain a ***medication history***.
- Ask about other possible ***symptoms of adrenal insufficiency*** (*see Box 21.2*).

BOX 21.1   MECHANISMS OF HYPONATREMIA

Hyponatremia implies that there is an excess of free water in the extracellular fluid in relation to sodium (rather than an absolute reduction in total body sodium).

Anti-diuretic hormone (ADH) increases the reabsorption of free water from renal collecting ducts. Hence, any excess free water in the extracellular compartment (and hyponatremia) is due to increased release of ADH, which could be appropriate or inappropriate.

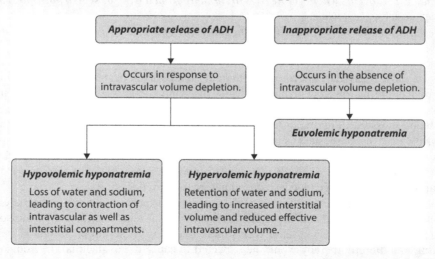

The usual causes of hypovolemic hyponatraemia are diarrhoea, vomiting and diuretic therapy, and those of hypervolemic hyponatraemia are oedematous states like cardiac failure, liver cirrhosis and nephrotic syndrome. Adrenal insufficiency causes euvolemic hyponatremia.

*He feels **tired**, **weak** and **exhausted**. He has **lost about 3–4 kg** in the last two to three months. He has **lost interest in food** because of a **constant sick feeling**. He denies fever, sweats, abdominal pain, diarrhoea or vomiting. He says his family members and friends have commented that he is **getting tanned**.*

His medical history is unremarkable. He does not take any prescription medication or 'over-the-counter' preparation.

There are too many non-specific symptoms, but the clue is in the tanning, which points to primary adrenal sufficiency. The pigmentation is caused by adrenocorticotrophic hormone (ACTH), which possesses melanocyte-stimulating properties. In primary adrenal insufficiency, reduced production of cortisol by the adrenal glands leads to increased ACTH secretion by the pituitary gland (*see Figure 21.1*). Pigmentation is not a feature of secondary adrenal insufficiency, as ACTH secretion is reduced. Interestingly, Cushing's syndrome resulting from ectopic ACTH secretion can also cause pigmentation.

The most common cause of primary adrenal insufficiency is autoimmunity. Among the secondary causes, the two important ones are tuberculosis and adrenal metastases. Other causes are rare and usually present as acute adrenal insufficiency (e.g. cytomegalovirus adrenalitis in acquired immunodeficiency syndrome, thrombosis due to anti-phospholipid antibody syndrome, bleeding in the adrenal glands due to disseminated intravascular coagulation).

Further questions to ask

- Is he on **long-term steroid therapy**?
- Any **headache or visual symptoms**? Is he **bumping into objects**?

(These two questions on steroid therapy and headache or visual disturbance are not relevant in this patient, as the tanning points to primary adrenal insufficiency.)

- Any **cough or haemoptysis**?

Fever, loss of weight (which he has already denied), cough and haemoptysis may point to tuberculosis or lung cancer with adrenal metastasis.

He denies headache, visual symptoms, cough or haemoptysis. He does not bump into objects on his sides. He has not knowingly been in contact with anyone with tuberculosis. He has never taken steroid. He lives with his wife and two children. He does not smoke or drink. He is a software programmer. He has been struggling to cope at work.

WHAT SHOULD YOU LOOK FOR ON EXAMINATION?

Perform a *general examination*.

- Ask for his *blood pressure*, both lying and standing.

Note: Postural hypotension is present if there is a fall in [a] systolic BP by $\geq$20 mm Hg *or* [b] diastolic BP by $\geq$10 mm Hg *or* [c] systolic blood pressure to <90 mm Hg, after standing for ~3 min.

- Check his *fluid status*.

Is he volume depleted, overloaded or euvolemic?

- Examine the palmar creases, buccal mucosa or scars for *pigmentation*.

*He looks **tired**. His **blood pressure is 114/76 mm Hg in the supine and 92/66 mm Hg in the standing position**. He is euvolemic. He looks **tanned** and there is evidence of **pigmentation of palmar creases**. The buccal mucosa looks normal. The rest of the examination is normal.*

 Examination has confirmed the presence of postural hypotension. The pigmentation is in keeping with primary adrenal insufficiency.

HOW SHOULD THIS PATIENT BE EVALUATED FURTHER?

You should request

- **Short Synacthen test** [this is the key investigation].

Note: A blood sample is drawn for measurement of cortisol and ACTH, following which 250 µg of Synacthen (synthetic ACTH) is administered, either intravenously or intramuscularly. Further blood samples are drawn at 30 and 60 minutes to measure serum cortisol. In Addison's disease, baseline cortisol is low and it fails to rise with Synacthen. Cortisol level is checked twice after Synacthen, as some patients may have a sub-normal response at 30 minutes, which normalises at 60 minutes.

- **Thyroid function tests**.
- **21-hydroxylase adrenal antibodies** (usually requested by the endocrinologist).

Positive adrenal antibodies would suggest that adrenal insufficiency is due to autoimmunity.

- **Chest X-ray** (to look for evidence of tuberculosis or lung cancer).
- **Adrenal CT scan** (if adrenal antibodies are negative).

WHAT SHOULD YOU TELL THE PATIENT?

You should tell him that

- His giddiness is due to orthostatic hypotension.

'You feel giddy because your blood pressure falls when you stand up. When we checked your blood pressure while you were lying in bed, the reading was normal. When we measured it again after you stood up, the reading was lower'.

- His blood test result shows hyponatremia.

'The blood test result shows that your salt level is low'.

- You suspect his symptoms are due to adrenal insufficiency.

'We have a gland on top of each kidney called adrenal. The adrenal glands produce a small amount of steroid. I suspect your adrenals are not making enough steroid. Not having enough steroid can cause the blood pressure to fall when you stand up and lower the salt level in your blood. It can also make you lose weight and feel tired and weak'.

- He is getting tanned because of the low steroid level.

'A gland located below the brain produces a hormone in an attempt to increase the production of steroid. This hormone makes the skin darker'.

- The adrenal insufficiency is most likely due to autoimmunity.

'I suspect your immune system is mistakenly attacking your adrenal glands. We do not know why the immune system makes this mistake in some people'.

- You would like to arrange some blood tests to confirm this.

'I'll ask for a few blood tests, including one to check the level of steroid. After drawing a blood sample, the nurse will give you an injection to stimulate the production of steroid and draw further blood samples after 30 and 60 minutes'.

- If adrenal insufficiency is confirmed, it can be treated with hydrocortisone and fludrocortisone.

'If the results show that you are not making enough steroid, we can start you on steroid pills and another pill to stop you from losing salt. These medications will make you feel much better, but let's first see what the blood tests show'.

- You will update him once the results of the investigations are back and refer him to a *'hormone specialist'* if the blood test confirms that his *'steroid level is low'*.

OUTCOME

- His **short Synacthen test is positive**.
- Thyroid stimulating hormone and thyroxine are normal. Chest X-ray is normal.

*He is referred to an endocrinologist. His **21-hydroxylase adrenal antibody is positive**, which supports an autoimmune aetiology. He is commenced on hydrocortisone and fludrocortisone. He is advised to never stop the steroid and wear a bracelet or carry a steroid card with him so that the medical team becomes aware in case he develops an emergency. He is also advised to double to dose of hydrocortisone if he becomes ill or come to the hospital to receive parenteral steroid if he is unable to take orally.*

BOX 21.2   SYMPTOMS OF ADRENAL INSUFFICIENCY

- Giddiness due to orthostatic hypotension.
- Abdominal pain, nausea, vomiting and diarrhoea.
- Weight loss.
- Tiredness, exhaustion, weakness and low mood.
- Pigmentation or tanning (only occurs in primary adrenal insufficiency, *see text*).

The 64-Year-Old Woman Who Recently Fractured Her Wrist   **Case 22**

A 64-year-old woman is referred to the medical clinic, following a recent fracture of her distal radius. Her orthopaedic surgeon is concerned about osteoporosis.

HOW SHOULD THIS PROBLEM BE APPROACHED?

- First, ask **how she fractured her radius**, to determine if it was a fragility fracture (also known as low-trauma fracture).

*She tells you that she **fractured her right wrist** three months ago. She tripped on the kerb while walking her dog and fell on her outstretched hand.*

This is a fragility fracture, as it occurred after she fell from her own standing height. A fragility fracture should always raise the suspicion of osteoporosis. Fractures that are sustained after falling from a height (e.g. from a ladder) are not considered fragility fractures, as they can occur in those with healthy bones as well.

- Ask if she has **fractured any other bone before**. Also ask if she has experienced any **back pain** in the past or **lost height** (might suggest vertebral compression fracture).

Note: A loss of 2 ½ inches in height since young adulthood is considered significant.

*She **broke her collar bone when she was four years old**. She has never suffered with back pain. She doesn't think she is losing height.*

The clavicular fracture at the age of four is not relevant. Osteoporotic fractures are common at sites where there is abundance of trabecular bone (e.g. neck of femur, distal radius, vertebrae, proximal humerus). Vertebral compression fractures are silent in more than two-thirds of patients, so a negative back pain history would not exclude this. Loss of height could result from either vertebral compression fracture *or* age-related shrinking of intervertebral discs. If in doubt, a plain radiograph of the spine should be requested.

    The history should explore possible risk factors for osteoporosis or fragility fractures. The skeleton undergoes remodelling throughout life to maintain the strength of bones. This involves removal of 'old' bone by *osteoclasts* and formation of 'new' bone by *osteoblasts*. Until the age of 30, osteoblasts are more

DOI: 10.1201/9781003430230-22

active than osteoclasts, resulting in a net gain of bone and progressive increase in bone density. Thereafter, osteoclasts become slightly more active, resulting in a net loss of about 0.5–1% of the skeleton every year. Thus, the risk of osteoporosis is increased by factors that affect the acquisition of peak bone mass and/or those that accelerate the subsequent loss.

You should

- Obtain details of **her medical problems** (*see Box 22.1*).

BOX 22.1   SOME MEDICAL CONDITIONS THAT MAY CAUSE OSTEOPOROSIS[†]

- **Endocrine** conditions (e.g. hyperthyroidism, hyperparathyroidism, hypogonadism, Cushing's syndrome, type I diabetes).
- Inflammatory **rheumatic** conditions (e.g. rheumatoid arthritis, ankylosing spondylitis).
- **Gastrointestinal** diseases (e.g. coeliac disease, inflammatory bowel disease).
- **Chronic liver** or **kidney disease**.
- **Haematological** malignancies (e.g. multiple myeloma).
- **Anorexia nervosa**.

[†] Rheumatoid arthritis, hyperthyroidism and multiple myeloma increase the risk of osteoporosis by activating the osteoclasts.
[†] Calcium absorption is reduced in coeliac disease (because of small bowel inflammation) and chronic kidney disease (because of reduced production of the activated form of vitamin D).
[†] Oestrogens (in women) and testosterone (in men) help to strengthen the bone by stimulating the osteoblasts, thus explaining the increased risk of osteoporosis with hypogonadism and anorexia nervosa.

- Obtain a detailed **medication history**, including preparations that can be bought across the counter.

Several medications increase the risk of osteoporosis. For example, (a) corticosteroids and heparin directly inhibit osteoblasts and stimulate osteoclasts, (b) gonadotrophin-releasing hormone analogues inhibit pituitary gonadotrophins, thereby reducing the production of testosterone or oestrogen and (c) aromatase inhibitors reduce the conversion of androgens to oestrogens.

- Ask how old she was at the **time of menarche and menopause**, and whether she took hormone replacement therapy (HRT) after menopause.

Late menarche and/or early menopause (<45 years of age, especially with no HRT thereafter) increase the risk of osteoporosis by reducing the exposure of bones to oestrogens.

- Obtain a **family history**. Ask particularly about **parental history of hip fracture**.

Genetic factors increase the risk of osteoporosis by affecting the peak bone mass.

- Ask about **smoking habit** and **alcohol consumption** (both can increase bone loss).
- Check her **dietary habits** to estimate her intake of calcium and ask **how active** she is.

Inadequate intake of calcium-containing foods and sedentary lifestyle are risk factors for osteoporosis.

- Assess her **future risk of falling**.

Several factors such as cognitive dysfunction, visual impairment, dizziness, muscle weakness, peripheral neuropathy, previous stroke, frailty and unfavourable environmental factors can increase the risk of falls.

*Her **uterus and both ovaries were removed at the age of 41**, as her menses was heavy from fibroids. She did not receive HRT. Her medical history is otherwise unremarkable. She does not take any medication. She s**mokes about five to ten cigarettes/day** and drinks alcohol socially.*

*Her **deceased mother fractured her hip** at the age of 80. She does not consume any dairy products but thinks her diet is otherwise healthy. She walks her dog every day and considers herself an active person. She is a retired civil servant. She lives with her husband.*

 The history has uncovered several risk factors for osteoporosis, such as [a] her early menopause, [b] maternal history of hip fracture and [c] smoking habit. Additionally, she has already sustained a low-trauma fracture, which would place her at a higher risk of developing further fractures.

WHAT SHOULD YOU LOOK FOR ON EXAMINATION?

- Ask for her **height and weight** measurements.

Height and weight measurements are useful for fracture risk assessment (FRAX) (*see below*). Low body mass index is a risk factor for osteoporosis.

- Perform a **general examination** to look for evidence of medical conditions that are known to cause osteoporosis (e.g. hyperthyroidism, Cushingoid features).

Her body mass index is 22. Examination is completely unremarkable.

HOW SHOULD THIS PATIENT BE INVESTIGATED?

The aim of investigating her is to assess her bone mineral density (BMD) and check for possible secondary causes. You should request

- **Dual energy absorptiometry** (DEXA) **scan** of the hip and spine to measure the BMD. This will be reported as T and Z score (*see Box 22.2*).

DEXA scan is not only helpful to diagnose osteoporosis but also assess her future risk of fracture and monitor her response to treatment.

BOX 22.2   THE T AND Z SCORES

The T score is a measure of the deviation of the patient's BMD from the mean BMD of a young adult population (aged about 30 years). Based on the World Health Organisation definition, a T score of up to −1.0 is considered normal, while a score between −1.0 and −2.5 is considered 'low bone mineral density' (or osteopenia) and a score below −2.5 is defined as osteoporosis.[†] These T score thresholds were fixed on the basis of the correlation with fracture risk, with the risk progressively increasing in continuum with declining T scores. In patients who have already had a fragility fracture, osteoporosis can be diagnosed, irrespective of the T score.

The Z score is a measure of the deviation of the patient's BMD from the average BMD of those in her age group, sex and ethnic background. The Z score is mainly useful in younger patients. It is not useful in patients >50 years of age, as the score does not decline with age and some patients with osteoporosis will have 'normal' Z scores. A Z score below −2.0 means that 'the BMD is below the expected range for age', which should prompt a search for secondary causes.

† The spinal BMD may be falsely elevated in the presence of degeneration, ankylosing spondylitis, vertebral fracture or scoliosis. Femoral neck BMD is therefore more reliable for initial diagnosis.

- **Blood tests**, including full blood count, erythrocyte sedimentation rate, liver function tests, serum creatinine, thyroid stimulating hormone, calcium and 25(OH) vitamin D level.

Further investigations such as serum parathyroid hormone level, serum testosterone, myeloma screen and coeliac screen may be indicated in some patients, depending on the results of initial investigations.

Note: Up to a third of the women and half of the men with osteoporosis may have an underlying medical cause.

A **plain radiograph of the thoracolumbar spine** should be requested in those with suspected vertebral compression fracture.

WHAT SHOULD YOU TELL THE PATIENT?

You should explain to her that

- She fractured her wrist most likely because of osteoporosis.

'I suspect you fractured your wrist because of thinning of the bones. We call this osteoporosis'.

- Osteoporosis is a medical condition that increases the risk of fracture.

'If bones are thin, they can break more easily when you fall'.

- Early menopause and maternal history of hip fracture are risk factors for developing osteoporosis.

'In women, ovaries produce the hormone oestrogen, which helps to strengthen bones. The level of oestrogen starts to decline from the time of menopause, which is usually around the age of 50. Because you had your ovaries removed at the age of 41, you must have lost the support of oestrogen much earlier. Additionally, I suspect your mother broke her hip bone because of osteoporosis and you probably inherited the risk from her'.

- You would arrange a bone density scan.

'I'll arrange a scan to check the strength of your bones. It is called a bone density test'.

- You would ask for some blood tests to check for underlying medical conditions that can predispose to osteoporosis.

'I'll ask for some blood tests to check for medical conditions that can increase the risk of osteoporosis'.

- Effective treatments are available to reduce her future risk of fracture.

'We have very effective medications to strengthen the bones and reduce the risk of further fractures. I'll discuss this once I have seen the results of your scan and the blood tests'.

- She should '*stop smoking, as it can weaken her bones*'.
- She should '*take vitamin D supplementation daily, consume a healthy diet to ensure adequate calcium intake and exercise on a regular basis*'. Weight-bearing exercise, like walking, is ideal.

Note: Some common foods that contain calcium include dairy products like milk, cheese and yoghurt, green leafy vegetables like spinach, broccoli, beans and okra, soya and fish like salmon and sardines.

- You will talk to her after she has had the tests.

OUTCOME

The results of her investigations are as follows:

- BMD scan reports **T score of −2.1 in the lumbar spine** and **−2.4 in the left femoral neck**.
- Blood counts, serum creatinine, vitamin D and calcium are normal.

 Although her BMD result shows osteopenia, she can be diagnosed with osteoporosis based on her fragility fracture. Her FRAX shows a ten-year probability of 31% for major osteoporotic fracture and 7.4% for hip fracture (*see Box 22.3*).

Before commencing an anti-resorptive agent for treatment of osteoporosis, it is important to ensure that vitamin D deficiency is corrected. It is also important to check her renal function (alendronate should not be used in patients with creatinine clearance below 35 mL/min) and serum calcium (anti-resorptive agents can aggravate pre-existing hypocalcemia by inhibiting osteoclasts and reducing the release of calcium from bones). Bisphosphonates are associated with a very small risk of osteonecrosis of the jaw (usually seen with higher doses of intravenous bisphosphonates used for cancer), especially when invasive dental procedures are performed. Long-term use of bisphosphonates is also associated with a small risk of atypical femoral fractures, hence the need for a 'drug holiday' after five to ten years of continuous treatment.

BOX 22.3 FRACTURE RISK ASSESSMENT

The aim of treating osteoporosis is to *prevent a* fracture, not just improve the BMD. The decision to treat is straightforward in patients with osteoporosis and previous fragility fractures, but in other cases, a risk assessment to estimate the ten-year probability of fracture would be helpful. This estimate is based on whether or not there are other factors that can *independently* increase the risk of fracture. An analogy could be drawn with hyperlipidemia, where the aim of treatment is to reduce the risk of myocardial infarction or stroke. The threshold for starting statin therapy would be lower in those with other independent cardiovascular risk factors.

Independent risk factors for fragility fractures include increasing age, low body mass index, previous fragility fractures, parental history of hip fracture, rheumatoid arthritis, use of corticosteroids, smoking habit, alcohol consumption and secondary causes of osteoporosis like premature menopause, insulin-dependent diabetes mellitus, hyperthyroidism, hypogonadism, malabsorption and chronic liver disease. The World Health Organisation has developed a fracture risk assessment score (FRAX score, see www.sheffield.ac.uk/FRAX) that enables us to input these risk factors with or without the femoral neck T score, and calculate the ten-year risk of fracture.

A ten-year risk of >3% for hip fracture *or* >20% for major osteoporotic fracture (hip, clinical spine, proximal humerus or forearm) is generally considered the threshold for starting pharmacological treatment. Clinical judgement should still take precedence, as there are some shortcomings with the FRAX calculation.

The 43-Year-Old Man with Hypercalcaemia

Case 23

A 43-year-old man presents to the emergency department with renal colic. Plain X-ray of the abdomen shows a radio-opaque calculus in the right kidney. His pain resolves with intramuscular diclofenac.

His serum calcium is 3.12 mmol/L (normal 2.1–2.6). Full blood count, serum creatinine and urinalysis are normal. Your opinion is sought for the hypercalcaemia.

His temperature is 36.8°C, pulse rate 76/min, blood pressure 122/78 mm Hg, respiratory rate 16/min and O_2 saturation 95% on room air.

HOW SHOULD THIS PROBLEM BE APPROACHED?

Hypercalcaemia is the most likely cause of his renal stone. After greeting the patient, ask how he is and ensure that he is well enough to talk to you.

- Ask only briefly about the ***renal colic***, as the focus of this consultation is hypercalcaemia.

*He says he is well and the pain has resolved. He suddenly developed **pain in his right loin** a few hours ago. The pain radiated to the groin. The pain was so bad that he couldn't stay still in one place. He has never experienced something like this before. There was no fever, burning sensation on passing urine or blood in the urine. The doctor in A and E has just told him that the X-ray shows a kidney stone.*

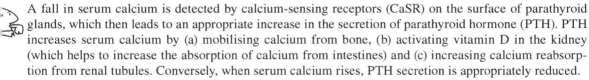

A fall in serum calcium is detected by calcium-sensing receptors (CaSR) on the surface of parathyroid glands, which then leads to an appropriate increase in the secretion of parathyroid hormone (PTH). PTH increases serum calcium by (a) mobilising calcium from bone, (b) activating vitamin D in the kidney (which helps to increase the absorption of calcium from intestines) and (c) increasing calcium reabsorption from renal tubules. Conversely, when serum calcium rises, PTH secretion is appropriately reduced.

The causes of hypercalcaemia are listed in *Box 23.1*, of which hyperparathyroidism (~80–90% of the cases) and malignancy are the most common. Hyperparathyroidism can be

- Primary (usually due to parathyroid adenoma, and rarely, hyperplasia or carcinoma).
- Secondary (due to chronic kidney disease, as deficiency of activated vitamin D reduces calcium absorption, which then leads to increased PTH secretion via negative feedback).
- Tertiary (autonomous secretion of PTH in chronic kidney disease after long-standing secondary hyperparathyroidism).

DOI: 10.1201/9781003430230-23

Hypercalcaemia occurs in primary and tertiary hyperparathyroidism (increased PTH in secondary hyperparathyroidism usually only restores serum calcium to normal).

In patients with malignancy, hypercalcaemia occurs because of PTH-related peptide secretion by cancer cells (e.g. non-metastatic solid tumours like lung cancer) or direct stimulation of osteoclasts by cytokines (e.g. multiple myeloma, bone metastases).

Thiazides cause hypercalcaemia by increasing the reabsorption of calcium from renal tubules, while lithium promotes increased PTH secretion. In hyperthyroidism, there is increased bone resorption, and in sarcoidosis, the granulomatous tissues secrete $1,25(OH)_2$ cholecalciferol. Familial hypocalciuric hypercalcaemia (FHH) is a rare autosomal dominant condition, in which CaSRs do not sense the rise in serum calcium. The secretion of PTH is therefore not suppressed. Hypocalciuria occurs because the CaSRs that are present in renal tubules are unable to sense the hypercalcaemia and appropriately increase calcium excretion in the urine.

BOX 23.1   CAUSES OF HYPERCALCAEMIA

- Hyperparathyroidism.
- Malignancy (e.g. solid tumours like lung cancer, multiple myeloma, bone metastases).
- Hypervitaminosis D (usually from administration of large doses of parenteral vitamin D).
- Medications (e.g. thiazides, lithium).
- Hyperthyroidism.
- Sarcoidosis.
- Familial hypercalciuric hypercalcaemia.

Apart from renal colic due to stone, symptoms of hypercalcaemia include loss of appetite, nausea, abdominal pain, constipation, polyuria (due to nephrogenic diabetes insipidus), lethargy and decline in cognition, hence the pneumonic *'bones, stones, abdominal groans and psychic moans'*. Some patients present with hypercalcaemic crisis, which is characterised by severe abdominal pain, altered mental state, vomiting, polyuria and intravascular volume depletion. Patients who present with crisis nearly always have an underlying malignancy.

Before proceeding further, tell him that his blood test shows hypercalcaemia. *'Your blood test shows that your calcium level is high. This may be the cause of the kidney stone. Please allow me to ask you a few questions and I will then explain why your calcium level might be high and what we can do about it'.*

- Ask about other **symptoms of hypercalcemia**, like loss of appetite, nausea, abdominal pain, constipation, polyuria, lethargy and problems with memory or concentration.
- Ask if he has ever **fractured a bone**.
- Ask if he **smokes** and check for **symptoms of cancer**, like cough, haemoptysis and loss of weight.
- Ask about **symptoms that may suggest sarcoidosis**, like joint pain, skin rashes, swollen lymph glands and breathlessness.
- Ask about **symptoms of hyperthyroidism**, like palpitations, tremors, diarrhoea, weight loss and swelling over the neck.
- Complete the **rest of the history**.

Ask about his past medical problems, medications taken (e.g. thiazide, lithium, vitamin D injections) and family history.

*His **bowel habit has been a bit irregular for the last six months**, with a bowel movement only occurring about once every two to three days. He was moving his bowels every day prior to that. Of late, he has also been **getting tired very easily**. He denies nausea, loss of appetite, polyuria or problems with memory or concentration. He has never fractured a bone. Review of systems is unremarkable, with no symptoms of cancer, sarcoidosis or hyperthyroidism.*

His past medical history is unremarkable except for childhood asthma and hepatitis A many years ago. He does not take any medication and has never received vitamin D. He does not smoke or drink. He is a social worker. He lives with his wife and three children. His family history is unremarkable.

Although non-specific, the recent change in his bowel habit and tiredness may be due to hypercalcaemia. The history has not provided any leads to an underlying cause of his hypercalcaemia. Medication-induced hypercalcaemia can be excluded. FHH is also less likely in the absence of a positive family history.

WHAT SHOULD YOU LOOK FOR ON EXAMINATION?

You should

- Check for signs of intravascular *volume depletion* (dryness of mucous membranes and reduced skin turgor).
- Perform a *general examination* to check for possible clues that may suggest an underlying cause of hypercalcaemia (e.g. finger clubbing, supraclavicular lymphadenopathy, skin rashes of sarcoidosis).
- *Listen to the lungs* and *palpate the abdomen* for hepatomegaly or mass.
- Check his *thyroid status*.

He is comfortable at rest. His mucous membranes are moist and skin turgor is not reduced. General examination is unremarkable. His lungs are clear and abdomen is soft, with no mass or organomegaly. He is clinically euthyroid.

HOW SHOULD HE BE EVALUATED?

You should request

- *Blood tests*, including serum PTH, phosphate, vitamin D and thyroid function tests.

Notes:

1. In patients with asymptomatic hypercalcaemia, it may be prudent to first repeat the serum calcium without a tourniquet to draw the blood sample.
2. Serum PTH is the crucial investigation. PTH is elevated or normal in primary hyperparathyroidism, and low in malignancy, hypervitaminosis and sarcoidosis. Normal PTH indicates primary hyperparathyroidism because high serum calcium would be expected to suppress PTH level.
3. PTH reduces the reabsorption of phosphate from renal tubules, so serum phosphate levels are low in primary hyperparathyroidism.
4. Concomitant vitamin D deficiency may mask hypercalcaemia in some patients with hyperparathyroidism. Following correction of vitamin D deficiency, serum calcium level rises further in these patients.

- *Chest X-ray* may reveal lung cancer or hilar lymphadenopathy of sarcoidosis.
- A *12-lead ECG* may show short QT interval.

The *following investigations are indicated in selected patients*, depending on the clinical presentation and serum PTH level.

- Serum angiotensin-converting enzyme and 1,25(OH)$_2$ vitamin D, if available (in suspected sarcoidosis).
- Myeloma screen and computed tomography of the chest, abdomen and pelvis (for cancer screening).
- 24-hour urine calcium (in suspected FHH).
- Bone mineral density (BMD) scan in patients with hyperparathyroidism.

Note: Forearm BMD is preferred, as hyperparathyroidism tends to affect cortical bone, which is predominant in the radius.

- Plain X-rays of hands may show sub-periosteal bone resorption, and X-rays of long bones, skull or pelvis may show osteitis fibrosa cystica ('brown tumour') in hyperparathyroidism.

WHAT SHOULD YOU TELL THE PATIENT?

Having already told him that his serum calcium level is high, you should now tell him that

- There are a number of causes for hypercalcaemia.

'There are a number of possible causes for a high calcium level in the blood. Based on my assessment, I am unable to say at present which one of those is causing the high calcium'.

- The recent change in his bowel habit and tiredness could be due to the hypercalcaemia.

'A high calcium level can affect the bowel movement and make you constipated. Because your bowel habits have been irregular for more than six months, I suspect your calcium level has been high for quite some time. High calcium can also make you feel tired'.

- You would like to arrange a few investigations.

'I'll first ask for a few blood tests and an X-ray of your chest. Depending on what these show, you may need some more tests later'.

- Treatment depends on the underlying cause of the hypercalcaemia.

'We'll discuss the treatments once we find out what is causing the high calcium. In the meantime, make sure you drink enough fluids to keep yourself hydrated'.

- You would talk to him when the results are back.
- The urologist (*'kidney specialist'*) will discuss the plan for the renal stone.

OUTCOME

His results are as follows:

- **Serum PTH 98 pg/mL** (normal 11–50).
- **Serum phosphate 0.84 mmol/L** (normal 1–1.45).

- Vitamin D 36 ng/mL (normal >30).
- Thyroid-stimulating hormone and thyroxine normal.
- Chest X-ray normal.

*He is referred to an endocrinologist. Bone density scan shows T scores of −0.4 in the spine, −0.8 in the femoral neck and −1.4 in the distal radius. Neck ultrasound and sestamibi scan show a **solitary parathyroid adenoma**. He is referred to an endocrine surgeon to consider parathyroidectomy. The urologist performs lithotripsy and removes the renal stone.*

His results are in keeping with primary hyperparathyroidism, as serum PTH is elevated and phosphate is low. This is not tertiary hyperparathyroidism, as his kidney function is normal. As mentioned earlier, hypercalcaemia with normal PTH should also make you suspect hyperparathyroidism, as the elevated calcium would normally be expected to suppress PTH level. Some patients may have normal calcium and high PTH due to concomitant vitamin D deficiency.

Ultrasound and sestamibi scan are useful to localise the parathyroid adenoma before surgery.

Parathyroidectomy was indicated in this patient because of his young age and presence of renal calculus. Other indications for surgery include reduced bone density and neuropsychiatric symptoms. Parathyroidectomy is likely to significantly reduce his risk of renal stone formation, and also improve his bowel habit and energy levels.

The 36-Year-Old Woman with Amenorrhoea

Case 24

A 36-year-old woman presents with a four-month history of amenorrhoea.

HOW SHOULD THIS PROBLEM BE APPROACHED?

---

*She tells you that she **hasn't had a period for nearly four months**. She has previously never missed a period except during her two pregnancies.*

 Amenorrhoea or absence of menstruation may be *primary* (never started menstruating) or *secondary* (cessation of menstruation for more than three months, after previous regular menses). The amenorrhoea in this patient is clearly secondary, as her menstruation only ceased four months back, having been regular prior to that.

- It is important to first establish that she is not **pregnant** or **breastfeeding**. Also ask if she is taking (or recently came off) the **oral contraceptive pill**.
- Check for functional causes of amenorrhoea, like athletic activity and anorexia nervosa.

Ask about her **eating and exercise habits**, **change in body weight** and **stressors**.

She has been sexually inactive for the last three years since divorcing her ex-husband. Her GP performed the urine pregnancy test anyway and it was negative. She has never been on the oral contraceptive pill.

She is a journalist. She lives with her two teenage daughters. She denies recent stresses at home or work. She goes for a brisk walk about two to three times a week. Her exercise routine and eating habits have not changed recently. Her weight has been steady. She does not play any sports.

 Having excluded physiological and functional causes, you should now look for features that may suggest a medical cause.

Amenorrhoea occurs due to low oestrogen. The production of oestrogen by the ovaries is stimulated by luteinising hormone (LH) and follicle-stimulating hormone (FSH) from the anterior pituitary, which in turn are stimulated by gonadotrophin-releasing hormone (GnRH) from the hypothalamus (*see Figure 24.1*). Hence, amenorrhoea may result from (a) ovarian insufficiency, (b) hypothalamus or pituitary disorder, (c) excess prolactin, (d) excess androgen *or* (e) thyroid disease (both hypo as well as hyperthyroidism).

DOI: 10.1201/9781003430230-24

Excess prolactin or androgen causes amenorrhoea by reducing the release of GnRH via negative feedback inhibition. In hypothyroidism, amenorrhoea occurs because of elevated prolactin (*see Box 24.1*), while in hyperthyroidism, the increased sex hormone binding globulin enables more oestrogen to be bound, thus effectively reducing the level of 'free' oestrogen.

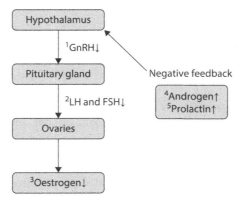

FIGURE 24.1 Hypothalamic-pituitary-ovarian axis and causes of amenorrhoea. GnRH = Gonadotrophin-releasing hormone, LH = Luteinising hormone, FSH = Follicle-stimulating hormone.

Further questions to ask:

▪ Any **headache** or **visual disturbance** (would suggest pituitary tumour)?

Even if she says that her eyesight is normal, ask if she is **bumping into objects** on her sides.

▪ Any **milk discharge from the nipple** (would suggest excess prolactin)?
▪ Any **abnormal hair growth or acne** (would suggest excess androgen)?

Note: The causes of excess androgen secretion include polycystic ovarian syndrome (the most common cause of secondary amenorrhoea), late-onset congenital adrenal hyperplasia, and adrenal and ovarian tumours that produce androgens.

▪ Any **symptoms of thyroid disease**, such as weight gain or loss, change in bowel habits, cold or heat intolerance, tremors, and palpitations?
▪ Any **menopausal symptoms** (caused by low oestrogen due to any cause), such as hot flashes, vaginal dryness, headache or low mood?
▪ What **medications** does she take (e.g. ovarian failure due to chemotherapeutic agents, increased prolactin due to dopamine antagonists)?
▪ Are there **risk factors for osteoporosis**, such as previous fragility fractures, family history of osteoporosis, smoking habit and alcohol consumption?

Note: Low oestrogen due to any cause increases the risk of osteoporosis (although her absolute risk of fracture would be low because of her young age).

*She denies headache. Her eyesight is normal, and she does not bump into objects on her sides. She has recently noticed an intermittent **milk discharge from both her nipples**. There is no acne, abnormal hair growth or symptoms of thyroid disease. Her past medical history is unremarkable, and she is on no regular medication. There is no personal or family history of low trauma fractures. She has never smoked and seldom drinks alcohol. She denies menopausal symptoms.*

The milk discharge from her nipples (galactorrhoea) suggests that her amenorrhoea is due to elevated prolactin (*see Box 24.1*).

BOX 24.1   CAUSES OF ELEVATED PROLACTIN

Prolactin is secreted by the anterior pituitary gland. As the name suggests, its main function is to promote lactation. Dopamine that is produced in the hypothalamus inhibits the release of prolactin, while thyrotrophin-releasing hormone has the opposite effect and stimulates the release of prolactin. Thus, excess prolactin could be due to

- ***Prolactin-secreting tumour***[†, ††].
- ***Dopamine antagonists*** (e.g. chlorpromazine, domperidone, metoclopramide).
- ***Tumour that compresses the pituitary stalk*** (the part that connects the hypothalamus and pituitary gland).

These tumours, although non-functional, prevent dopamine from reaching the pituitary by compressing the pituitary stalk.

- ***Hypothyroidism***.

Low thyroxine increases the production of thyrotrophin-releasing hormone by the hypothalamus.

[†] In a small number of patients with prolactinoma, there may be features of acromegaly because of co-secretion of growth hormone by the pituitary tumour.
[††] Macroprolactinomas (>1 cm) may compress the normal pituitary tissue and present with features of hypopituitarism.

High prolactin due to medication can be ruled out. Although there are no features suggestive of hypothyroidism, a simple blood test should help to exclude this. It is very likely that she has got a pituitary tumour, possibly a microadenoma (<1 cm). Interestingly, headache and bitemporal hemianopia are more common in men than in women with prolactinoma. This is because of the non-specific nature of symptoms in men (e.g. erectile dysfunction, loss of libido, fatigue), which delays their presentation and allows the tumour to grow larger. Women present much earlier with amenorrhoea and galactorrhoea.

WHAT SHOULD YOU LOOK FOR ON EXAMINATION?

Examination should be based on the history. You should

- Check her ***thyroid status***.
- Look for ***hirsutism and acne***.
- Check for ***bitemporal hemianopia***, especially in patients with headache or visual disturbance.

General examination is unremarkable. She is clinically euthyroid. There is no evidence of hirsutism or acne. Her visual fields are normal.

HOW SHOULD THIS PATIENT BE EVALUATED FURTHER?

- ***Serum prolactin*** is the key investigation in this patient.
- ***Serum LH and FSH***.

Note: Think of ovarian insufficiency or natural menopause if LH and FSH are elevated, and hypothalamic or pituitary disorder if LH and FSH are both reduced.

- ***Thyroid function tests***.
- ***Pituitary MRI scan*** (if serum prolactin is high).
- ***Serum testosterone***, ***dehydroepiandrosterone and 17-OH progesterone*** (in patients with features of virilisation or androgen excess).

WHAT SHOULD YOU TELL THE PATIENT?

You should tell her that

- The amenorrhoea is most likely due to elevated prolactin.

'I suspect your periods have stopped because you are producing too much of a hormone called prolactin'.

- The galactorrhoea is also caused by the elevated prolactin.

'The milk discharge from your breasts is also caused by excess prolactin. Prolactin helps the breasts to produce milk and it should only be produced after childbirth, not at other times'.

- The cause of excess prolactin is most likely a pituitary tumour.

'Prolactin is made by a small gland called pituitary that is located below the brain. We often find a small growth in this gland in people with high prolactin'.

- You would ask for some blood tests, including serum prolactin level.

'I'll ask for some blood tests, including one to check your prolactin level'.

- If prolactin is elevated, you will refer to an endocrinologist and ask for a scan of the pituitary.

'If the blood tests confirm that your prolactin level is high, I'll ask a hormone specialist to see you. I'll also arrange a scan of the pituitary gland to check if there is a growth'.

- The endocrinologist will plan the treatment depending on the results of the investigations.

'Once the results of these tests are available, the specialist will discuss the treatment options with you. There are medications that can shrink the growth and bring the prolactin level back to normal. This will restore your periods and stop the milk discharge as well'.

- You will update her when the results of the tests are back.

OUTCOME

Her blood test results are as follows:

- **Serum prolactin 324 μg/dL** (normal range for non-pregnant women 4–24).
- Serum LH and FSH low.
- TSH and thyroxine normal.
- Full blood count, liver and renal function are normal.
- MRI scan of the pituitary shows a **microadenoma**.

She is commenced on cabergoline (dopamine agonist), following which the serum prolactin returns to normal, and the amenorrhoea and galactorrhoea resolve.

The 51-Year-Old Man with Polyuria

Case 25

A 51-year-old man is referred to the medical clinic with a three-month history of excessive urination. Two recent fasting blood glucose values and HbA₁c have been normal.

HOW SHOULD THIS PROBLEM BE APPROACHED?

---

*He tells you that he has been **passing a lot of water** for the last six months. He drinks several jugs of water every day because he is **thirsty all the time**. This is causing a lot of inconvenience for him in his job as a lorry driver, as he is forced to take frequent toilet breaks during long-distance drives. He also wakes up about two to three times at night to go to the toilet. His GP tested him for diabetes on two separate occasions and told him that his **blood sugar result was normal**.*

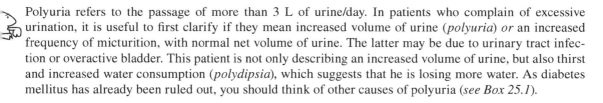

Polyuria refers to the passage of more than 3 L of urine/day. In patients who complain of excessive urination, it is useful to first clarify if they mean increased volume of urine (*polyuria*) or an increased frequency of micturition, with normal net volume of urine. The latter may be due to urinary tract infection or overactive bladder. This patient is not only describing an increased volume of urine, but also thirst and increased water consumption (*polydipsia*), which suggests that he is losing more water. As diabetes mellitus has already been ruled out, you should think of other causes of polyuria (*see Box 25.1*).

BOX 25.1   CAUSES OF POLYURIA

- Diabetes mellitus.
- Medications (e.g. diuretics) and alcohol.
- Chronic kidney disease.
- Hypercalcaemia or hypokalaemia.
- Diabetes insipidus.[†, ††,†††]
- Psychogenic polydipsia.

[†] Diabetes insipidus (DI) occurs due to [a] reduced secretion of anti-diuretic hormone (ADH) by the posterior pituitary gland (central DI) *or* [b] reduced responsiveness of the renal collecting ducts to the action of ADH (nephrogenic DI). Free water reabsorption from the kidneys is reduced as a result, leading to the passage of large amounts of dilute and insipid (tasteless) urine.

[††] Central DI may be idiopathic *or* secondary to pituitary tumour, hypothalamic-pituitary surgery, trauma, infections like tuberculosis or infiltrative diseases like sarcoidosis.

[†††] Nephrogenic DI may be familial *or* secondary to lithium, hypokalaemia or hypercalcaemia.

DOI: 10.1201/9781003430230-25

You should ask about:

- **Headache** and **visual symptoms** (may suggest pituitary tumour).

Even if he says that he can see normally, ask if he is **bumping into objects** on his sides.

- **Difficulty in raising his arms or rising from a seated position** (proximal weakness due to hypokalaemia).
- **Loss of appetite, nausea, constipation and abdominal or back pain** (symptoms of hypercalcaemia).
- His past **medical problems**.

A previous diagnosis of renal or neurological disease, surgery or trauma to the head, psychiatric problems and tuberculosis are particularly relevant.

- **Medications taken** and **alcohol** intake.

He denies headache. His eyesight is normal, and he does not bump into objects on his sides. He is able to raise his arms and rise from the seated position without any difficulty. He denies loss of appetite, nausea, abdominal pain, constipation and back pain.

*His past medical history is blameless, with no previous diagnosis of renal, neurological or psychiatric disease. He has never been diagnosed or knowingly been in contact with anyone with tuberculosis. There is no history of previous trauma or surgery to the head. He does not take any medication. He seldom dinks alcohol but **smokes about 20 cigarettes/day**. He lives with his wife.*

Medication and alcohol-induced diuresis can be excluded based on the history. Although there are no features suggestive of hypercalcaemia, hypokalaemia or chronic kidney disease, some simple blood tests should help to exclude these possibilities. Diabetes insipidus (DI), although rare, is a possible differential. The absence of headache or visual symptoms makes it unlikely that he has a large pituitary tumour. Psychogenic polydipsia (compulsive water drinking, leading to low plasma osmolality and appropriate suppression of ADH secretion) should not be considered at this stage.

WHAT SHOULD YOU LOOK FOR ON EXAMINATION?

- Check for signs of **intravascular volume depletion** (e.g. reduced skin turgor, dryness of mucous membranes).
- Examine his **visual fields** for evidence of bitemporal hemianopia.

His vital parameters are normal. There are no signs of volume depletion. Visual fields are normal, with no evidence of bitemporal hemianopia. Rest of the examination is unremarkable.

HOW SHOULD THIS PATIENT BE EVALUATED?

You should request

- **Serum creatinine, electrolytes** and **calcium**.

These tests would help to confirm or rule out chronic kidney disease, hypokalaemia or hypercalcaemia.

- *Plasma and urine osmolality.*

DI is characterised by elevated plasma osmolality and low urine osmolality, as there is less free water reabsorption from renal tubules.

- *Magnetic resonance imaging (MRI) scan of the pituitary* (in patients with central DI).

WHAT SHOULD YOU TELL THE PATIENT AT THIS STAGE?

You should tell him that

- The cause of his polyuria is not diabetes mellitus.

'Diabetes is the most common cause for passing too much water. You do not have diabetes because your blood sugar results are normal'.

- Apart from diabetes, there are other causes of polyuria. You would like to arrange some investigations to check for these causes, as the history has not provided any leads.

'There are a few other possible causes. You can pass a large amount of water if the kidneys are not working well, or there is too much calcium or not enough potassium in the blood. I'll ask for a few blood tests to check for these causes'.

- DI is another type of diabetes that can cause polyuria.

'There is a less common type of diabetes that can make you pass a lot of water. This has got nothing to do with sugar. We have a tiny gland below the brain called pituitary, which makes a hormone that helps to retain water in the body. If the pituitary gland does not produce enough of this hormone or the hormone does not work properly, water cannot be retained in the body and a large amount will be lost in the urine. When you lose more water in the urine, it makes you thirsty and forces you to drink more fluids. I'll ask for some blood and urine tests to check for this as well'.

- You will refer him to a *'hormone specialist'* after the initial test results are back. The specialist will discuss the treatment options.
- You will update him once the results of the tests are back.

OUTCOME

The results of the investigations are as follows:

- Serum creatinine 78 μmol/L, **sodium 148 mmol/L** and potassium 4.1 mmol/L.
- Corrected serum calcium 2.36 mmol/L (normal 2.2–2.7).
- **Plasma osmolality 316 mOsm/kg** (normal 275–295) and **urine osmolality 140 mOsm/kg** (normal 500–800).

The high plasma osmolality and low urine osmolality point to DI. He should be referred to an endocrinologist. MRI of the pituitary should be requested to exclude a pituitary tumour. The water deprivation test is useful to differentiate between central and nephrogenic DI (*see Table 25.1*).

The results have excluded chronic kidney disease, hypercalcaemia and hypokalaemia. Psychogenic polydipsia can also be excluded, as plasma osmolality would be expected to be low in this condition.

TABLE 25.1   The water deprivation test[a]

	BASELINE PLASMA OSMOLALITY	*BASELINE URINE OSMOLALITY*	*FOLLOWING WATER DEPRIVATION*
Cranial DI	Increased.	Decreased.	Plasma osmolality increases further. ADH is not released in response to a rise in plasma osmolality, so urine osmolality remains low. Urine osmolality rises after administration of desmopressin.
Nephrogenic DI	Increased.	Decreased.	As above, but no change in urine osmolality even after administration of desmopressin.
Psychogenic polydipsia	Decreased, as a result of compulsive water drinking (ADH release is inhibited because of reduced plasma osmolality).	Appropriately decreased.	Plasma and urine osmolality become normal.

[a] Normal response to water deprivation is a rise in plasma osmolality, which stimulates the secretion of ADH. This causes reabsorption of free water from the kidneys and rise in urine osmolality.

The endocrinologist arranges the water deprivation test. **Following water deprivation, urine osmolality fails to rise**, *confirming the diagnosis of DI.* **After administration of desmopressin**, **urine osmolality rises**, *suggesting that the DI is central. MRI scan of the pituitary gland is normal, with no evidence of tumour. The other pituitary hormones are checked and found to be normal, thus excluding pan-hypopituitarism.*

In the absence of any of the known causes, the DI is presumed to be idiopathic. He is commenced on desmopressin, which results in significant improvement of his symptoms.

The 28-Year-Old Woman with High Blood Pressure   **Case 26**

A 28-year-old woman is referred to the medical clinic, as her blood pressure has been consistently over 160/100 mm Hg for the last three months.

HOW SHOULD THIS PROBLEM BE APPROACHED?

- Find out **why her blood pressure was checked** in the first place.

*She says she first consulted her GP about three months ago for pain in her right elbow. Her GP diagnosed tennis elbow and advised a splint and topical anti-inflammatory cream, which helped to improve the pain over the next few weeks. It was during these consultations that her **blood pressure readings were noted to be high**. She then bought a blood pressure machine and the readings have been similar at home too.*

- Ensure that she is well, with no features of **hypertensive emergency** (*see Box 26.1*).

Ask about headache, focal neurological symptoms, seizures, visual symptoms, breathlessness, chest pain and reduced urine output.

Note: Both hypertensive emergency and urgency are characterised by significantly elevated blood pressure (systolic >180 mm Hg *or* diastolic >120 mm Hg). While the former is associated with end-organ injury (brain, eyes, heart and kidney), the latter is not.

BOX 26.1   MANIFESTATIONS OF HYPERTENSIVE EMERGENCY

- Hypertensive encephalopathy or stroke.
- Retinopathy.
- Left heart failure.
- Acute coronary syndrome.
- Aortic dissection.
- Acute kidney injury.
- Thrombotic microangiopathy.

She feels well. There are no features of hypertensive emergency.

Although blood pressure transiently increases when patients visit the hospital or clinic ('white coat hypertension'), she could be labelled as hypertensive on the basis that repeated blood pressure measurements have been consistently high for several weeks, not only in the clinic but also at home. Having established that there are no features of hypertensive emergency, a detailed history should be obtained to uncover a possible secondary cause for her hypertension because of her young age.

In general, a secondary cause should be suspected in:

- Patients younger than 35 years of age.
- Those who develop hypertension after the age of 55.
- Those who are resistant to three or more anti-hypertensive drugs.

BOX 26.2   SECONDARY CAUSES OF HYPERTENSION†

- ***Renal causes*** (e.g. acute or chronic glomerulonephritis, polycystic kidney disease, renal artery stenosis).
- ***Endocrine causes*** (e.g. Cushing's syndrome, primary aldosteronism, phaeochromocytoma, hyperparathyroidism, hyperthyroidism).
- ***Drugs*** (e.g. corticosteroids, non-steroidal anti-inflammatory drugs, cyclosporine, illicit drugs like cocaine and amphetamines).
- ***Pregnancy-related hypertension*** (pre-eclampsia, eclampsia).
- ***Coarctation of aorta***.
- ***Obstructive sleep apnoea***.

† Underlying mechanisms include (a) increased peripheral vascular resistance due to vasoconstriction, (b) increased blood volume due to sodium and water retention and (c) increased cardiac output. In renal artery stenosis, for example, reduced renal blood flow activates the renin-angiotensin-aldosterone axis, which leads to increased levels of angiotensin II and aldosterone. The angiotensin II causes vasoconstriction, and aldosterone retains sodium and water.

Further questions to ask (*see Box 26.2*):

- ***Features that may suggest renal disease*** (e.g. change in the colour of urine or frothing, ankle swelling, previous diagnosis of kidney disease, history of recurrent urinary tract infections, family history of kidney disease).
- ***Features that may suggest endocrine disease*** (e.g. change in weight, easy bruising, proximal limb weakness, tremors, palpitations, diarrhoea, heat intolerance, 'panic attacks').

Note: 'Panic attacks' (brief episodes of headache, palpitations, sweating and tremors) are a feature of phaeochromocytoma.

- ***Snoring*** and ***daytime sleepiness*** (obstructive sleep apnoea).

You should ask if her bed partner or roommate complains that she snores!

- ***Leg claudication*** or ***cold feet*** (coarctation of aorta).
- ***Medications taken***, including the use of 'over-the-counter' preparations and illicit drugs.
- Her ***last menstrual period***.

She denies symptoms of renal or endocrine disease, leg claudication, cold feet and daytime sleepiness. Her past medical history is unremarkable. She does not take any prescription medication or 'over-the-counter' preparation or use illicit drugs. She does not smoke or drink. She is single and has never been pregnant. Her last menstrual period was ten days ago. She works as a checkout clerk at the local super-market and lives alone.

WHAT SHOULD YOU LOOK FOR ON EXAMINATION?

You should

- Check her *peripheral pulses* and ask for her *blood pressure in both arms*.
- Check for *radio-femoral delay*.

Note: If radio-femoral delay is present, ask for the blood pressure in upper and lower limbs, as coarctation of aorta is characterised by upper limb hypertension and lower limb hypotension.

- Examine the heart and check for *murmurs* and *signs of heart failure* (e.g. basal lung crackles, ankle oedema).
- Examine the abdomen for *palpable kidneys* and audible *renal bruit*.
- Look for *signs that may suggest an endocrine cause* (*see Box 26.3*).

> ### BOX 26.3   SIGNS THAT MAY SUGGEST SECONDARY HYPERTENSION
>
> - Cushingoid appearance, moon facies, abdominal striae (*Cushing's syndrome*), proximal limb weakness (*Cushing's syndrome, Conn's syndrome or hyperthyroidism*).
> - Tachycardia, atrial fibrillation, tremor, goitre, exophthalmos (*hyperthyroidism*).
> - Palpable kidneys (*polycystic kidney disease*).
> - Renal artery bruit (*renal artery stenosis*).
> - Unequal pulses, difference in blood pressure of >10 mm Hg between the upper limbs or evidence of peripheral arterial bruits (*Takayasu's arteritis*).
> - Radio-femoral delay and murmur of aortic coarctation.
> - Neurofibromas or *café-au-lait* spots (associated with hypertension).

*She weighs 53 kg. Her blood pressure is **162/102 mm Hg in her right arm and 156/98 in her left arm**. Cardiovascular examination is otherwise normal. All her peripheral pulses are felt equally. There is no radio-femoral delay. There are no bruits over the carotid, subclavian or renal arteries. Her kidneys are not palpable. There are no stigmata of endocrine disease.*

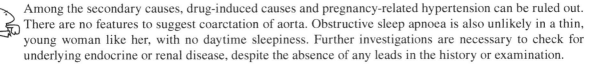

Among the secondary causes, drug-induced causes and pregnancy-related hypertension can be ruled out. There are no features to suggest coarctation of aorta. Obstructive sleep apnoea is also unlikely in a thin, young woman like her, with no daytime sleepiness. Further investigations are necessary to check for underlying endocrine or renal disease, despite the absence of any leads in the history or examination.

HOW SHOULD THIS PATIENT BE INVESTIGATED?

An age-based approach is useful. You should think of (a) coarctation of aorta, renal parenchymal disease, renal artery stenosis due to fibromuscular dysplasia and Takayasu's arteritis in adolescents and young adults, (b) endocrine causes and sleep apnoea in the middle aged *and* (c) atherosclerotic renal artery stenosis in the elderly.

In this patient, you should ask for

- **Blood tests**, including full blood count, serum creatinine and electrolytes, and fasting glucose.
- **Urinalysis** (microscopic examination and protein-creatinine ratio).
- **Urine pregnancy test**.
- **12-lead ECG** (left ventricular hypertrophy or strain would suggest long-standing hypertension).
- **Chest X-ray** (might reveal signs of heart failure, notching of the ribs in patients with coarctation of the aorta).
- **Duplex ultrasound scan of the kidneys**.

The ultrasound scan is useful to look for structural problems in the kidneys (e.g. contracted kidneys, renal outflow obstruction *or* polycystic kidneys), and Doppler helps to assess renal arterial flow, which is useful to diagnose renal artery stenosis.

- **Aldosterone-renin ratio**.

Aldosterone is elevated and renin is suppressed in primary aldosteronism, while both aldosterone and renin are elevated in secondary aldosteronism (e.g. renal artery stenosis).

The following tests should be requested in selected patients:

- **Screening tests for Cushing's syndrome** (dexamethasone suppression test, 24-hour urinary cortisol, late-night salivary cortisol) and **24-hour urinary catecholamines and metanephrines** (for phaeochromocytoma).
- **Serum calcium** and **thyroid-stimulating hormone**.
- **Erythrocyte sedimentation rate** in patients with suspected Takayasu's arteritis (although non-specific).
- **CT or MR angiogram of aorta** in patients with suspected coarctation of aorta or Takayasu's arteritis.
- **Sleep studies** in patients with suspected obstructive sleep apnoea.

WHAT SHOULD YOU TELL THE PATIENT AT THIS STAGE?

You should tell her that

- She is hypertensive.

'I am concerned that your blood pressure has been persistently high for more than three months'.

- A secondary cause should be excluded.

'In the majority of people with high blood pressure, we do not know what causes it. Because high blood pressure is not so common in someone of your age, we should look for an underlying medical problem. This is particularly important because if we can find out what the underlying problem is and treat it, the blood pressure will return to normal'.

- Some renal and endocrine conditions can lead to hypertension.

'Inflammation of the kidneys, narrowing of blood vessels that supply the kidneys and hormone-related problems are some of the medical conditions that can cause a high blood pressure'.

- You haven't picked up any leads for a secondary cause from your clinical assessment. Further investigations are therefore necessary.

'So far, I haven't found any evidence of an underlying medical problem. I'll arrange some blood and urine tests, a scan of your kidneys, a tracing of your heart and an X-ray of your chest. You may need further tests depending on the results of these initial ones. These tests will hopefully tell us why your blood pressure is high'.

- You would refer her to a specialist depending on the results of these tests.
- You would prescribe amlodipine to lower her blood pressure in the meantime.

'I'll prescribe a medication called amlodipine to lower your blood pressure. This medication may occasionally cause side effects like giddiness, constipation and swelling around the ankles'.

- You will update her when the results of these tests are back.

OUTCOME

Her results show.

- Haemoglobin 120 g/L, white cell count 5.6×10^9/L and platelet count 218×10^9/L.
- Serum creatinine 68 µmol/L.
- Serum K^+ 4.1 mmol/L.
- Urinalysis shows no protein, blood, casts or active sediments.
- Urine pregnancy test negative.
- Renin and aldosterone are both elevated.
- Chest X-ray shows normal heart size and clear lung fields.
- 12-lead ECG is normal, with no evidence of left ventricular hypertrophy.

*Renal ultrasound scan shows a difference in size between the two kidneys. The **right kidney measures 11 cm and the left kidney measures 8.2 cm**. There is no evidence of hydronephrosis or polycystic kidneys. Doppler shows **left renal artery stenosis**.*

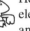 Her renal duplex scan results are suggestive of left renal artery stenosis. This is also supported by the elevated renin and aldosterone (secondary aldosteronism). The normal renal function is reassuring. CT and MR angiogram are other imaging modalities that can help to diagnose renal artery stenosis. The most likely cause in a woman of her age is fibromuscular dysplasia.

Her renal artery stenosis is unlikely to be due to Takayasu's arteritis, as all her peripheral pulses are felt, and there is no difference in blood pressure between the two arms (difference in systolic BP of >10 mm Hg) or evidence of involvement of other blood vessels. She should be referred to a vascular surgeon to consider angioplasty. If angioplasty is successful, she should be able to discontinue anti-hypertensive medications.

The 27-Year-Old Woman Who Is Passing Very Little Urine

Case 27

A 27-year-old woman presents to the acute medical unit with oliguria.
Her temperature is 36.8°C, pulse rate 72/minute, BP 154/102 mm Hg, respiratory rate 16/minute and oxygen saturation 98% on room air.

HOW SHOULD THIS PROBLEM BE APPROACHED?

---

*She tells you that she has been **peeing very little for the last three days**, despite drinking enough water. Her **urine looks very dark**.*

You should

- First, ask about **symptoms that may suggest fluid overload**, like shortness of breath, orthopnoea and leg swelling or facial puffiness.

    The most important concern in patients with oliguria is fluid overload, which could potentially result in life-threatening acute pulmonary oedema.

- Ask **what she means by 'dark urine'**.

*She is not breathless or orthopneic. Her **ankles have been swollen** for the last one week. Her face has not been puffy. She says her **urine looks like coke**.*

 In adults, oliguria is defined as the passage of less than 400 mL of urine/day (the minimum volume that is required to excrete the waste products of metabolism). In this patient, the presence of associated features such as [a] 'coke-coloured urine' (which suggests haematuria), [b] ankle oedema (which is most likely due to proteinuria) and [c] elevated blood pressure, point to acute glomerulonephritis (GN). The absence of features of acute pulmonary oedema, such as breathlessness, tachypnoea and low oxygen saturation, is reassuring.

DOI: 10.1201/9781003430230-27

GN is usually immune mediated. The antibodies either target a self-antigen in the glomerulus (e.g. glomerular basement membrane antigen as in Goodpasture's syndrome) *or* a foreign antigen that is planted in the glomerulus (e.g. hepatitis B virus antigen). Alternatively, immune complexes may form elsewhere and then get deposited in the glomerulus (e.g. systemic lupus erythematosus or SLE). Clinically, patients with GN present with acute nephritis, nephrotic syndrome, asymptomatic proteinuria or haematuria, acute kidney injury *or* chronic kidney disease.

In acute nephritis, the immune system targets the *endothelial side of the glomerulus* (unlike in nephrotic syndrome, where the *epithelial side* is targeted). The inflamed endothelium is unable to produce enough glomerular filtrate, which leads to a fall in the urine output (*oliguria* and *acute kidney injury*). The renin-angiotensin-aldosterone system is activated in an attempt to increase the glomerular filtrate, and this causes efferent arteriolar constriction (*elevated blood pressure*). The capillary inflammation allows red blood cells and protein to appear in the urine (*haematuria and proteinuria*). Proteinuria leads to hypoalbuminemia, which lowers the oncotic pressure (*oedema*).

Acute GN results from [a] immune complex deposition (the immune complexes may contain bacterial antigens, as in post-infectious GN, *or* self-antigens, as in SLE) *or* [b] direct antibody-mediated inflammation, as in anti-neutrophil cytoplasmic antibody (ANCA)-associated vasculitis or Goodpasture's syndrome (*see Box 27.1*).

BOX 27.1   SOME UNDERLYING CAUSES OF ACUTE GLOMERULONEPHRITIS

- Post-infective causes (e.g. post-streptococcal GN, IgA nephropathy).
- Systemic lupus erythematosus (SLE).
- Systemic vasculitis (e.g. ANCA-associated vasculitis, Henoch-Schonlein purpura).
- Goodpasture's syndrome.
- Idiopathic rapidly progressive GN.

Further questions should explore the features that may suggest a possible underlying cause for her acute nephritis. You should ask about:

- *Recent infective symptoms*, particularly skin or pharyngeal infection.

Note: Post-streptococcal GN and IgA nephropathy are caused by deposition of IgG and IgA immune complexes in the glomerulus, respectively. While the former manifests about three weeks after the infection (the time it takes to form IgG antibodies), the latter occurs at the same time or within a day of the infection (as IgA antibodies are already present on mucosal surfaces).

- *Symptoms that may suggest an underlying autoimmune condition*, like SLE, vasculitis or Goodpasture's syndrome (*see Table 27.1*). A full review of systems is essential.

The clinical features of SLE or vasculitis result from antibodies or immune complexes targeting the other organ systems.

- Her other *medical problems*.
- *Medications* taken (current as well as recent past, including those that can be purchased across the counter).
- *Family history* of kidney disease.
- *Obstetric* and *menstrual history*.

TABLE 27.1   General screening questions for autoimmune connective tissue disease[a]

Musculoskeletal	Joint pain.
Mucocutaneous	Skin rashes, photosensitivity, hair loss, mouth ulcers, dry eyes and mouth.
Constitutional	Fever, weight loss, fatigue.
Vascular	Raynaud's phenomenon, previous thrombosis (due to anti-phospholipid syndrome).
Ocular	Red eyes (iritis or scleritis).
ENT	Sinusitis, nasal crusts, epistaxis, hearing loss (due to ANCA-associated vasculitis).
Neurological	Headache, altered mental status, focal neurological symptoms like weakness or numbness (e.g. proximal muscle weakness, mononeuritis multiplex).
Cardiorespiratory	Cough, breathlessness (e.g. interstitial lung disease), haemoptysis (e.g. diffuse alveolar haemorrhage), pleuritic chest pain (due to pleurisy or pericarditis).
Abdominal	Abdominal pain, rectal bleeding (due to mesenteric vasculitis).
Obstetric	Previous pregnancy morbidity (recurrent miscarriages or still births due to anti-phospholipid syndrome).

[a] Clues may also be obtained from the results of blood tests (e.g. haemolytic anaemia, leucopenia, lymphopenia or thrombocytopenia due to SLE).

*Her **joints have been painful** for the last three months, particularly hands, wrists, elbows and feet. She usually feels stiff in the mornings for the first 30 minutes. She has not noticed any swelling in her joints. She feels **tired all the time**. She denies skin rashes, photosensitivity, mouth ulcers, hair loss, sicca symptoms, Raynaud's phenomenon, fever or weight loss. Review of systems is unremarkable. There is no history of recent illnesses, travel or infectious contacts.*

Her past medical history is blameless. She does not take any medication. Her family history is unremarkable. She has never been pregnant. She has been sexually inactive for more than six months, since breaking up with her boyfriend. Her last menstrual period was two weeks ago. She has never smoked and drunk alcohol only socially. She works as a receptionist in a hotel.

Post-infectious GN seems less likely in the absence of recent illnesses. Her joint pain and tiredness, although non-specific, point to an autoimmune problem like SLE. ANCA-associated vasculitis is a differential diagnosis, despite the absence of clinical involvement of other organs.

WHAT SHOULD YOU LOOK FOR ON EXAMINATION?

Apart from ***vital signs***, you should

- Check for ***signs of fluid overload***.
- Perform a thorough ***general examination*** to pick clues that may suggest SLE or systemic vasculitis.
- Ask for ***urine dipstick*** examination.

*She appears comfortable at rest. There is **bilateral pitting oedema** in her legs up to the level of her mid-shins. Her jugular venous pressure is not elevated. The **proximal interphalangeal**, **metacarpophalangeal and wrist joints are tender**, but not swollen. There are no skin rashes. Her heart sounds are normal and lungs are clear. Abdomen is soft and non-tender, with no organomegaly. Urine dipstick shows **2+ protein and 3+ blood**.*

HOW SHOULD THIS PATIENT BE EVALUATED?

You should request

- *Urine microscopic examination* and *protein-creatinine ratio*.

The microscopic examination is useful to look for active sediments such as red blood cells, white blood cells and casts.

Note: If red blood cells are reported on ordinary microscopy, you should ask for *phase contrast examination* to localise the source of bleeding. Isomorphic red cells (red cells with uniform morphology) are predominant in lower urinary tract bleeding, while dysmorphic red cells (red cells of varying morphology) of >20% would suggest glomerular bleeding. Dysmorphism occurs because the red cells have to squeeze past the glomerular basement membrane to get into Bowman's space.

- Full blood count, liver function tests, serum creatinine and electrolytes, blood glucose, lipid panel, prothrombin time and activated partial thromboplastin time (in anticipation of the need for renal biopsy) and vitamin D.
- *Autoantibodies*, including ANA, anti-double-stranded DNA antibody, antibodies to extractable nuclear antigens or anti-ENA, ANCA and anti-GBM antibody.

Note: Anti-ENA antibodies include anti-Ro, La, Sm and RNP. They are named after the person in whom they were first discovered (e.g. Robert, Lavaine, Smith) or the antigen that is targeted (e.g. ribonucleoprotein). Anti-Sm is highly specific for SLE, although not very sensitive.

- *Erythrocyte sedimentation rate* and *complement levels*.

Low complement levels (C3 and C4) would suggest an immune complex-mediated GN (e.g. post-streptococcal GN, SLE), as immune complexes consume complements.

- *Anti-streptolysin titre* (elevated level would support a diagnosis of post-streptococcal GN) and *screening tests for hepatitis B and C*.
- *Urine pregnancy test*.
- *Chest X-ray* may reveal signs of fluid overload or pulmonary shadows suggestive of vasculitis or Goodpasture's syndrome.
- *Ultrasound scan of the kidneys* (to confirm the presence of two kidneys, exclude structural abnormalities and estimate the size of the kidneys).

A *renal biopsy* may be necessary depending on the results of the initial investigations.

WHAT SHOULD YOU TELL THE PATIENT?

You should tell her that

- Her oliguria is due to GN.

'I suspect your kidneys are inflamed. We have tiny filters in our kidneys which help to produce urine and get rid of the wastes and excess fluids. When these filters are inflamed, they are unable to produce enough urine and the excess fluids and wastes start to accumulate in the body'.

- Her blood pressure is high.

'*Your blood pressure is high. When the kidneys are inflamed, some hormones are produced by the body in an attempt to increase the volume of urine. These hormones raise the blood pressure*'.

- Her urine dipstick shows proteinuria and haematuria.

'*The kidneys normally do not allow protein or blood cells to get into the urine. We found some protein and blood in your urine, which again suggests that your kidneys are inflamed*'.

- The joint pain and tiredness may be related to her nephritis.

'*I suspect your immune system is mistakenly attacking the kidneys. In some people, the immune system also attacks the joints. This would explain why your joints hurt and you feel so tired*'.

- You would recommend admission to hospital.
- You would arrange some investigations.

'*I'll ask for some blood and urine tests, a scan of your kidneys and an X-ray of your chest. These tests will tell us if your kidneys are working normally and why they are inflamed*'.

- You would ask a nephrologist ('*kidney specialist*') to see her.

'*The kidney specialist might arrange a biopsy. A biopsy is a minor procedure in which a small piece of tissue is taken from the kidney so that it can be examined under a microscope. The kidney specialist will explain this to you*'.

- You would commence her on diuretics and an anti-hypertensive.

'*I'll start you on medications to remove the excess fluid and lower your blood pressure. You should also restrict your intake of water and salt*'.

- You will update her when the results of these tests are available.

OUTCOME

The results of her initial tests are as follows:

- Estimated proteinuria based on **urine PCR is 1.2 g/day**.
- Microscopic examination shows **56 red cells/high power field** and **red cell casts**. Phase contrast microscopy shows **34% dysmorphic and 66% isomorphic red cells**.
- **Haemoglobin 106 g/L, white cell count 3.2×10^9/L** (neutrophils 1.8×10^9/L, **lymphocytes 0.4 10^9/L**) and **platelet count 118×10^9/L**.
- **Serum creatinine 152 µmol/L** (normal range 70–120). Electrolytes normal.
- Liver function tests, blood glucose, lipid panel, vitamin D, PT and APTT normal.
- **Erythrocyte sedimentation rate 68 mm/hour**.
- ASO titre normal.
- Hepatitis B surface antigen, anti-hepatitis B core IgG and hepatitis C antibody negative.
- **ANA 1/320. Anti-double-stranded DNA >10 IU/mL.**

- Anti-ENA, ANCA and anti-GBM negative.
- **C3 complement 56 mg/dL** (normal 82–160) and **C4 complement 9 mg/dL** (15–44).
- Urine pregnancy test negative.
- Chest X-ray normal.
- Ultrasound of the kidneys shows two normal-sized kidneys, with no evidence of obstruction.

The test results have shown numerous abnormalities. Her urine PCR result has confirmed the presence of significant proteinuria. The presence of red cell casts and dysmorphic red cells in the urine suggests glomerular bleeding. There is evidence of acute kidney injury. The positive ANA and anti-double-stranded DNA are in keeping with a diagnosis of SLE, the latter being highly specific for this diagnosis. The depressed complement level indicates immune complex formation, which is also a feature of SLE. The elevated anti-double-stranded DNA and depressed complement levels indicate active SLE, and higher risk of renal involvement. Leucopenia, lymphopenia and thrombocytopenia are also in keeping with SLE.

Renal biopsy should be arranged, not only to *confirm* the diagnosis of lupus nephritis, but also to assess the severity of histological changes and decide the appropriate treatment strategy.

*She is referred to the nephrologist, who arranges a renal biopsy. Renal biopsy shows **diffuse proliferative nephritis**. Immunofluorescence microscopy shows the presence of IgG, IgM, IgA, C3, C4 and C1q in the glomerulus (known as **full house staining**, which is characteristic of lupus nephritis).*

Her anti-phospholipid antibodies are negative. She is commenced on high dose prednisolone, mycophenolate mofetil and hydroxychloroquine along with frusemide and ramipril. She is advised not to get pregnant, as her lupus is active and drugs like mycophenolate and ramipril are teratogenic. The nephrologist decides to follow her in the outpatient clinic.

The 46-Year-Old Man with Swelling of His Legs

Case 28

A 46-year-old gentleman presents with a two-week history of swelling of his legs.
His pulse rate is 76/minute, BP 116/72 mm Hg, respiratory rate 16/minute and oxygen saturation 97% on room air.

HOW SHOULD THIS PROBLEM BE APPROACHED?

---

*A quick examination reveals **bilateral pitting leg oedema up to the level of his shins**.*

- Explore his principal complaint and establish the **extent of swelling**.
- Ask if he gets **breathless** (pulmonary oedema due to fluid overload *or* pleural effusion).
- Ask if his **abdomen is distended** (due to ascites).

*He tells you that he first noticed the **swelling around his ankles** about two to three weeks ago. The swelling has since progressively increased, and it now extends to the level of mid-shins. His **face looks 'puffy'** in the mornings. There is no swelling in his arms or hands. He hasn't exerted much recently, but he does not get breathless at rest or at night while lying in bed. His abdomen is not distended.*

Oedema occurs because of an increase in the volume of fluid in the interstitial compartment. Fluid that is filtered from the high-pressure arterial end of the capillary into interstitial compartment is reabsorbed at the low-pressure venous end of the capillary. Any excess fluid that is not reabsorbed is returned to the circulation via lymphatics. The plasma proteins maintain the oncotic pressure and hold the fluid back in the vascular compartment. Thus, oedema may result from [a] increased hydrostatic pressure, [b] reduced oncotic pressure or [c] lymphatic obstruction (*see Figure 28.1*).

A local cause like lymphatic obstruction or deep vein thrombosis can be ruled out, as both his legs are swollen, and his face is puffy in the mornings.

The next set of questions should explore the features of possible underlying causes of oedema:

- Is there a history of **heart, liver or kidney disease**?
- Is he **passing less urine**? Any **frothing** (bubbles in the urine) **or change in colour of the urine**?
- Any **diarrhoea** or **steatorrhoea** (malabsorption)?

DOI: 10.1201/9781003430230-28

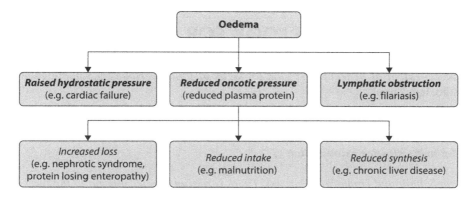

FIGURE 28.1   Mechanisms and underlying causes of oedema.

*His past medical history is blameless, with no previous diagnosis of heart, liver or kidney disease. He is not passing less urine than usual. He has noticed **bubbles in the urine**, but there is no change in colour. He denies diarrhoea or steatorrhoea.*

The frothy urine suggests proteinuria (although not all patients may report this). It appears that the oedema is due to hypoalbuminemia.

BOX 28.1   CAUSES OF PROTEINURIA[†]

- Diabetic nephropathy.
- Hypertensive nephropathy.
- Autoimmune disease (e.g. systemic lupus erythematosus).
- Infections (e.g. hepatitis B or C, human immunodeficiency virus infection).
- Drugs (e.g. non-steroidal anti-inflammatory drugs, gold, penicillamine).
- Pregnancy.

[†] Some non-renal causes (usually transient and unlikely to cause heavy proteinuria) include orthostatic proteinuria (protein is not present in the early morning urine sample), urinary tract infection, exfoliative skin diseases and congestive cardiac failure.

Further questions to ask to determine the possible cause of proteinuria (*see Box 28.1*):

- Is he a known **diabetic** or **hypertensive**?
- Any **joint pain** or **skin rashes**?
- Are there **risk factors for infections**, such as hepatitis B or C and HIV?
- What **medications** does he take?
- Any **family history of kidney disease** (e.g. polycystic kidney disease)?

He is not a known diabetic or hypertensive. He last had his fasting blood glucose checked about six months ago and was told that it was normal. He denies joint pain or skin rashes. There are no risk factors for hepatitis or HIV. He does not take any medication. The relevant family history is unremarkable. He lives with his wife and three teenage children. He has never smoked and seldom drinks alcohol. He works as a sales representative for a pharmaceutical company.

WHAT SHOULD YOU LOOK FOR ON EXAMINATION?

- Check the **extent of oedema**, and look for **signs of fluid overload** (elevated jugular venous pressure, lung crepitations).
- Look for signs that may suggest an **underlying cause** (e.g. skin rashes or synovitis due to auto-immune connective tissue disease).
- Palpate the abdomen to check for **enlarged kidneys**.
- Ask for **urine dipstick examination**.

*He is moderately built and comfortable at rest. There is **pitting leg oedema** up to the level of his mid-shins. There is no oedema in his upper limbs or face. His jugular venous pressure is not elevated. Heart sounds are normal and lungs are clear. Abdominal examination reveals no free fluid or organomegaly. Rest of the examination is normal. **Urine dipstick shows 4+ protein** and no blood.*

HOW SHOULD HE BE EVALUATED FURTHER?

You should request

- **Urine protein-creatinine ratio** or **24-hour urine protein measurement** for quantification of the proteinuria (*see Box 28.2*).
- **Urinalysis**, including microscopic examination for red cells and casts.
- **Blood tests**, including full blood count, liver function tests, serum creatinine and electrolytes, fasting blood glucose, HbA_1c, lipid panel, tests for hepatitis B and C, HIV test (*with his consent*) and vitamin D.
- **Anti-nuclear antibody** (screening test for SLE).

All patients with glomerulonephritis should be screened (even in the absence of extra-renal features), as it could be the sole manifestation of SLE.

- **Chest X-ray** may reveal signs of fluid overload or pleural effusion.
- **Renal ultrasound** (useful before planning a renal biopsy and to looking for evidence of polycystic kidney disease).

BOX 28.2   MEASUREMENT OF PROTEINURIA

During health, less than 150 mg of protein (or 30 mg of albumin) is passed in the urine every day. Urine dipsticks only provide an estimate of the *protein concentration* in the tested sample. A dipstick reading of 1+, for example, corresponds to a protein concentration of ~30 mg/100 mL, which roughly equates to a 24-hour proteinuria of 300–450 mg/day (assuming that the urine volume is 1000–1500 mL/day).

Although considered the gold standard, a timed collection of urine over 24 hours is inconvenient, cumbersome and subject to collection errors. Hence, the urine protein/creatinine ratio (PCR) is widely used in practice. A 24-hour proteinuria of 500 mg/day roughly corresponds to a urine PCR of 50 mg/mmol (as the urine creatinine excretion is constant around 10 mmol/day).

The albumin/creatinine ratio (ACR) is more sensitive than PCR for lower levels of proteinuria and is used to screen for diabetic nephropathy (where the aim is to detect evidence of nephropathy, very early). An ACR between 2.5 and 30 mg/mmol in men or 3.5 and 30 mg/mmol in women is considered micro-albuminuria (level of >30 mg/mmol is macro-albuminuria).

WHAT SHOULD YOU TELL THE PATIENT?

You should tell him that

- His leg swelling is due to hypoalbuminemia.

'I suspect your legs are swollen because your blood protein level is low. Proteins in the blood help to keep fluids inside blood vessels. When there is not enough protein, fluids move from the blood vessels into surrounding tissues and initially tend to collect around the ankles'.

- His hypoalbuminemia is due to proteinuria.

'Your blood protein level is low because you are passing a lot of protein in your urine. The urine test has confirmed this. The bubbles that you see is because of protein in the urine'.

- You suspect his proteinuria is due to glomerulonephritis.

'I suspect you are losing protein in the urine because your kidneys are inflamed'.

- The underlying cause of her glomerulonephritis is not clear.

'Based on my assessment so far, I am unable to say why your kidneys are inflamed. There are a few possible reasons, like diabetes, some infections, certain medications and autoimmune disease, which means the immune system mistakenly attacks the kidneys'.

- You will arrange some investigations.

'I'll ask for some blood and urine tests, an X-ray of your chest and a scan of the kidneys. These tests will tell us how your kidneys are working, how much protein you are passing in the urine and if you have any of the medical conditions that can cause inflammation of the kidneys'.

- You would ask a nephrologist (*'kidney specialist'*) to see him.

'The kidney specialist might arrange a biopsy. A biopsy is a minor procedure in which a small piece of tissue is taken from the kidney so that this could be examined under the microscope. The kidney specialist will explain this to you'.

- You would commence him on diuretics and angiotensin-converting enzyme inhibitor.

'I'll start you on medications to remove the excess fluid and reduce the loss of protein in the urine. You should also restrict your intake of water and salt'.

- You will update him when the test results are back.

OUTCOME

His results are as follows:

- **The estimated 24-hour urine protein excretion by urine PCR is 7.24 g**. Microscopic examination of the urine shows four white cells, two red cells and no casts.
- Full blood count and liver function tests normal.
- **Serum albumin is 16 g/L** (normal range 35–55).
- Serum creatinine is 82 μmol/L, fasting glucose 5.6 mmol/L and **total cholesterol 8.4 mmol/L**.
- Anti-nuclear antibody is negative.
- Tests for hepatitis B and C are negative.
- Chest X-ray is normal, with no evidence of pulmonary congestion or pleural effusion.

Renal ultrasound shows two normal-sized kidneys, with no evidence of obstruction or cysts.

His results are in keeping with nephrotic syndrome. In nephrotic syndrome, there is loss of podocytes in the glomerular basement membrane (GBM). The diseased GBM leaks protein, as the negative charge is lost (the GBM normally repels the albumin, as they are both negatively charged). Patients with nephrotic syndrome present with (a) heavy proteinuria (>3.5 g of proteinuria/24 hours), (b) hypoalbuminemia, (c) oedema and (d) hypercholesterolemia (as the liver produces more LDL cholesterol in an attempt to maintain the oncotic pressure).

Among the underlying causes (*see Box 28.3*), diabetes, SLE, and hepatitis B and C can be excluded on the basis of the blood test results. He is not obese. He hasn't been taking any medications that are known to cause nephrotic syndrome. The renal ultrasound has not revealed evidence of polycystic kidney disease or other structural lesions. Hence, the cause of his nephrotic syndrome is not clear. All adults with nephrotic syndrome should be referred for a renal biopsy. In children, nephrotic syndrome is usually presumed to be due to minimal lesion glomerulonephritis, and empirical steroid therapy is often commenced even in the absence of biopsy evidence.

BOX 28.3   CAUSES OF NEPHROTIC SYNDROME

PRIMARY

The underlying cause is not known, hence labelled on the basis of the histological changes found on light microscopy (e.g. minimal lesion glomerulonephritis, idiopathic membranous glomerulonephritis, membranoproliferative glomerulonephritis, focal segmental glomerulosclerosis).[†]

SECONDARY

- Diabetes mellitus.
- Systemic lupus erythematosus.
- Drugs (e.g. NSAIDs, gold, penicillamine).
- Infections (e.g. hepatitis B, hepatitis C, HIV).
- Obesity-related glomerulopathy.
- Amyloidosis.
- Malignancy.

[†] Membranous glomerulonephritis means there is thickening of the basement membrane; membranoproliferative means there is thickening of the basement membrane plus proliferation of the mesangial cells; focal segmental glomerulosclerosis means there is hardening of a part of the glomerulus (segmental), involving less than 50% of the glomeruli (focal).

*He is referred to the nephrologist. Renal biopsy is reported as showing **membranous glomerulonephritis**. He is commenced on furosemide, lisinopril and atorvastatin. He is advised to restrict the intake of fluids and salt, receive the pneumococcal vaccine because of increased risk of infection (due to loss of complements and immunoglobulins in the urine) and start prophylactic anticoagulation because of the risk of thrombosis (due to loss of anti-thrombin III in the urine). The nephrologist decides not to commence immunosuppressive therapy straightaway and instead closely monitor him.*

The 34-Year-Old Man with Haematuria

Case 29

A 34-year-old gentleman presents to the emergency unit with a two-day history of haematuria. His urine dipstick examination shows 4+ blood, but no protein.

HOW SHOULD THIS PROBLEM BE APPROACHED?

*He tells you that his **urine has been bright red coloured** for the last two days. This has never happened before. He feels well otherwise.*

Patients who describe a change in the colour of the urine to pink, brown or red may or may not be passing blood (*see Figure 29.1*). Porphyria, myoglobinuria, haemoglobinuria and consumption of beetroot can also cause a change in the colour of urine. Although his urine dipstick shows 4+ blood, a microscopic examination should be done to check if this is true haematuria.

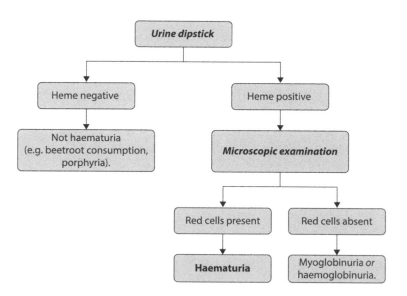

FIGURE 29.1 Urine examination for blood.

DOI: 10.1201/9781003430230-29

True haematuria can be gross (visible to the patient) *or* microscopic (≥3 red blood cells/high power field). It is classified as 'glomerular' or 'non-glomerular'. The presence of hypertension, elevated serum creatinine and red cell casts in the urine or dysmorphic red cells on phase-contrast microscopic examination would suggest glomerular haematuria.

Some common causes of haematuria are listed in *Box 29.1*. Of these, glomerulonephritis, trauma, infection, calculus and inherited renal disease are the possible causes to consider in this man.

BOX 29.1   SOME UNDERLYING CAUSES OF HAEMATURIA

Glomerular causes (glomerulonephritis)

- Post-infective (e.g. IgA nephropathy, post-streptococcal glomerulonephritis).
- Systemic lupus erythematosus.
- ANCA-associated vasculitis.
- Anti-glomerular basement membrane disease.

Non-glomerular causes

- Trauma (e.g. catheterisation, prostate biopsy).
- Renal tract calculus.
- Urinary tract infection (e.g. bacterial, tuberculosis, schistosomiasis).
- Malignancy (e.g. renal cell carcinoma, bladder or prostate cancer).
- Benign prostatic hypertrophy.
- Inherited renal disease (e.g. polycystic kidney disease, Alport syndrome).

Further questions to ask:

- Any recent *trauma* (e.g. urological procedures, catheterisation or prostate biopsy)?
- Any *frothing of the urine* and *leg swelling* (due to proteinuria), *recent throat infection* (e.g. IgA nephropathy or post-streptococcal nephritis), *joint pains*, *skin rashes*, *breathlessness*, *haemoptysis*, *ENT symptoms or ocular inflammation* (glomerulonephritis due to vasculitis or systemic lupus erythematosus)?
- Any *pain in the abdomen or back*?

In patients with painful haematuria, think of calculus (colicky pain in the loin radiating to the groin) or infection (back pain in pyelonephritis or supra-pubic pain in cystitis).

- Any *dysuria, urgency or frequency of micturition*?

Obtain a *sexual history*, if appropriate.

- Any *family history* of renal disease?

Note: In older men, it is important to enquire about symptoms of prostatism, like hesitancy, poor stream and terminal dribbling.

He denies urinary symptoms like frothing, pain on micturition, hesitancy, urgency or increased frequency, abdominal or back pain, ankle swelling, fever or weight loss. There are no features of glomerulonephritis. Both his parents died in a road traffic accident when he was only four years old, and he was brought up by his aunt. He is not aware of any medical problems in his parents.

His medical history is unremarkable, except for childhood asthma. He lives with his wife and three-year-old son. His wife is his only sexual partner. He has never smoked and been teetotal all his life. He works as a cashier for a private bank.

Although the history has not offered any leads to the underlying cause of his haematuria, certain conditions can be ruled out. Benign prostatic hypertrophy and malignancy are unlikely because of his young age. Renal calculus is unlikely, as this usually presents with episodes of colicky pain. Urinary tract infection (UTI) need not be considered because of the absence of suggestive symptoms. Moreover, UTI is uncommon in men, unless there is an underlying structural problem.

Glomerulonephritis should still be considered as it cannot be excluded based on the history alone. An inherited renal disease is also possible.

WHAT SHOULD YOU LOOK FOR ON EXAMINATION?

You should

- Ask for his ***vital parameters***.
- Examine his ***abdomen*** and check for renal angle tenderness, mass and enlarged kidneys.
- Perform a ***general examination***.

Look for clues that may suggest an underlying medical condition, like autoimmune connective tissue disease.

*His vital parameters are normal. Blood pressure is 124/82 mm Hg. There is no leg oedema. Abdominal examination reveals **palpable masses in both flanks**. The masses are bimanually palpable, ballotable and resonant on percussion. There is no flank tenderness. Rest of the examination is unremarkable.*

The bilateral flank masses are most likely enlarged kidneys, as they are bimanually palpable and ballotable. The most likely cause is adult polycystic kidney disease (APKD). Haematuria occurs in APKD because of cyst rupture. A detailed family history should be obtained. Renal cysts can also occur in some rare multi-system diseases like tuberous sclerosis and von Hippel-Lindau disease, but they usually present much earlier in life.

*He is not aware of any kidney problems in his parents or grandparents. His aunt, who brought him up, was his father's only sibling. She **died of brain haemorrhage** when she was only 45. Her two daughters are well, with no known medical problems, as far as he is aware.*

The history of brain haemorrhage in his aunt is relevant, as there is an association between APKD and cerebral berry aneurysms. Other associations of APKD are hepatic, splenic and pancreatic cysts, valvular heart disease (aortic or mitral incompetence) and diverticular disease. APKD is an autosomal dominant condition, with most of them occurring due to mutation on chromosome 16 (risk of transmission to the offspring is therefore 50%). Complications of APKD include hypertension, chronic kidney disease, haemorrhage into the cyst, infection and calculi.

HOW SHOULD THIS PATIENT BE INVESTIGATED?

The general approach to haematuria is outlined in *Figure 29.2*. In this patient, you should ask for

- *Abdominal ultrasound or CT scan* (to confirm the presence of polycystic kidneys and look for cysts in other organs).
- *Full blood count* and serum *creatinine*.

Interestingly, patients with APKD may be polycythaemic even after developing advanced chronic kidney disease because of erythropoietin production by interstitial tissues of the kidneys.

- *Urinalysis*, including microscopic examination and *protein-creatinine ratio* (PCR).
- *Magnetic resonance angiogram (MRA) of the brain* (because of the family history of cerebral haemorrhage in his aunt) if the diagnosis of APKD is confirmed by imaging.

An *echocardiogram* should also be requested, especially in those with heart murmurs.

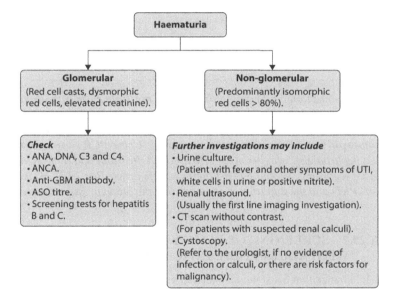

FIGURE 29.2   Approach to haematuria.

ANA = anti-nuclear antibody, anti-DNA = anti-double-stranded deoxyribonucleic acid, ANCA = anti-neutrophil cytoplasmic antibody, anti-GBM = anti-glomerular basement membrane antibody, ASO = anti-streptolysin O.

WHAT SHOULD YOU TELL THE PATIENT AT THIS STAGE?

You should tell him that

- His kidneys are enlarged, most likely due to polycystic kidney disease.

'When I examined your tummy, I found that both your kidneys are enlarged. I suspect you have developed cysts in your kidneys, which have made them bigger. Cysts are small areas of fluid collection, like bubbles. We call this polycystic kidney disease. I'll ask for a scan of your kidneys to confirm this'.

- The haematuria is possibly due to cyst rupture.

'You are passing blood in your urine because one or more of these cysts may have ruptured'.

- Polycystic kidney disease is *'an inherited condition, which means it occurs because of a faulty gene'.*
- His aunt, who suffered the brain haemorrhage, possibly had polycystic kidneys.

'You probably inherited this condition from your father. I wonder whether your aunt had a similar problem in her kidneys. Some people with this problem develop areas of weakness in blood vessels of the brain. We call them aneurysms. These aneurysms can rupture and cause bleeding in or around the brain'.

- Apart from the scan of the kidneys, you will arrange *'some blood tests to see how the kidneys are working and also a urine test'.*
- The *'bleeding will hopefully stop soon'.* There is no need for any specific intervention.
- If the scan confirms polycystic kidney disease, you will *'refer him to a kidney specialist, arrange a scan of his brain to check for aneurysms and talk about screening of his family members for this condition'.*

OUTCOME

*Abdominal ultrasound examination confirms the presence of **multiple cysts in both kidneys**, **in keeping with adult polycystic kidney disease**. There are no cysts in the liver, pancreas or spleen. His full blood count and renal function are normal. Microscopic examination of the urine shows **numerous red cells**, of which **93% are isomorphic** on phase-contrast examination. Urine PCR shows no proteinuria.*

He is referred to a nephrologist, who arranges MRA scan of the brain and a 2D echocardiogram. He is given appropriate advice regarding screening of his family members (see Box 29.2). He is told about the possible complications of APKD and the importance of monitoring the blood pressure and renal function.

BOX 29.2   SCREENING OF FAMILY MEMBERS OF PATIENTS WITH ADULT POLYCYSTIC KIDNEY DISEASE

- There is a 1:2 chance that his son has inherited the condition, as it is autosomal dominant.
- His future children also have a 1:2 chance of inheriting the condition.
- His son should get an ultrasound scan during his late teens. If the scan is normal, it should be repeated when he is 30. APKD can be virtually excluded if there are no cysts at the age of 30.
- Genetic testing is problematic because a large number of mutations are associated with APKD.
- His son should get his blood pressure, renal function and proteinuria monitored on an annual basis.
- Both his cousins should be screened for APKD.
- If he wishes to discuss this further, he should be referred to a geneticist.

The 55-Year-Old Man with Dysuria

Case 30

A 55-year-old man presents with a two-day history of pain during micturition.

HOW SHOULD THIS PROBLEM BE APPROACHED?

---

*He tells you that he feels a **burning discomfort when he pees**. This started two days ago. He **feels the urge to pee all the time** and has been **going to the toilet more often**. He has also been experiencing a **discomfort in the lower part of his tummy**.*

He is describing dysuria, urinary urgency, frequency and lower abdominal discomfort, which suggest possible urinary tract infection (UTI). UTI can affect the lower urinary tract (cystitis, urethritis) *or* involve the kidneys (pyelonephritis). It is known as 'complicated UTI' if there is an underlying structural or functional problem of the urinary tract. Identifying complicated UTI is important because treatment is difficult and there is a risk of recurrence. UTI in men is considered complicated, as there is nearly always an underlying predisposing factor (*see Box 30.1*). UTIs are not common in men because of the longer length of urethra, making it difficult for bacteria to travel to the bladder.

BOX 30.1   SOME RISK FACTORS FOR MALE UTI

- Structural problems of urinary tract (e.g. calculus, tumour, prostate hypertrophy, urethral stricture, adult polycystic kidney disease, horseshoe kidney).
- Functional problems (e.g. neurogenic bladder, vesicoureteric reflux).

Structural and functional problems increase the risk of infection by causing stasis of urine.

- Catheterisation (long-term use of indwelling catheter or intermittent self-catheterisation) *or* recent instrumentation (e.g. cystoscopy, nephrostomy).
- Diabetes mellitus.
- Immunosuppression.

DOI: 10.1201/9781003430230-30

Further questions to ask:

- Ask about *other possible symptoms of UTI*, such as fever, chills, rigors, nausea and vomiting, back pain, cloudy or foul-smelling urine, and blood in the urine.

Note: The presence of fever, chills, vomiting and back pain should alert you to possible pyelonephritis.

- Ask if he has had *UTIs in the past*.

In patients with recurrent UTIs, it would be prudent to check previous culture and sensitivity results to guide empirical antibiotic therapy.

- Look for *features that may suggest the presence of an underling problem*, such as renal colic, passage of stones in the urine, urinary hesitancy and poor stream, urinary catheterisation and recent instrumentation of urinary tract.
- Ask if he is a *diabetic* or has any *osmotic symptoms* like polyuria and polydipsia.
- Ask about his *past medical history* and *regular medications*.

Particularly check for diabetes, neurological conditions that affect the bladder and immunosuppression.

- Obtain a *family history*.

Ask if there is anyone in his family with kidney problems (e.g. polycystic kidney disease).

- Obtain a *sexual history*.

Be tactful. Start with '*I hope you won't mind if I ask you some sensitive questions*'.

He has been feeling feverish but did not measure his temperature. His right loin has been painful since the day before. There is no blood in the urine, and it is not cloudy or foul smelling. He feels sick but has not vomited. He denies polyuria and polydipsia, and his weight is steady. He has never had urine infection before. He has had some problems with urination for more than a year. He must wait a while for urine to come out and the stream is usually weak. He does not use a catheter and has not undergone any procedures in his urinary tract.

Apart from high cholesterol for which he takes a statin, his medical history is unremarkable. His blood sugar was normal when it was last checked about a year ago. The relevant family history is unremarkable. He is in a monogamous relationship with his wife and has never had sexual partners outside his marriage. He does not smoke. He drinks a glass of whiskey or wine nearly every day before going to bed. He is allergic to amoxicillin. He is a policeman.

- You should *clarify what the allergic reaction to penicillin was*.

It is important to clarify if he developed anaphylaxis or it was only a skin rash. Some patients use the word 'allergy' for non-allergic reactions. This is important to decide the choice of antibiotic.

He says he developed an itchy skin rash when he took amoxicillin many years ago, for a chest infection. There was no swelling of the eyes, lips or tongue, and he did not faint or become breathless. The reaction subsided within a couple of days.

 The loin pain suggests possible involvement of the kidney. Hesitancy and poor stream are obstructive symptoms, which suggest prostate enlargement.

WHAT SHOULD YOU LOOK FOR ON EXAMINATION?

You should

- Ask for his *vital signs* and check his *hydration status*.
- *Palpate the renal angle* to check for tenderness.
- *Examine the abdomen* to check for suprapubic tenderness and enlarged kidneys.

Offer to perform a *per-rectal examination* to check for an enlarged prostate.

*He looks comfortable at rest. His **temperature is 37.8°C**, **pulse rate 84/minute**, blood pressure 124/88 mm Hg, respiratory rate 16/minute and oxygen saturation 98% on room air. He is tender at the **right renal angle**. His abdomen is soft. His kidneys are not palpable.*

HOW SHOULD HE BE EVALUATED?

You should request

- *Blood tests*, including full blood count, liver function tests, serum creatinine and glucose.

In patients with suspected renal calculus, you should also ask for serum calcium and uric acid.

- *Urinalysis and microscopic examination*.

Look for the presence of nitrites, pyuria and red blood cells.

Note: The presence of white cells in the urine may not always indicate infection. A positive nitrite indicates the presence of bacteria in urine (usually *Escherichia coli*, *Proteus* and *Klebsiella*).

- Ask for *urine culture*.

In patients with suspected pyelonephritis and those who are systemically unwell, ask for *blood cultures*.

- *Imaging* (ultrasound of the kidneys, ureter and bladder *or* CT scan of the abdomen and pelvis).

Imaging is indicated in [a] patients with suspected renal stone or obstructive lesion, [b] all men with UTI, [c] patients who do not respond well to initial antibiotic therapy and [d] those with recurrent UTI.

WHAT SHOULD YOU TELL THE PATIENT?

You should tell him that

- His symptoms are possibly due to UTI.

'I suspect you have developed a urine infection'.

- UTI is not so common in men.

'Urine infections are much more common in women. In men, they usually occur because of an underlying problem that obstructs the free flow of urine'.

- His prostate may be enlarged.

'From your description, it appears that your prostate gland may be enlarged. An enlarged prostate can obstruct the flow of urine and increase the risk of infection (draw a diagram to explain). *Prostate trouble can make it harder to pee, which would explain why your urine stream is weak and it takes time for urine to come out'.*

- You would recommend admission to hospital for a few days.
- You would arrange a few tests.

'I'll ask for some blood and urine tests. I'll also arrange for a scan to check for prostate enlargement'.

- You would start him on an antibiotic, which he should take for about seven to ten days. You would recommend *'giving this through the vein'* to begin with.
- He should drink plenty of fluids.
- Once the infection is treated, you would refer him to a urologist (*'prostate specialist'*).

OUTCOME

His **white cell count is 14.2 × 10⁹/L** (normal 4–11), with neutrophilia. Haemoglobin, platelet count, liver function tests, serum creatinine and blood glucose are normal. **Urinalysis shows positive nitrite, 12 red blood cells and 74 white blood cells**. Urine culture **is positive for E. coli**. CT scan of the abdomen and pelvis confirms **enlargement of the prostate**, but there are no other abnormal findings.

He responds well to ceftriaxone. The urologist requests prostate-specific antigen, which is normal. He starts him on tamsulosin and arranges to follow him in clinic.

The 40-Year-Old Man with Acute Kidney Injury

Case 31

A 40-year-old man presents to the acute admissions unit with complaints of tiredness and exhaustion. His oxygen saturation is 96% on room air, pulse rate 76/minute, BP 124/82 mm Hg, respiratory rate 16/minute and temperature 37°C.

His blood test results show normal full blood count, serum creatinine 324 μmol/L (normal 70–120), serum sodium 142 mmol/L, potassium 5.3 mmol/L and bicarbonate 20 mmol/L. The 12-lead ECG is normal. His serum creatinine was 74 μmol/L, when it was checked during his annual health screening six months ago.

HOW SHOULD THIS PROBLEM BE APPROACHED?

The most striking abnormalities are the elevated serum creatinine, hyperkalaemia and low serum bicarbonate. The serum creatinine was normal six months ago, which establishes that this is acute kidney injury (AKI) and not chronic kidney disease (CKD) (*see Box 31.1*).

BOX 31.1   KEY QUESTIONS TO ASK WHEN FACED WITH A PATIENT WITH AKI

- Are there any life-threatening complications (e.g. acute pulmonary oedema due to volume overload, severe hyperkalaemia or metabolic acidosis)?
- Is there an indication for urgent dialysis?
- What is the underlying cause of the kidney injury (pre-renal, intrinsic renal or post-renal)?

---

*He looks **tired** but is alert. He denies breathlessness or orthopnoea.*

There are no features of acute pulmonary oedema, such as breathlessness, low oxygen saturation or tachypnoea, and the hyperkalaemia and metabolic acidosis are mild. Hence, there is no indication for urgent dialysis (*see Box 31.2*).

BOX 31.2   INDICATIONS FOR DIALYSIS IN PATIENTS WITH ACUTE KIDNEY INJURY

- Refractory pulmonary oedema.
- Refractory hyperkalaemia.
- Severe metabolic acidosis (pH <7.2).
- Symptomatic uraemia (encephalopathy or pericarditis).

Having ensured that he is stable, a detailed history should be obtained, bearing in mind the possible underlying causes of AKI (*see Box 31.3*).

BOX 31.3   UNDERLYING CAUSES OF ACUTE KIDNEY INJURY

Pre-renal (inadequate blood flow to the kidneys):

- Intravascular volume depletion (e.g. diarrhoea, vomiting or blood loss).
- Hypotension due to cardiogenic shock or sepsis.
- Drugs[†] (e.g. non-steroidal anti-inflammatory drugs [NSAIDs], angiotensin-converting enzyme inhibitors [ACEIs]).

Post-renal (obstruction to the free flow of urine):

- Benign prostatic hypertrophy.
- Stones, tumours and strictures.

Intrinsic renal (pathology in glomeruli, tubules, interstitium or vasculature):

- Glomerulonephritis.
- Acute tubular necrosis (due to prolonged renal hypoperfusion,[††] toxins like aminoglycosides and radiographic contrast media, immunoglobulin light chains or myoglobin).
- Interstitial nephritis (usually caused by an allergic reaction to NSAIDs, proton pump inhibitors or antibiotics).
- Vascular (e.g. systemic vasculitis, malignant hypertension, thrombotic thrombocytopenic purpura, haemolytic uraemic syndrome).

[†] NSAIDs cause AKI by blocking the action of prostaglandins, which help to keep the renal blood vessels open. When renal perfusion is reduced, as in patients with renal artery stenosis, the renin-angiotensin-aldosterone system is activated. Angiotensin II causes efferent arteriolar constriction, which helps to increase glomerular pressure and maintain urine output. The administration of ACEI reduces the formation of angiotensinogen II, thus preventing the constriction of efferent arterioles and leading to a reduction in glomerular pressure, oliguria and rise in serum creatinine.

[††] The blood vessels that supply the renal tubules arise from efferent arterioles. When efferent arteriolar constriction is prolonged, as in patients with prolonged renal hypoperfusion, blood supply to the tubules is compromised, leading to tubular necrosis.

You should ask about:

- His *urine output*. Is he passing less urine than usual?
- *Symptoms that may suggest a pre-renal cause* (e.g. diarrhoea, vomiting, recent blood loss, fever or other symptoms of infection).
- *Obstructive symptoms*, like urinary hesitancy, poor stream and terminal dribbling.

- *Symptoms of glomerulonephritis*, like ankle swelling or facial puffiness, frothy urine and 'coke-coloured' urine.
- Features that may suggest an *underlying cause of glomerulonephritis* (e.g. recent pharyngitis, joint pain, skin rashes, haemoptysis, mononeuritis multiplex, ENT symptoms).
- Recent *contrast procedures* (e.g. computed tomography, coronary angiogram).
- His background *medical problems* (e.g. hypertension, diabetes, systemic lupus erythematosus, hepatitis B or C, human immunodeficiency virus infection).
- *Medications* taken, including 'over-the-counter' preparations.
- *Family history* of renal disease.

*He says he has been feeling **tired and exhausted** since **running a 21-km marathon**, two days ago. All his **muscles have been aching**. He is not sure if he is passing less urine than usual, but the **urine looks brownish**. He goes for a brisk walk about two to three times a week, but he has never participated in a marathon before. He hasn't played any sport since his teenage years.*

He thinks he drank enough fluids on the day of marathon. He denies vomiting, diarrhoea, blood loss or recent infective symptoms. There are no symptoms suggestive of glomerulonephritis or urinary outflow obstruction. His medical history is blameless, and there is no one in his immediate family with kidney disease. His blood sugar and cholesterol results were normal, when last checked about six months ago. He does not take any prescription medication or 'over-the-counter' preparation. He does not smoke or drink. He is an investment banker. He lives with his wife and two children.

The widespread muscular aching and passage of brown-coloured urine, soon after the severe unaccustomed physical exertion, points to rhabdomyolysis as the cause of his AKI. Additionally, it is quite possible that he did not consume enough fluids on the day of marathon. The hyperkalaemia is likely due to both AKI as well as muscle injury (release of potassium from muscle cells). There are no features of intrinsic renal disease or urinary outflow obstruction.

Apart from potassium, rhabdomyolysis leads to release of other contents of the muscle, like creatine kinase (CK), myoglobin, lactate dehydrogenase, aspartate aminotransferase (AST) and phosphate into blood. Rhabdomyolysis causes AKI because myoglobin is toxic to renal tubules. Causes of rhabdomyolysis, apart from severe physical exertion, include muscle crush injuries, compartment syndrome, seizures and toxins like statin, alcohol and cocaine.

WHAT SHOULD YOU LOOK FOR ON EXAMINATION?

You should

- Assess the *hydration status*.

Pulse rate, blood pressure (including postural drop), skin turgor, dryness of mucous membranes, jugular venous pressure and lung crepitations should help with this assessment.

- Examine the abdomen. Percuss over the suprapubic area to check for *bladder enlargement*.
- Look for clues that may suggest an *underlying cause* (e.g. vasculitis).
- Examine the *muscle power* in all groups and check for *muscle tenderness*.

*There are no signs of volume depletion or overload. His abdomen is soft and non-tender. There is no suprapubic dullness. There is mild **generalised tenderness of his muscles**, but the power is grade 5 in all muscle groups. The rest of the examination is normal.*

HOW SHOULD THIS PATIENT BE INVESTIGATED FURTHER?

You should request

- Serum *CK*, *liver function tests*, *calcium and phosphate*.
- *Urinalysis* to check for proteinuria, haematuria and casts.

Note: Presence of 'blood' in the urine, without red cells is indirect evidence of myoglobinuria. Testing for myoglobin itself is expensive and not necessary.

- *Chest X-ray*.
- *Ultrasound of the kidneys, ureters and bladder* (KUB) to assess the size of kidneys (small kidneys would suggest CKD) and exclude urinary outflow obstruction.

The following investigations are indicated in selected patients, depending on clinical presentation.

- *Urine phase-contrast microscopy* (in patients with haematuria) and *urine protein-creatinine ratio* (to quantify proteinuria).
- *Screening tests for an underlying cause of glomerulonephritis* (e.g. anti-nuclear antibody, anti-double-stranded DNA, anti-neutrophil cytoplasmic antibody, anti-glomerular basement membrane antibody, C3 and C4, hepatitis B and C screen, HIV test).

A *renal biopsy* may be required in patients with suspected glomerulonephritis.

- *Myeloma screen* (in patients >40 years of age, with unexplained AKI).
- *Peripheral blood film* (in patients with suspected thrombotic microangiopathy).

WHAT SHOULD YOU TELL THE PATIENT AT THIS STAGE?

You should tell him that

- His blood tests show evidence of AKI.

'Your blood tests show that your kidneys are not working well'.

- You suspect his kidney injury is due to rhabdomyolysis.

'After severe physical exertion, muscle cells can break down and release some proteins into the blood. These proteins can harm the kidneys'.

- The kidney injury is reversible.

'This does not mean that your kidneys are permanently damaged. We should be able to reverse this by giving you fluids to flush out the muscle proteins'.

- The serum potassium is mildly elevated. You would commence him on calcium resonium and continue to monitor this.

'When the kidneys don't work well, potassium level in the blood can go up. Your potassium is slightly high. High potassium can cause the heartbeat to become irregular or slow, but the tracing of your heart shows that your heartbeat is fine. We will give you a medication to reduce the potassium level and closely monitor this. You should avoid bananas, oranges and fruit juices for now, as they contain a lot of potassium'.

- You would be asking for a blood test to *'check the level of muscle protein in the blood'* and a *'scan of the kidneys to check if there are other possible reasons for the reduced kidney function'*.
- You would recommend admission to hospital, as his kidney function needs to be closely monitored.
- If the kidney function is not improving as expected, you would seek an opinion from a *'kidney specialist'*.

OUTCOME

His results are as follows:

- Urine is **positive for haem**. There are no red blood cells.
- **Serum CK 11346 IU/mL** (normal <200).
- **Serum corrected calcium 2.12 mmol/L** (normal 2.2–2.7).
- **Serum phosphate 1.56 mmol/L** (normal 1.1–1.45).

*Liver function tests show **AST 182 U/L (10–44)**, **alanine aminotransferase (ALT) 76 U/L** (10–34), alkaline phosphatase 98 U/L (40–150) and γ-glutamyl transferase 32 U/L (12–64).*

Ultrasound KUB is reported as 'The right kidney measures 10.4 cm and the left kidney 10.1 cm. No evidence of outflow obstruction or renal parenchymal disease'.

Chest X-ray shows normal heart size and clear lung fields.

The elevated CK confirms our clinical impression of rhabdomyolysis. Rhabdomyolysis, by definition, is elevation of CK level to >10 times the upper limit of normal. The presence of haem in the absence of red blood cells is indirect evidence of myoglobin in the urine. His AST and ALT are elevated, most likely due to muscle injury rather than liver disease. Phosphate that is released from muscle cells binds to calcium, causing hypocalcaemia. His kidney injury is likely to improve with hydration.

He is given 3 L of intravenous fluids/day and closely monitored. The hyperkalaemia is managed with calcium resonium and dietary restriction of potassium. His myalgia gradually improves over the next few days. A week later, his serum creatinine is 78 μmol/L and serum CK 916 IU/mL. His serum potassium, bicarbonate, calcium and phosphate, all return to normal.

The 51-Year-Old Man with Impaired Renal Function

Case 32

A 51-year-old gentleman seeks your advice, as his blood test results show some abnormalities. He recently had these blood tests as part of a routine health screening package.

Haemoglobin 114 g/L, MCV 85 fl.
White cell count 5.2 × 10⁹/L.
Platelet count 318 × 10⁹/L.
Liver function tests normal.
Serum creatinine 228 μmol/L (normal range 70–120).
Estimated glomerular filtration rate (eGFR) 28 mL/min/1.73 m².
Serum electrolytes (sodium, potassium, chloride and bicarbonate) normal.
Serum corrected calcium 2.28 mmol/L (normal 2.2–2.7).
Serum phosphate 1.42 mmol/L (normal 1.1–1.45).
Thyroid stimulating hormone and free thyroxine normal.
Fasting glucose 5.4 mmol/L.
HbA₁c 36 mmol/mol.
Low-density lipoprotein 3.8 mmol/L (target <2.7).
Triglycerides 4.1 mmol/L (target <1.7).
High-density lipoprotein 0.8 mmol/L (target >1.0).
Urinalysis shows 1+ protein. No blood, casts or active sediments.
Screening tests for hepatitis B and C, and HIV negative.

HOW SHOULD THIS PROBLEM BE APPROACHED?

The most striking abnormalities are [a] the elevated serum creatinine, with low eGFR, [b] normocytic anaemia, [c] proteinuria and [d] deranged lipid panel results. Because he had these tests routinely, as part of a health screening package, the impairment of renal function is most likely due to chronic kidney disease (CKD) rather than acute kidney injury (AKI). It is indeed quite possible that there was a recent acute deterioration ('acute on chronic kidney disease').

The distinction between AKI and CKD is important because the former is usually reversible, while the latter is not (*see Box 32.1*).

DOI: 10.1201/9781003430230-32

BOX 32.1   DISTINGUISHING ACUTE KIDNEY INJURY FROM CHRONIC KIDNEY DISEASE

▪ *Previous lab test results*.

Demonstration of a normal serum creatinine in the recent past is strong evidence in favour of acute kidney injury.

▪ *The size of the kidneys*.

The presence of bilateral contracted kidneys on ultrasound imaging would suggest CKD. However, there are exceptions because CKD due to certain aetiologies (e.g. diabetic nephropathy, amyloidosis or polycystic kidney disease) may not lead to a reduction in size of the kidneys.

▪ *Anaemia, hypocalcaemia and hyperphosphatemia*.

They do not help to distinguish AKI and CKD, but a normal haemoglobin or serum phosphate would be somewhat unusual in CKD.

An e-GFR of 28 mL/min would place this patient in stage 4 CKD (*see Box 32.2*).

BOX 32.2   STAGES OF CKD

STAGE	EGFR (IN ML/MIN/1.73 M²)	COMMENTS
1	≥90	In the presence of urinary abnormalities *or* structural or genetic kidney disease.
2	60–89	
3	30–59	
4	15–29	
5	<15 or on dialysis	End-stage renal disease.

*He says he had these blood tests a week ago. He is particularly **very concerned about the kidney test result**. He is not sure what that means. He did not expect these results, as he feels well.*

Say something reassuring. '*The results suggest that your kidneys are not working well, but please allow me to first ask you a few questions and I will then explain what these results mean and what we can do about this*'.

Obtain a detailed history (*see Box 32.3*). After confirming that he is indeed asymptomatic, ask about:

▪ *Blood tests done in the past* to check his kidney function.
▪ *His medical history*, particularly diabetes (although not relevant in this man, as his fasting blood glucose and HbA$_1$c are normal), hypertension, peripheral vascular disease, previous stroke or heart attack, and autoimmune connective tissue disease.
▪ Symptoms that suggest *volume overload* (e.g. breathlessness, orthopnoea, ankle swelling), *volume depletion* (e.g. recent diarrhoea, vomiting or blood loss) or *anaemia* (tiredness).
▪ Symptoms of *urinary outflow obstruction* (e.g. hesitancy, poor stream, terminal dribbling).
▪ *Medications taken* (including 'over-the-counter' preparations).

It is particularly important to check if he is taking nephrotoxic medications or preparations.

- *Family history of kidney disease* (e.g. adult polycystic kidney disease, Alport syndrome).
- *Smoking habit*, *alcohol intake*, *personal background* and *occupation*.

BOX 32.3   SOME UNDERLYING CAUSES OF CHRONIC KIDNEY DISEASE[†]

- Diabetic nephropathy.
- Hypertensive nephropathy.
- Chronic glomerulonephritis.
- Chronic or recurrent urinary tract infection.
- Adult-onset polycystic kidney disease.
- Renovascular disease.
- Urinary tract obstruction.

[†] The three most common causes are diabetes, hypertension and chronic glomerulonephritis.

---

*He is **asymptomatic**. He says the last time he had a blood test prior to this was probably more than ten years ago. There is no history of diabetes, hypertension, peripheral vascular disease, stroke, ischemic heart disease or autoimmune connective tissue disease. He denies recent vomiting, diarrhoea, blood loss, breathlessness, orthopnoea, ankle swelling or obstructive urinary symptoms.*

*He does not take prescription medications or 'over-the-counter' preparations. The relevant family history is unremarkable. He **smokes ten cigarettes a day** and drinks a glass of wine most evenings. He lives with his wife and 16-year-old daughter. He is a chartered accountant.*

WHAT SHOULD YOU LOOK FOR ON EXAMINATION?

You should

- Ask for his *blood pressure* and check his *peripheral pulses*.
- Check his *volume status*.

Signs of volume overload include ankle oedema, elevated jugular venous pressure and basal lung crepitations, and those of volume depletion are hypotension, reduced skin turgor and dryness of mucous membranes.

- Look for *signs that may suggest an underlying cause* (e.g. synovitis or skin rashes of autoimmune connective tissue disease) although the history does not point to this.
- Palpate the abdomen for *enlarged kidneys* and listen for *renal artery bruits*.

*He is moderately built, comfortable at rest and well nourished. His **blood pressure is 174/102 mm Hg**. The other vital parameters are satisfactory, and there are no signs of volume overload or depletion. All his peripheral pulses are felt well. His kidneys are not palpable and there are no renal artery bruits. The rest of the examination is unremarkable.*

The elevated blood pressure may be the cause or consequence of his CKD. The absence of a positive family history would not exclude polycystic kidney disease or Alport syndrome, although it would be unusual for these conditions to present for the first time at the age of 51 with CKD. The history has not uncovered any reversible factors that can worsen renal function in CKD, such as renal outflow tract obstruction, volume depletion or ingestion of nephrotoxic medications.

CKD is a risk factor for cardiovascular disease. It is therefore important to address his other risk factors, such as hypertension, hyperlipidaemia and smoking habit. Based on the urine albumin-creatinine ratio, patients are classified as A1 (<3 mg/mol), A2 (3–30 mg/mol) or A3 (>30 mg/mol), with higher levels of albuminuria being associated with increased risk of CKD progression.

WHAT SHOULD YOU TELL THE PATIENT?

You should tell him that

- The test results suggest CKD.

'Although we do not have any previous blood test results for comparison, I suspect your kidney function has gradually declined over many years'.

- His blood pressure reading is high, and this may be the cause of his CKD.

'Your blood pressure reading is high. It is quite possible that your kidneys were affected because of the high blood pressure, but it is difficult to be sure about this because the kidney problem could have started first and led to the rise in blood pressure. It is often not possible to precisely pinpoint a reason for the decline in kidney function'.

- The blood tests show that he is anaemic.

'Your blood results also show that you are anaemic. Anaemia simply means that you have less haemoglobin, the protein that carries oxygen around in the blood. Our kidneys make a hormone that helps with the production of haemoglobin. When the kidney function declines, this hormone is not produced in sufficient amounts. I suspect your anaemia is due to the kidney problem, but I'll ask for some blood tests to rule out other possible causes'.

- You will organise an ultrasound scan of his kidneys.

'I'll arrange for a scan of your kidneys. If the scan shows that your kidneys are smaller in size, it would confirm my suspicion that your kidney function has declined slowly over many years. The scan will also tell us if there is any blockage that is obstructing the free flow of urine. If we find a blockage, it is important to relieve this, as it might help to improve the kidney function, at least partially'.

- You will arrange *'an X-ray of the chest, an electrical tracing of the heart and a urine test to check the amount of protein'.*
- Several measures could help to slow down further progression of his kidney disease (this is the most important message to get across to him).

'Although we won't be able to reverse your kidney function to normal, several measures can help to reduce the rate at which it progresses. You might eventually need dialysis or transplantation, but we can certainly delay this for as long as possible by following these measures'.

- It is important to treat the hypertension.

'One would be to keep your blood pressure under control. I would recommend starting a medication to lower the blood pressure'.

- CKD increases the risk of heart disease. This can be reduced by following healthy lifestyle measures.

'Your blood tests show that your cholesterol level is high, for which I would recommend starting a medication. You should stop smoking, cut down the intake of sugars, fats and salt, and exercise on a regular basis'.

- He should not take any medication without seeking medical advice.

'You shouldn't take any medication without asking a doctor. Several medications are excreted by kidneys, and can accumulate in the body when the kidneys don't work well'.

- He will need blood and urine tests to monitor his kidney function and proteinuria, at least every six months.
- You would refer him to a nephrologist (*'kidney specialist'*) and give him some information booklets to read in the meantime (or suggest some useful websites).

OUTCOME

---

*The ultrasound scan of his kidneys shows **bilateral contracted kidneys**. His right kidney measures 8.4 cm and left kidney 8.6 cm. There are no features of renal outflow tract obstruction.*

- His serum ferritin, vitamin B_{12} and folate are normal.
- **Vitamin D 24 ng/mL** (normal >30).
- **Parathyroid hormone level 84 ng/L** (normal 10–65).
- **Urine ACR 18 mg/mol**.
- His 12-lead ECG shows changes in keeping with **left ventricular hypertrophy**.
- Chest X-ray is normal.

 The finding of bilateral contracted kidneys is in keeping with CKD (normal kidney size is about 10–12 cm). His CKD is most likely due to hypertensive nephropathy, as his 12-lead ECG shows features of left ventricular hypertrophy. His anaemia could be attributed to CKD, as his haematinics are normal. He will need erythropoietin if he becomes symptomatic. He should be commenced on lipid-lowering therapy and anti-hypertensive medication(s), aiming to keep the blood pressure below 130/80 (an angiotensin-converting enzyme inhibitor would be the first choice, as he has proteinuria).

He should receive vitamin D replacement but patients with advanced CKD may not respond to 25(OH) cholecalciferol, as this needs to be activated by the kidneys to form $1,25(OH)_2$ cholecalciferol. If there is no response to cholecalciferol or ergocalciferol, he should therefore be commenced on either calcitriol *or* 1α-calcidol (the latter is converted to calcitriol in the liver by the enzyme 25-hydroxylase). When calcitriol formation is reduced, there is reduced calcium absorption from the gut, resulting in hypocalcaemia. The parathyroid glands are stimulated to produce more parathormone (secondary hyperparathyroidism), which helps to restore normal serum calcium levels by [a] reabsorbing calcium from renal tubules and [b] shifting calcium from bones to the blood (thus increasing the risk of osteoporosis or osteomalacia). Patients with advanced CKD may develop hyperphosphatemia because of reduced excretion, so they should be advised to reduce the intake of phosphates and commenced on phosphate-binding agents such as sevelamer or calcium acetate.

The 56-Year-Old Woman with **Case 33**
Dysphagia

A 56-year-old woman presents with a three-month history of difficulty in swallowing.

HOW SHOULD THIS PROBLEM BE APPROACHED?

- First, ask the patient to *clarify what she means by 'difficulty in swallowing'*.

Is it difficulty in swallowing (dysphagia), pain on swallowing (odynophagia) or simply the sensation of a lump in the throat without actual difficulty in swallowing (globus hystericus)?

- What is the *level of dysphagia* (oropharyngeal or oesophageal)?

In oropharyngeal dysphagia, the difficulty is in initiating swallowing, while in oesophageal dysphagia, the 'food gets stuck' a few seconds after initiating swallowing (*see Box 33.1* and *Figure 33.1*). Oropharyngeal dysphagia may be accompanied by dysarthria, choking, nasal regurgitation or lower cranial nerve palsies.

BOX 33.1   CAUSES OF DYSPHAGIA

Oropharyngeal dysphagia

- Stroke.
- Parkinson's disease.

Rare causes include polymyositis or dermatomyositis (*muscle*), myasthenia gravis (*neuromuscular junction*), Guillain-Barre syndrome (*nerve roots and peripheral nerves*) and motor neurone disease (*cranial nerve nuclei*).

Oesophageal dysphagia

- Benign stricture due to gastro-oesophageal reflux disease.
- Malignant stricture due to cancer in the oesophagus or gastric fundus.
- Achalasia cardia.

DOI: 10.1201/9781003430230-33

Rare causes include extrinsic compression (e.g. goitre, bronchogenic carcinoma, mediastinal lymph node, aortic aneurysm, enlarged left atrium), systemic sclerosis, diffuse oesophageal spasm, oesophageal web and Schatzki ring (narrowing of the lower oesophagus caused by a ring of mucosal tissue).

■ Is the dysphagia caused by a *mechanical or a motility problem*?

A short history of progressively worsening dysphagia (weeks to months), mainly to solids, would suggest mechanical dysphagia, while a longer history of intermittent dysphagia (months to years) to both solids and liquids would suggest a motility problem.

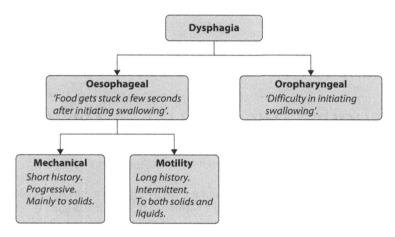

FIGURE 33.1   Approach to dysphagia.

*She tells you that eating has become a real ordeal for her. The problem **started about three months ago** and it is **getting worse** by the day. She can get the food bolus past the throat, but it gets **stuck behind the breastbone** a few moments later. There is no pain on swallowing or feeling of a lump in her throat. She does not choke or cough while eating, and there is no change in her speech. The **difficulty is mainly with solid foods** like meat, fruits or vegetables. She is still able to manage liquids and porridge.*

Her dysphagia appears to be at the level of the oesophagus. The short history of progressively worsening dysphagia, mainly to solids, is concerning. It must be presumed to be due to cancer of the oesophagus until proven otherwise. Benign oesophageal stricture resulting from long-standing gastro-oesophageal reflux disease is a differential diagnosis.

Further questions to ask:

■ Has she *lost weight*? If so, how much has she lost and over how long?

Weight loss can result from any cause of dysphagia because of reduced intake of food.

■ Any *fever, cough, expectoration or breathlessness*?

Stasis of food in oesophagus increases the risk of aspiration pneumonia.

■ Does she get *heartburn* or *a sour taste in the mouth*?

These symptoms may suggest gastro-oesophageal reflux disease (GORD).

Note: Long-standing GORD may be complicated by [a] oesophagitis, [b] Barrett's oesophagus, [c] oesophageal stricture and [d] oesophageal cancer.

- Ask about her other ***medical problems*** and regular ***medications***.

Non-steroidal anti-inflammatory drugs and bisphosphonates can cause oesophagitis, while calcium channel blockers and nitrates can worsen acid reflux by relaxing the lower oesophageal sphincter.

- Ask about ***smoking habit and alcohol consumption***.

Both smoking and alcohol increase the risk of carcinoma of oesophagus.

*She says she has **lost about 5 kg in the last three months** without trying. She has suffered with **heart-burn** for many years but never sought medical advice for this. She occasionally takes ranitidine, which she buys across the counter. Her medical history is otherwise unremarkable, and she does not take any regular medication. She has **smoked 20 cigarettes/day for the last 35 years**. She drinks a glass of wine at least three to four times a week. She works for a travel agency and lives with her husband.*

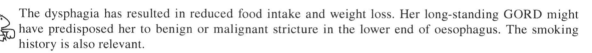

The dysphagia has resulted in reduced food intake and weight loss. Her long-standing GORD might have predisposed her to benign or malignant stricture in the lower end of oesophagus. The smoking history is also relevant.

WHAT SHOULD YOU LOOK FOR ON EXAMINATION?

You should

- Check her ***nutritional state***.
- Look for ***signs that may point to an underlying cause*** of her dysphagia (e.g. goitre, right supra-clavicular lymph node enlargement).
- Palpate the ***abdomen*** to particularly check for hepatomegaly (metastasis) and epigastric mass.
- ***Listen to the base of her lungs*** for crepitations.

In patients with oropharyngeal dysphagia, the nervous system should be examined to check for signs of stroke, Parkinson's disease and lower cranial palsies.

*She is **thin**, but not cachectic or malnourished. She weighs 46 kg. Vital signs are normal. Her blood pressure is 112/72 mm Hg. There is no pallor, supraclavicular lymph node enlargement or goitre. Her abdomen is soft and non-tender, with no palpable masses or organomegaly. Her lungs are clear.*

HOW SHOULD THIS PATIENT BE INVESTIGATED?

- She should be referred for urgent ***upper gastrointestinal (GI) endoscopy***.

Endoscopy may help to directly visualise the pathology causing her dysphagia, and obtain biopsies.

- ***Blood tests***, including full blood count, liver function tests, and serum creatinine and electrolytes.
- A ***chest X-ray*** may show air-fluid level in patients with achalasia cardia or reveal conditions that compress the oesophagus (e.g. lung cancer, pericardial effusion, aortic aneurysm, enlarged left atrium, retrosternal goitre).

WHAT SHOULD YOU TELL THE PATIENT?

You should tell her that

- Her dysphagia appears to be at the oesophageal level.

(Take a piece of paper and draw a simple diagram to explain.)

'The food that we eat moves from the mouth to the back of our throat, and then along the food pipe to the stomach. I suspect you have trouble swallowing because food is not easily moving along the food pipe'.

- The dysphagia is mechanical.

'This may be due to narrowing or blockage of the food pipe'.

- The cause of obstruction is not clear. You will refer her to a gastroenterologist, who will organise an endoscopic examination.

'I am not sure what is causing this narrowing or blockage. I'll ask a stomach specialist to see you. It is very likely that he would suggest a camera test, which involves passing a long tube with a camera down your throat to look inside your food pipe and stomach. This will tell us if your food pipe is narrowed or blocked, and what is causing this'.

- You will arrange *'some blood tests and an X-ray of her chest'* in the meantime.
- You will refer her to a dietician.

'I am concerned that you have lost so much weight. I'll ask a dietician to see you so that they can suggest some liquid diets to increase your nutritional intake'.

- (If she directly asks if this could be something serious.)

Do not brush off her concerns, but bear in mind that the diagnosis of cancer has not been confirmed yet. Be sympathetic.

'It is possible that there is a growth in the food pipe, but it is difficult to be sure about this without doing the camera test to directly look inside. I'll ask the specialist to see you as soon as possible so that we can get the answers quickly. Apart from a growth, there are other possible causes too. The heart burn that you have been experiencing for a long time suggests that the acid in your stomach has been leaking back up into the food pipe. Sometimes, the acid can cause inflammation of the lower end of the food pipe, and over time, it can lead to narrowing'.

OUTCOME

The chest X-ray shows a normal cardiac shadow and clear lung fields. Her Hb is 128 g/L. Rest of the blood counts, and her liver and renal function are normal.

*The gastroenterologist sees her urgently and arranges an upper GI endoscopy, which shows a **growth in the lower end of the oesophagus**. Biopsy is reported as showing **adenocarcinoma**. The staging computed tomography scan does not show any metastases. She is referred to the upper GI surgeon and oncologist.*

The 46-Year-Old Man with Epigastric Pain

Case 34

A 46-year-old man presents with a six-month history of intermittent upper abdominal pain.

HOW SHOULD THIS PROBLEM BE APPROACHED?

*He tells you that for the last six months, he has been experiencing an **intermittent discomfort in the upper part of his tummy** (and points to the epigastric region).*

- Start with an open-ended question and *explore his main complaint of epigastric pain*, bearing in mind the underlying causes (*see Figure 34.1*).

Ask about the onset and progression of symptoms, site of pain and radiation, character and aggravating and relieving factors.

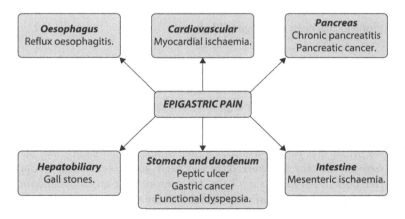

FIGURE 34.1   Causes of long-standing epigastric pain.

*The pain does not radiate to the chest, arm or back. When the problem started six months ago, he was only experiencing this discomfort about once or twice a week, but of late, it has been **troubling him nearly every day**. It is particularly **worse after a heavy meal**. He **feels bloated and full** even before he completes a meal. The pain is not related to exertion. He once went to A and E when the pain was bad. He had a CT scan of his heart at the time, and the doctor told him that it was fine.*

His description fits with dyspepsia (indigestion). The term dyspepsia includes epigastric pain, abdominal bloating, post-prandial fullness and early satiety. Although heartburn due to gastro-oesophageal reflux disease (GORD) is not considered dyspepsia, it often co-exists with dyspepsia. The most common *or* important diagnoses to consider in patients with dyspepsia are (a) peptic ulcer, (b) non-steroidal anti-inflammatory drug (NSAID)-induced dyspepsia, (c) gastric cancer and (d) functional dyspepsia. Of these, functional dyspepsia accounts for more than 70% of the cases, but it should be diagnosed only after exclusion of organic causes. It appears that he had a CT coronary angiogram, which excluded coronary artery disease.

Further questions to ask:

- Ask about *associated symptoms*, such as loss of appetite, dysphagia, nausea, vomiting, hematemesis and melena, weight loss, change in bowel habits and jaundice.
- Ask if he gets *heartburn*.

Is it accompanied by a sour taste in the mouth or cough?

- Ask if the *discomfort is worse with specific foods* (e.g. milk in lactose intolerance, wheat in coeliac disease, fat in gall stones).
- Ask about his *diet and eating habits*.

What kind of foods does he tend to eat? What is the portion size?

- What *medications* does he take?

Ask particularly about NSAIDs and aspirin.

- Complete the *rest of the history*.

Ask about his medical problems, family history (e.g. stomach cancer), smoking habit, alcohol intake, occupation and lifestyle.

- Ask if this problem has been *investigated before*.

*He denies loss of appetite, problem with swallowing, heartburn, sour taste in the mouth, cough, nausea, vomiting, hematemesis or yellowing of the skin or eyes. He moves his bowels once daily, passing solid stools. There is no recent change in bowel habits, melena or rectal bleeding. The discomfort is not brought on by milk, wheat or fatty foods. He says **he is a** 'foodie' and particularly fond of fried chicken, burgers and spicy Indian curries. He weighs 93 kg and thinks he has **gained at least 25 kg over the last 15–20 years**.*

*He was diagnosed with **high blood pressure** two years ago, for which he takes 5 mg of **amlodipine** once daily. His blood pressure is well controlled on amlodipine. When he last had his blood tests about eight months ago, he was told that his **cholesterol was high**, and glucose was borderline. A statin was suggested by a private doctor, but he was not keen. He does not take any anti-inflammatory medication or aspirin. He drinks **one or two glasses of wine with his dinner every day** but often exceeds this amount during weekends. He **smokes about 20 cigarettes/day**. His family history is unremarkable. He lives with his wife and two boys, aged 15 and 12. He is an accountant. He says his **job is quite stressful**. He considers himself **sedentary**. So far, he has not consulted anyone for this problem.*

There are no alarm symptoms to suggest cancer (*see Box 34.1*), which is reassuring. Possible causes of his dyspepsia are peptic ulcer and functional dyspepsia. Peptic ulcers are usually caused by *Helicobacter pylori* or NSAIDs, of which the latter can be excluded in this patient.

H. pylori is also associated with chronic gastritis, gastric cancer and gastric mucosa-associated lymphoid tissue (MALT) lymphoma. The association with functional dyspepsia is controversial. The strategy in younger patients (<55 years, but the age threshold is lower in countries with higher incidence of gastric cancer) without alarm symptoms is to 'test and treat' (*see Figure 34.2*). Eradication of *H. pylori* will (a) cure most patients with peptic ulcer, (b) reduce the risk of developing gastric cancer and (c) improve the symptoms in a small number of patients with functional dyspepsia.

BOX 34.1   ALARM FEATURES IN PATIENTS PRESENTING WITH DYSPEPSIA

- Dysphagia.
- Persistent vomiting.
- Gastrointestinal bleeding or iron deficiency anaemia.
- Unintentional weight loss.
- Mass in the epigastrium.

There are several lifestyle factors that need to be addressed in this man, including his unhealthy diet, lack of exercise, smoking habit, consumption of excess amounts of alcohol and stress at work.

WHAT SHOULD YOU LOOK FOR ON EXAMINATION?

You should

- Ask for his **body mass index** and **blood pressure**.
- Check for **pallor**.
- Examine the **abdomen** to check for epigastric tenderness, mass and organomegaly.

*His **body mass index** is 33 kg/m². He is **centrally obese**. There is no conjunctival pallor. Examination of his abdomen is unremarkable, with no tenderness, mass or organomegaly.*

HOW SHOULD HE BE EVALUATED FURTHER?

You should ask for

- **Blood tests**, including full blood count, liver function tests and renal function.
- Non-invasive **test for H. pylori** (*see Figure 34.2*).

The urea breath test (UBT) is the test of choice in adult patients because of its excellent sensitivity and specificity (the stool antigen test is preferred in children). A capsule of urea with radiolabelled carbon is administered to the patient. The test relies on the production of urease enzyme by *H. pylori*, which breaks down urea into ammonia and carbon dioxide. The carbon dioxide (which contains radiolabelled carbon) is absorbed into blood and then exhaled. Thus, measuring radiolabelled carbon in the breath can help to determine the presence of *H. pylori* (radiolabelled carbon will not appear in the breath if there is no *H. pylori*). The UBT should be repeated at least four weeks after completing treatment to confirm the eradication of *H. pylori*.

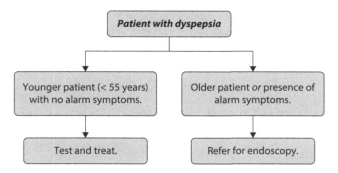

FIGURE 34.2   Diagnostic approach to dyspepsia.

WHAT SHOULD YOU TELL THE PATIENT?

You should tell him that

- His epigastric pain is due to dyspepsia.

'Your tummy discomfort is caused by indigestion'.

- Various conditions cause dyspepsia.

'In some people, indigestion is caused by inflammation of the stomach. However, in most people, we do not find a cause'.

- You would like to arrange some blood tests and test him for *H. pylori*.

'This kind of inflammation is often caused by bacteria that live in the stomach. I'll arrange a breath test to check if these bacteria are present in your stomach. For this, you will be asked to swallow a capsule and then blow into a balloon after a few minutes to collect your breath. Our nurse will explain this to you. I'll also ask for some blood tests to be done'.

- He will be treated for *H. pylori* if the UBT is positive.

'If the breath test shows that you have these bacteria in the stomach, I'll give you a couple of antibiotics to take for two weeks and a pill to reduce acid production in the stomach. We will then repeat the breath test after four weeks to check if the bacteria have been cleared'.

- You will refer him to the gastroenterologist if *H. pylori* eradication is not successful.

'If this treatment does not clear the bacteria, I'll refer you to a specialist'.

- It is important to follow healthy lifestyle measures.

'You should eat healthily and get some exercise to lose weight. It is also important to stop smoking and cut down the alcohol. Healthy habits will not only improve the indigestion, but also reduce your risk of getting heart problems in the future'.

OUTCOME

*His full blood count, liver function tests and renal function are normal. The **UBT is positive**. He is treated with omeprazole, amoxicillin and clarithromycin for two weeks. He is asked to return for the UBT in four weeks.*

The initial empirical regimen to treat *H. pylori* usually includes a proton pump inhibitor (PPI), amoxicillin and clarithromycin. A sequential regimen is followed, with amoxicillin given for the first five to seven days and clarithromycin for the next five to seven days. The PPI is given for 10–14 days. Antibiotic resistance is a problem, particularly to clarithromycin. In such patients, quadruple therapy (with the addition of metronidazole) or bismuth-based regimens can be tried.

No regimen is 100% effective, so the UBT should be repeated after four weeks to confirm eradication of *H. pylori*. If *H. pylori* are still present, second-line empirical therapy with PPI, bismuth, metronidazole and tetracycline can be tried. If the second course of treatment fails or the patient is still symptomatic, he should be referred to a gastroenterologist. If organic pathology is excluded with endoscopy, the patient would be diagnosed with functional dyspepsia and tried on long-term PPI, prokinetic drugs and tricyclic anti-depressants, but treatment is generally difficult.

The 53-Year-Old Man with Haematemesis

Case 35

A 53-year-old man presents to the emergency department with haematemesis.

HOW SHOULD THIS PROBLEM BE APPROACHED?

- You should assess and **stabilise the ABC first** and ensure that **intravenous access** has been secured.

If the vital parameters are unstable, the patient should be resuscitated first, before any history is obtained.

He is alert and oriented. His oxygen saturation is 95% on room air, pulse 76/minute, blood pressure (lying) 124/76 mm Hg, respiratory rate 16/minute and temperature 37°C. His peripheries are warm.

 Although his vital parameters are satisfactory, it is worth noting that hypotension may not be an early sign, especially in younger patients, and patients receiving β-blockers for portal hypertension may not develop tachycardia.

*He tells you that he **was sick with a small amount of blood** that morning. This happened around 8 am, soon after he had his breakfast. He thought he'll wait and see, but because he was **sick again with blood** around 11 am, he decided to come to the emergency department.*

- **Confirm that he is describing haematemesis** and not haemoptysis.

This distinction can be made based on (a) the colour of blood (coffee ground in haematemesis *versus* bright red in haemoptysis), (b) preceding symptoms (cough *versus* nausea), (c) appearance of the expelled contents (mixed with food *versus* frothy) and (d) history of melena.

- Ask **how much blood he vomited** (generally measured in cup sizes).

The history may underestimate the blood loss, as a large amount may be concealed within the gastrointestinal tract.

- Ask if he feels **faint, giddy or weak** (symptoms of hypovolemia).
- Ask if this has **happened before**.

DOI: 10.1201/9781003430230-35

*He shows you a picture of the vomitus and it looks **coffee ground** and **mixed with some undigested food**. He last moved his bowels on the day before. The stools were brown in colour and not black and tarry. He is unable to precisely say how much blood he vomited, but he does not feel faint, giddy or weak. This has never happened before.*

Further questions should explore the features of possible underlying causes (*see Box 35.1*). Ask about

- The *timing of haematemesis*.

Did the blood appear after a few episodes of vomiting or retching, *or* was it mixed with the vomitus right from the beginning?

Note: In patients with Mallory-Weiss tear, blood appears after prolonged vomiting or retching.

- *Abdominal pain* (e.g. peptic ulcer).
- *Dysphagia* or *weight loss* (e.g. malignancy).
- His other medical problems, particularly a *previous diagnosis of chronic liver disease or peptic ulcer*.
- *Medications* taken (e.g. aspirin, NSAIDs, anticoagulants) and *alcohol consumption*.
- *Previous endoscopies* and results.

BOX 35.1   SOME UNDERLYING CAUSES OF UPPER GASTROINTESTINAL BLEEDING

- Peptic ulcer disease.
- Mallory-Weiss tear.
- Oesophageal or gastric varices.
- Oesophagitis.
- Oesophageal or gastric malignancy.
- Angiodysplasia.

---

*The blood did not appear after prolonged vomiting or retching. He denies abdominal pain, dysphagia, acid reflux symptoms and weight loss. He says he **used to drink heavily in the past** but stopped after he was **diagnosed with liver cirrhosis** about 18 months ago. The specialist whom he saw at the time arranged a camera test, but he defaulted and did not go back to see him again. He was prescribed some medications but did not take them.*

*His medical history is otherwise unremarkable. He does not take a non-steroidal anti-inflammatory drug, aspirin or anti-coagulant. He has **smoked about 10 cigarettes/day for the last 30 years**. He is unemployed and lives on his own.*

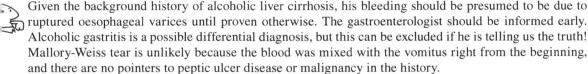

Given the background history of alcoholic liver cirrhosis, his bleeding should be presumed to be due to ruptured oesophageal varices until proven otherwise. The gastroenterologist should be informed early. Alcoholic gastritis is a possible differential diagnosis, but this can be excluded if he is telling us the truth! Mallory-Weiss tear is unlikely because the blood was mixed with the vomitus right from the beginning, and there are no pointers to peptic ulcer disease or malignancy in the history.

WHAT SHOULD YOU LOOK FOR ON EXAMINATION?

You should

- Look for signs of *chronic liver disease* (*see Box 35.2*).

BOX 35.2   SIGNS OF CHRONIC LIVER DISEASE

- Ascites.
- Splenomegaly (due to portal hypertension).
- Spider naevi (more than 2 is significant).
- Gynaecomastia/loss of axillary hair.
- Palmar erythema/Dupuytren's contracture/finger clubbing.

- Palpate the abdomen for *epigastric tenderness*.
- Check for *features of alcohol withdrawal* (e.g. delirium, tremor, sweating), especially if you think he is still drinking.

Offer to do a *digital rectal examination* to check for melena.

*He is moderately built and looks comfortable at rest. He is alert and oriented. There are several **spider naevi** over the chest and arms, but no finger clubbing, palmar erythema, Dupuytren's contracture, loss of axillary hair, gynaecomastia, jaundice or leg oedema. There is no asterixis or tremor. His abdomen is soft and non-tender. The **spleen is palpable**, about three fingerbreadths below the left costal margin. There is **positive shifting dullness**.*

The spider naevi, splenomegaly and ascites are in keeping with chronic liver disease. Gastrointestinal bleeding increases the risk of developing encephalopathy in patients with cirrhosis, but there are no pointers to this at present, as (a) he is alert and oriented and (b) there is no asterixis.

He should be kept nil by mouth and commenced on (a) intravenous fluids, (b) an intravenous proton pump inhibitor, (c) somatostatin (it reduces portal pressure by causing splanchnic vasoconstriction) and (d) a broad-spectrum antibiotic, like ceftriaxone, to provide Gram-negative cover (patients with variceal bleeding are at increased risk of infection, and the use of broad-spectrum antibiotics improves survival). (e) Blood transfusion should be considered in patients who are actively bleeding and haemodynamically unstable, but over-transfusion should be avoided. (f) Patients with platelet count <50 should be transfused platelets, and (g) those with coagulopathy (INR >1.5 or low fibrinogen) given fresh frozen plasma.

HOW SHOULD THIS PATIENT BE
INVESTIGATED FURTHER?

- *Blood tests*, including full blood count, liver function tests, prothrombin time, serum urea, creatinine and electrolytes.

Note: In patients with upper gastrointestinal bleeding, serum urea may be disproportionately elevated compared to creatinine because of increased protein absorption.

- *Group and cross match* 4–6 units (if actively bleeding).
- *Infection screen* (e.g. blood and urine cultures, chest X-ray) is mandatory in patients with fever or suspicion of infection.
- All patients with suspected variceal bleeding should undergo *upper gastrointestinal endoscopy*.

Endoscopy is useful to not only identify the source of blood loss, but also perform therapeutic procedures like variceal band ligation or sclerotherapy.

- *Ultrasound scan* of his abdomen (once he is stable).

This will help to show features of cirrhosis (splenomegaly, ascites and shrunken liver) and identify the obvious presence of hepatocellular carcinoma.

WHAT SHOULD YOU TELL THE PATIENT AT THIS STAGE?

You should tell him that

- The bleeding may be due to ruptured varices.

'I suspect you were sick with blood because of your liver problem. Liver cirrhosis causes blood vessels in the lower end of the food pipe to bulge. These blood vessels can sometimes burst and cause this kind of bleeding'.

- He needs admission to hospital for closer monitoring, as the bleeding may recur.
- You would request some blood tests.
- You would ask a gastroenterologist to see him.

'We will ask the liver specialist to see you. It is very likely that he would suggest passing a camera to look inside your food pipe and stomach. This will help to not only see where the bleeding is coming from, but also do something to stop the bleeding. The specialist will explain this to you'.

- He should not take anything by mouth.

'You should not eat or drink anything until you have had the camera test. This will help the specialist to clearly see the lining of your food pipe and stomach when he passes the camera'.

- You would be starting him on intravenous fluids, proton pump inhibitor, somatostatin and ceftriaxone.

'In the meantime, I'll start you on a drip and give you some medications to reduce the chance of further bleeding. I'll also start you on an antibiotic because liver problem can increase the risk of infection'.

- You may consider blood transfusion if he continues to bleed.
- You will keep him updated.

OUTCOME

The following results are obtained:

- Haemoglobin 122 g/L (previous values not available), white cell counts 6.4×10^9/L and **platelet count 134×10^9/L**.
- Liver function tests show aspartate aminotransferase 50 U/L (10–44 U/L), alanine aminotransferase 38 U/L (10–34 U/L), alkaline phosphatase 124 U/L (40–150 U/L), γ-GT 54 U/L (12–64 U/L) and **albumin 30 g/L** (34–48 g/L).
- Serum urea, creatinine and electrolytes normal.
- PT and APTT normal.

The low platelet count is most likely due to hypersplenism. The normal coagulation results are reassuring, but he should continue to be monitored. The low albumin is due to chronic liver disease.

His vital parameters are closely monitored. He is commenced on intravenous somatostatin, esomeprazole and ceftriaxone. Gastroscopy confirms the presence of oesophageal varices. The gastroenterologist performs variceal band ligation to prevent the recurrence of bleeding.

He remains stable and is discharged after a couple of days. He is commenced on spironolactone, carvedilol and B complex vitamins. The gastroenterologist arranges to follow him in his clinic and plans to refer him to the liver unit for an opinion regarding liver transplantation.

The 38-Year-Old Woman with Jaundice

Case 36

A 38-year-old woman presents with a two-day history of abdominal pain and yellowing of the eyes and skin.

She is alert and oriented. Her temperature is 37.1°C, pulse rate 60/minute, BP 116/72 mm Hg, respiratory rate 16/minute and oxygen saturation 98% on room air.

HOW SHOULD THIS PROBLEM BE APPROACHED?

*She tells you that her **tummy has been painful** for the last two days and her **skin and eyes have turned yellow**. She has been feeling **feverish and tired** for the last three to four days.*

The only cause for yellow discoloration of the eyes is jaundice! There are three important questions to ask when faced with a patient with jaundice:

- Is it pre-hepatic, hepatocellular or post-hepatic?
- Is there any evidence of acute decompensation (acute liver failure)?

Features of acute decompensation include (a) encephalopathy (impaired consciousness or altered mental state) and (b) coagulopathy (clinical evidence of bleeding or prolonged prothrombin time [PT]).

- Are there any features of chronic liver disease?

In this patient, jaundice is likely to be either hepatocellular or post-hepatic, as she complains of fever and abdominal pain. Features of post-hepatic jaundice (also known as cholestatic or obstructive jaundice) include pale stools, dark urine and pruritus. The obstruction to the free flow of bile from the liver to the intestine causes retrograde flow of conjugated bilirubin into the blood and then urine, explaining the pale stools and dark urine. Bile salts that escape from hepatocytes into the blood stream accumulate in the skin and cause itching.

Cholestasis is classified as intra- or extra-hepatic (*see Figure 36.1*) depending on the level of obstruction. Extra-hepatic cholestasis (disease involving extra-hepatic bile ducts) may be painful or painless. *Painful jaundice* is usually due to a benign cause like gall stone impacted in the common hepatic or bile duct, while *painless jaundice* should alert you to a sinister cause like cancer in the head of pancreas or cholangiocarcinoma. Intra-hepatic cholestasis (disease involving intra-hepatic bile ducts) may be caused by hepatitis (swollen liver cells compress the biliary canaliculi), primary biliary cholangitis or drugs (e.g. amoxicillin, erythromycin, chlorpromazine).

DOI: 10.1201/9781003430230-36

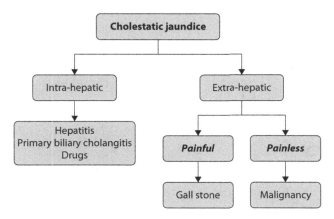

FIGURE 36.1   Simple approach to cholestatic jaundice.

Initial questions to ask:

- Is there any **change in the colour of her urine and stools**?
- Any **itching**?
- Explore her complaint of **abdominal pain**.

Ask about the site of pain, radiation, character of the pain, and aggravating and relieving factors.

Note: Abdominal pain in patients with jaundice may be due to hepatitis or gall stone impacted in the common hepatic or bile duct. Gall stones cause pain because of biliary colic, or a complication like cholecystitis, cholangitis or pancreatitis.

- Ask about the **fever**. Did she measure her temperature? Was it accompanied by **rigors**?

Cholangitis should be suspected in patients with (a) cholestatic jaundice, (b) right hypochondrial pain and (c) fever with rigors (*Charcot's triad*). Other probable causes of fever in a patient with jaundice are cholecystitis, pancreatitis and hepatitis.

*She noticed the yellow discoloration in her eyes and skin two days ago. There is no change in the colour of her urine or stools. She denies itching. She feels the **pain in the right upper part of her tummy** and it does not radiate anywhere. It is a dull ache, with no specific aggravating or relieving factors. Although she feels feverish, her temperature has been normal. She has not been shivering.*

 Cholestasis is less likely because of the absence of pruritus and the normal colour of her stools and urine. Further questions should explore the features of hepatitis. The most common causes of hepatitis are infections and toxins (*see Box 36.1*).

BOX 36.1   COMMON CAUSES OF HEPATITIS†

- **Infections** like viral hepatitis, Epstein-Barr virus (EBV), cytomegalovirus (CMV), malaria, yellow fever, leptospirosis and herpes simplex.
- **Toxic causes** like prescription drugs, alcohol, 'over-the-counter' preparations, recreational drugs, paracetamol overdose and mushroom poisoning.

† Less common causes include autoimmune hepatitis, sepsis, ischemic hepatitis, congestive cardiac failure, Budd-Chiari syndrome, Wilson's disease and pregnancy-related causes (e.g. acute fatty liver, pre-eclampsia or hyperemesis gravidarum).

Further questions to ask:

- Ask if she *travelled anywhere recently*.

If there is a positive travel history, ask where she stayed, what she did there and who accompanied her. Also ask if she received any vaccines prior to her trip or take any precautions against malaria (if she went to a country with high prevalence of malaria).

- Ask about *risk factors for hepatitis B or C*.

Risk factors include high-risk sexual behaviour, receipt of blood products and sharing of needles for intravenous drug abuse, tattoos or body piercings.

- Obtain a *detailed drug history* and ask about her *alcohol intake*.

Ask not only about prescription drugs, but also preparations taken across the counter, supplements and recreational drugs.

- Complete the *rest of the history*.

Ask if she has previously been diagnosed with liver disease, family history of liver disease, her occupation, date of her last menstrual period and obstetric history.

*She went on a **two-week holiday with her husband to India** and returned three weeks ago. She was born in India and migrated to the UK ten years ago. She and her husband visit their relatives in the southern part of India every year, but this time, they also went on a trip to Delhi, Agra and Rajasthan. They stayed in 4-star hotels, mostly ate in good restaurants and only drank bottled water. She did not consume raw seafood or come in contact with dirty water. She did not receive any vaccines prior to her travel or take any medication for malaria prophylaxis. She applied a mosquito repellent on her skin when she was in India. Her husband has been well.*

She has never received blood transfusion, used intravenous drugs or had tattoos or body piercings. Her husband is her only sexual partner. She does not take prescription drugs or supplements. She does not smoke or drink. She and her husband were investigated for primary infertility a few years ago, but no cause was found. They tried in vitro fertilisation, but it was not successful. Her medical history is otherwise unremarkable. She is not aware of anyone in her immediate family with liver disease. She works for the local council office. Her last menstrual period was ten days ago.

A trip to Asia or Africa poses a risk for hepatitis A or E, as both are transmitted faeco-orally. The incubation period is two to six weeks, so her recent trip to India is relevant. She should have ideally received vaccination to protect against hepatitis A, but it is not uncommon for people visiting their homeland to not do so. Malaria is a differential diagnosis, as it can cause both haemolysis and hepatitis, and the incubation period can range from a few days to several weeks (depending on the species). She should also be tested for hepatitis B or C although there are no risk factors.

Among the other infectious causes, Epstein-Barr virus (EBV) and cytomegalovirus (CMV) should be considered, especially if the markers for viral hepatitis are negative. India is not a 'yellow fever country' and she did not perform any activities that would place her at risk of developing leptospirosis (e.g. outdoor activities involving contact with dirty water), so there is no need to test for these two infections. The history does not suggest a toxic cause for her hepatitis.

Among the less common causes, autoimmune hepatitis can present acutely, but the relevant antibody tests can be held off pending the results of the viral markers. There are no pointers to ischemic hepatitis, cardiac failure or hepatic vein thrombosis. Pregnancy-related causes can be ruled out because her last menstrual period was only ten days ago and there is a background history of infertility. Wilson's disease need not be considered because it presents much earlier in life and there are no extra-pyramidal features.

WHAT SHOULD YOU LOOK FOR ON EXAMINATION?

You should

- Look for *icterus* in the sclera and skin.
- Check for signs of *encephalopathy* (although unlikely in this patient, as she is alert and oriented, and has given a good history).

Signs of encephalopathy include altered mentation, *fetor hepaticus* and hepatic flap.

- Look for *signs of chronic liver disease* (*see Box 36.2*).
- Examine the *abdomen*.

Check for hepatomegaly, splenomegaly and free fluid in the abdomen. Feel for tenderness, particularly in the right hypochondrium (tender hepatomegaly) and right costal margin (*Murphy's sign*).

BOX 36.2 SIGNS OF CHRONIC LIVER DISEASE

- Ascites.
- Splenomegaly (due to portal hypertension).
- Spider naevi (>2 is significant).
- Gynaecomastia/loss of axillary hair.
- Palmar erythema/Dupuytren's contracture/finger clubbing.

Examination confirms **icterus in the sclera and skin**. *There are no signs of chronic liver disease. The* **liver is palpable** *about 3 cm below the right costal margin, and it is* **tender**. *The spleen is not palpable and there is no free fluid. The rest of the examination is normal.*

HOW SHOULD THIS PATIENT BE INVESTIGATED?

You should ask for

- *Blood tests*, including full blood count, liver function tests, serum creatinine and electrolytes, PT and blood glucose.

Prolongation of PT occurs in severe liver disease because of reduced synthesis of clotting factors. It has prognostic value.

- Tests to *screen for infectious causes of acute hepatitis*, including [a] hepatitis A IgM, [b] hepatitis B surface antigen and anti-hepatitis B core IgM, [c] hepatitis C antibody and [d] blood films for malarial parasites.

Hepatitis E IgM, EBV IgM and CMV IgM can be requested if the above tests are negative.

- *Urine pregnancy test* (in all pre-menopausal women).
- *Ultrasound scan of the liver and biliary system*.

Ultrasound examination is useful to [a] look for bile duct dilatation (feature of extra-hepatic biliary obstruction), [b] look for features of chronic liver disease, like splenomegaly and ascites and [c] assess the patency of blood vessels (with Doppler).

- *Liver autoimmune screen* (if viral markers are negative).

This includes anti-smooth muscle antibody, anti-mitochondrial antibody, anti-liver-kidney-microsomal antibody, anti-nuclear antibody (ANA) and Ig levels.

WHAT SHOULD YOU TELL THE PATIENT?

You should explain to her that

- Her symptoms are due to acute hepatitis.

'You don't feel well because your liver is inflamed. We call this hepatitis. The yellowing of the skin and eyes is due to jaundice'.

- This is most likely due to a viral infection or malaria.

'This is most likely due to a virus. I suspect you caught this virus through food when you were in India. Another possible cause is malaria'.

- You would like to arrange some blood tests and an ultrasound scan.

'I'll ask for some blood tests and a scan of your liver. These tests will help to confirm the inflammation of the liver and tell us if this is due to a virus or malaria'.

- If her illness is due to the virus, it should hopefully settle soon.

'Most people who catch this virus get well in a few days'.

- You would prescribe a small dose of an analgesic to control the pain.
- She should not take any medications without medical advice.

'I'll give you a small dose of a painkiller to control the pain. You should not take any other medication without consulting a doctor. One of the main jobs of the liver is to break down the medications and supplements that we take. When the liver is inflamed, these substances can accumulate in the body and become toxic'.

- You will come back and talk to her when the test results are back.
- There is no need for admission to hospital. She can rest at home.

OUTCOME

Her blood test results show:

- Full blood count and serum creatinine are normal.
- Liver function tests show **serum bilirubin 62 mmol/L** (normal 5–23), **aspartate aminotransferase 502 U/L** (10–44), **alanine aminotransferase 812 U/L** (10–34), **alkaline phosphatase 194 U/L** (40–150) and **γ-GT 96 U/L** (12–64).
- Serum albumin 38 g/L (34–48).
- PT 13.2 seconds (normal 11–14 seconds).
- Blood glucose 5.2 mmol/L.
- **Hepatitis A IgM positive**.
- Hepatitis B surface antigen negative and anti-hepatitis B Core IgM negative. Hepatitis C antibody negative.
- Blood film for malarial parasites × 3 negative.
- **Ultrasound scan of the abdomen confirms hepatomegaly**. The bile ducts are not dilated. There is no splenomegaly or free fluid in the abdomen.

Her elevated alanine aminotransferase is due to hepatitis. The positive hepatitis A IgM is in keeping with acute hepatitis A infection (positive hepatitis A IgG would suggest remote infection). The synthetic function of the liver is not impaired, as her PT is normal. The normal albumin and platelet count, combined with the absence of relevant symptoms and signs, rule out chronic liver disease (the low serum albumin in chronic liver disease is due to reduced synthesis and thrombocytopenia due to hypersplenism).

The results have excluded acute hepatitis B, hepatitis C and malaria. There is no need to test for EBV or CMV or request an autoimmune screen. The ultrasound scan has excluded post-hepatic obstruction, as the bile ducts are not dilated. The normal haemoglobin would exclude haemolysis (cause of pre-hepatic jaundice). Gilbert's syndrome may co-exist with hepatitis, but the absence of previous episodes of jaundice would make this unlikely.

She is discharged home later that day. Her illness resolves within the next few days. Two weeks later, her liver function tests return to normal.

The 44-Year-Old Woman with Abnormal Liver Function Tests

Case 37

A 44-year-old woman is referred by the general surgeon because of abnormal liver function tests.
   Her serum aspartate aminotransferase is 96 U/L (10–44), alanine aminotransferase 118 U/L (10–34), alkaline phosphatase 114 U/L (40–150), γ-GT 36 U/L (12–64) and serum albumin 41 g/L (34–48). Full blood count and renal function are normal.

HOW SHOULD THIS PROBLEM BE APPROACHED?

*She tells you that she went to see the surgeon three weeks ago for a lump in her right breast. He biopsied the lesion and told her that it was a benign lump. He requested some blood tests at the time, and they showed that her **liver tests were abnormal**. He therefore suggested seeing the medical doctor. She **feels well** and doesn't understand why her liver tests are abnormal.*

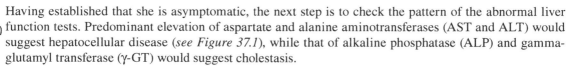

Having established that she is asymptomatic, the next step is to check the pattern of the abnormal liver function tests. Predominant elevation of aspartate and alanine aminotransferases (AST and ALT) would suggest hepatocellular disease (*see Figure 37.1*), while that of alkaline phosphatase (ALP) and gamma-glutamyl transferase (γ-GT) would suggest cholestasis.

In this patient, AST and ALT are elevated, while ALP and γ-GT are normal. The elevation is predominantly that of ALT. The most likely causes are (a) non-alcoholic fatty liver disease (NAFLD), (b) medication- or alcohol-induced liver disease, (c) chronic viral hepatitis and (d) autoimmune hepatitis. Her serum albumin and platelet count are normal, so it is unlikely that she has chronic liver disease (the low serum albumin in chronic liver disease is due to reduced synthesis and thrombocytopenia due to hypersplenism).

You should now ask about:

- Her other medical problems, particularly **diabetes** and **hyperlipidaemia**.
- Regular **medications**, and any that she took recently.

DOI: 10.1201/9781003430230-37

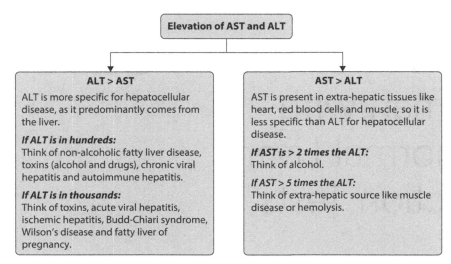

FIGURE 37.1   Causes of elevated AST and ALT.

Also ask about *preparations bought across the counter* and *use of illicit drugs*.

- Her *alcohol* intake.
- *Risk factors for viral hepatitis* (e.g. recent travel, infectious contacts, tattoos and body piercing, previous blood transfusions and sexual history).
- *Joint pain* and *skin rashes*.
- *Family history* of liver disease.

*Her **finger prick blood sugar readings were noted to be borderline** when she was tested three weeks ago. She has never had her cholesterol checked. She has **gradually gained over 20 kg in the last 15 years**. She admits that she is sedentary and tends to snack a lot. Her medical history is otherwise unremarkable. She does not take any prescription drug or 'over-the-counter' preparation. She has never used illicit drugs. She drinks a **glass of wine about two to three times a week** and has never exceeded this amount ever. She does not smoke.*

She has not travelled anywhere recently. She hasn't got any tattoos or body piercings. She has never received a blood transfusion. Her husband is her only sexual partner. Her last menstrual period was five days ago. She denies joint pain and skin rashes. Apart from diabetes in both parents, her family history is unremarkable. She is a primary school teacher. She lives with her husband and two children, aged 17 and 14.

 Non-Alcoholic Aatty Liver Disease (NAFLD) is the most likely diagnosis. She should be screened for diabetes and hyperlipidaemia. She should also be tested for hepatitis B and C. Medication- or alcohol-induced liver disease can be ruled out. Although less likely, she should be tested for autoimmune hepatitis if the initial investigations do not reveal a clear cause for her elevated liver enzymes.

WHAT SHOULD YOU LOOK FOR ON EXAMINATION?

You should

- Ask for her *body mass index*.
- Check for *markers of chronic liver disease* (*see Box 37.1*).

BOX 37.1   SIGNS OF CHRONIC LIVER DISEASE

- Ascites.
- Splenomegaly (due to portal hypertension).
- Spider naevi (>2 is significant).
- Gynaecomastia/loss of axillary hair.
- Palmar erythema/Dupuytren's contracture/finger clubbing.

- Examine the *abdomen* for palpable liver and spleen, and check for free fluid.

She is overweight. Her body mass index is 31. There are no markers of chronic liver disease. Examination of her abdomen is unremarkable, with no hepatosplenomegaly or free fluid.

HOW SHOULD SHE BE EVALUATED FURTHER?

You should request

- Fasting *blood glucose*, *HbA₁c* and *lipid panel*.
- *Screening tests for hepatitis B and C* (hepatitis B surface antigen and anti-hepatitis B surface antibody, anti-hepatitis B core IgG and hepatitis C antibody).
- *Ultrasound scan of her liver*.

WHAT SHOULD YOU TELL THE PATIENT?

You should tell her that

- Her liver function test abnormalities are most likely due to fatty liver disease.

'I suspect your liver tests are abnormal because of fat deposition in the liver'.

- Fatty liver disease occurs in those with obesity or metabolic syndrome.

'Fat deposition in the liver occurs in people who are overweight and those who have diabetes or high cholesterol'.

- You would request an ultrasound scan of the liver and screen for hepatitis, diabetes and hyperlipidaemia.

'I'll ask for a scan of your liver and blood tests to check for diabetes and high cholesterol. I'll also check for viruses that can cause inflammation of the liver'.

- She should lose weight and follow healthy lifestyle measures to reduce the progression of her liver disease.

'You should start eating healthily and cut down the intake of sugars and fats. You should also try to get some exercise. You can start with gentle walking and then gradually increase the pace. These healthy

habits will help you lose weight and reduce further fat accumulation in the liver. Over time, too much fat could lead to scarring of the liver, but you can greatly reduce this risk if you lose weight'.

- She should avoid hepatotoxic medications.

'You should not take any medication or supplement without seeking medical advice, as some of them can affect the liver'.

- You would refer her to a hepatologist (*'liver specialist'*) once the test results are back.

OUTCOME

- Ultrasound of the liver shows **bright echotexture in keeping with fatty liver disease**. There is no splenomegaly or free fluid in the abdomen.
- Hepatitis B and C screen negative.
- **Fasting glucose 6.8 mmol/L**.
- **HbA$_1$C 52 mmol/mol**.
- Serum **total cholesterol 6.1 mmol/L, low-density lipoprotein 4 mmol/L** (target <2.7 mmol/L), high-density lipoprotein 1.1 mmol/L (target >1 mmol/L) and **triglycerides 3.8 mmol/L** (target <1.7 mmol/L).

An oral glucose tolerance test is performed. **Her blood glucose, two hours after 75 g of glucose is 9.1 mmol/L.** *The hepatologist arranges liver transient elastography scan (see Box 37.2), which shows a liver stiffness measurement of 5 kPa. She is commenced on atorvastatin.*

BOX 37.2   LIVER TRANSIENT ELASTOGRAPHY SCAN: THE BASICS

Liver fibrosis may not cause any symptoms, and liver function tests may be deceptively normal even in advanced fibrosis. Although considered the gold standard to diagnose fibrosis, liver biopsy is not ideal, as it is invasive and associated with complications such as bleeding. Transient elastography is a non-invasive method for the assessment of liver fibrosis. It is painless and not associated with any known complications. An ultrasound probe is placed on the skin in the liver area to generate a vibration wave (shear wave), and the time taken for the shear wave to travel to a particular depth inside the liver is measured. Fibrous tissue is harder than normal liver tissue, so the extent of liver fibrosis is estimated based on the shear wave velocity. To improve the test reliability, the median of ten readings is reported. Most healthy adults without liver disease will have a liver stiffness measurement of <7 kPa.

The ultrasound findings are in keeping with fatty liver. There are no features of chronic liver disease. Her blood glucose readings are in keeping with impaired glucose tolerance. Her lipid profile is deranged. Her overall presentation is in keeping with NAFLD and metabolic syndrome.

Hepatic fibrosis and cirrhosis are potential long-term complications of NAFLD. NAFLD scoring systems are available, which help to estimate the risk of fibrosis. The scoring system takes into account the following factors: age, body mass index, diagnosis of diabetes, AST, ALT, serum albumin and platelet count. A transient elastography scan should be requested in patients at higher risk of developing liver fibrosis.

The 22-Year-Old Woman Who Took an Overdose of Paracetamol

Case 38

A 22-year-old woman is brought to the emergency department by her boyfriend, as she had taken 20 tablets of paracetamol a little while ago.

She is conscious and alert. Her temperature is 36.5°C, pulse rate 72/minute, BP 112/76 mm Hg, respiratory rate 16/minute and oxygen saturation 97% on room air.

HOW SHOULD THIS PROBLEM BE APPROACHED?

After checking that she is well enough to talk to you, ask what happened.

*She tells you that she feels fine. She had an argument with her boyfriend and **took 20 tablets of paracetamol**. She keeps paracetamol at home, as she occasionally gets migraine.*

Initial questions to ask:

- Check for ***symptoms of overdose***.

Patients may be asymptomatic or experience gastrointestinal symptoms like abdominal pain and nausea or vomiting in the acute phase. Liver damage usually occurs after 72–96 hours, when patients can become comatose or develop right upper quadrant pain, oliguria and bleeding.

Vomiting immediately after ingesting the overdose might reduce the amount of paracetamol that is absorbed, so it is important to enquire about this.

- At ***what time*** did she take the tablets?

This information will help to interpret the nomogram and decide whether N-acetylcysteine (NAC) should be given (*see below*).

- Did she ***take all the tablets together or was the ingestion staggered***?

DOI: 10.1201/9781003430230-38

The nomogram cannot be interpreted if the ingestion was staggered over several hours.

- ■ ***Did she take anything else*** along with the paracetamol?

Check if she took codeine (e.g. compound preparations containing codeine and paracetamol), benzo-diazepine or alcohol.

*She is asymptomatic. She **took all the tablets together** over about 15–20 minutes, **two hours earlier**. She did not take any other tablet or consume alcohol. She did not vomit after taking the tablets.*

Paracetamol is the most common drug used for overdose, and the leading cause of fulminant liver cell failure in many countries. Paracetamol is normally metabolised to glucuronide and sulphate in the liver. A small amount is metabolised to N-acetyl p-benzoquinone imine (NAPQI), which is detoxified by glutathione. When more than 150 mg/kg of paracetamol is consumed over a short span of time, either together or staggered over several hours, hepatic glutathione stores will not be sufficient to detoxify NAPQI. The NAPQI that is not detoxified can potentially cause fulminant hepatic failure and acute kidney injury. Patients with pre-existing glutathione depletion states (e.g. chronic alcoholism, malnutrition, receiving enzyme-inducing drugs like phenytoin, carbamazepine or rifampicin) are prone to developing paracetamol toxicity at lower doses.

The aim of treatment is to replenish glutathione so that NAPQI can be detoxified. The antidote of choice is NAC, which is converted to glutathione in the liver (glutathione itself cannot be given because it does not cross the liver cell membrane). In patients who develop severe allergic reactions with NAC, oral methionine is an option, but this is less effective than NAC and not widely available.

Further questions to ask:

- ■ How is her ***mood*** now and does she still ***feel suicidal***?

As she is in the acute phase, keep this brief. A detailed screening for depressive symptoms can be deferred to a later time when she is medically stable and more settled. It is however important to check if she still '*wishes to end her life*' so that appropriate suicidal precautions can be taken (although it appears that she acted impulsively and did not plan this over several days).

- ■ Check her ***medical history***.

A history of chronic liver or kidney disease and psychiatric illness is particularly relevant.

- ■ Ask what ***medications*** she takes.

Enzyme-inducing drugs like phenytoin, carbamazepine and rifampicin increase the risk of paracetamol toxicity.

- ■ Ask about ***smoking habit, alcohol consumption and use of illicit drugs***.
- ■ Check her ***social background*** and ***occupation***, and ***obstetric and menstrual history***.

*She says she feels ashamed and embarrassed. She fought with her boyfriend, as he was getting close to another girl. She **does not feel suicidal**. Her past medical history is blameless, except for childhood asthma and migraine. She does not take any regular medication. She has never smoked and seldom drinks alcohol. She does not use illicit drugs. She lives with her boyfriend in a flat. She is a waitress in a restaurant. She has never been pregnant. Her last menstrual period was five days ago.*

WHAT SHOULD YOU LOOK FOR ON EXAMINATION?

Having already ensured that her *vital signs* are satisfactory, and she is *conscious and alert*, you should

- Ask for her *capillary blood glucose*.
- Check her *pupils*.

Think of opioid overdose in patients with small pupils.

- Examine her *abdomen for tenderness*, and check for *hepatic flap* and *markers of chronic liver disease*.
- Ask for her *body weight* (to calculate the paracetamol taken in mg/kg) and see if she looks *malnourished*.

Her pupils are normal in size and reactive to light. Her capillary blood glucose is 7.8 mmol/L. Her abdomen is soft and non-tender. There is no hepatic flap or markers of chronic liver disease. She weighs 48 kg. She looks well nourished.

HOW SHOULD THIS PATIENT BE INVESTIGATED?

You should request

- *Blood tests*, including full blood count, liver function tests, renal panel, venous blood glucose, lactate and salicylate levels.
- *Prothrombin time or international normalised ratio* (INR).
- *Serum paracetamol level*.

Paracetamol level should be checked only if the tablets were taken together. The level should not be checked before 4 hours from the time of overdose (as the absorption may not be complete) *or* after 24 hours. The result should be plotted on a nomogram to decide if treatment with NAC is necessary. There are two treatment lines on the nomogram. For patients with pre-existing glutathione depletion states, the high-risk treatment line should be used.

If the initial paracetamol level is normal, it may be repeated after some hours if (a) there is discordance between the reported amount ingested and the initial serum paracetamol level, (b) there is doubt about the reported time of ingestion or (c) the patient took a sustained release preparation.

- *Arterial blood gases* are indicated in patients with high anion gap and those with fulminant liver failure to decide on the need for liver transplantation.
- *Urine pregnancy test*.

Notes:

1. The four key investigations are serum paracetamol level, INR, serum alanine aminotransferase and creatinine.
2. Serious harm is unlikely if the liver function tests and serum creatinine are normal after 24 hours *and* paracetamol level is below the treatment line.

WHAT SHOULD YOU TELL THE PATIENT?

You should tell her that

- You would like to admit and closely monitor her.
- There is a risk of hepatotoxicity, kidney injury and coagulation abnormality with paracetamol overdose. You would like to start her on NAC to reduce this risk.

'Taking too much paracetamol can affect the liver, kidneys and clotting of blood. I would like to start you on an antidote medication to reduce this risk. This medication will be given through the vein'.

- You would request some blood tests now and draw another blood sample two hours later to check the paracetamol level.

'I'll first ask for some blood tests now to check your blood counts, liver, kidneys and blood clotting. After a couple of hours, we will draw another blood sample to check the paracetamol level in your blood. We must wait at least four hours after you took the tablets to check the paracetamol level, hence the second blood test'.

- If the paracetamol level is high, you will *'continue the antidote medication for 24 hours'*. She will be monitored closely during this time.
- You would seek the opinion of a hepatologist (*'liver specialist'*) depending on her progress and results of her blood tests.
- You would recommend seeing a psychiatrist (*'mental health specialist'*) for some counselling before she is discharged.

She tells you that she feels fine and asks if she can be discharged if the blood tests are normal. She is happy to sign the form and go home at her own risk. After asking why she wants to leave, you should tell her that

- She has taken a large amount of paracetamol and the blood level is unlikely to be 'normal'.
- Even if the blood tests are normal, the toxic effects could be delayed, and you would prefer to monitor her in hospital and repeat the blood tests later.
- Paracetamol overdose can damage the liver. She may potentially need a liver transplant or even die without treatment. The risk can be greatly reduced with timely treatment.

An overdose patient refusing treatment *or* insisting on getting discharged against medical advice poses a difficult ethical dilemma (*autonomy versus duty of care*), often requiring the inputs of the senior most clinician, psychiatrist and the clinical ethics team.

If you allow her to go home and she dies later, you will have to justify your decision during the inquest. On the other hand, if you treat her against her wishes, you risk being sued by her for battery. Opinions may be divided on what exactly should be done in this situation, but in general, her capacity and suicidal risk should first be assessed (*get the psychiatrist*). It should not be assumed that she lacks capacity just because her decision is unwise or irrational.

- If she lacks capacity, she can be treated in her best interests.
- If she has capacity but is suicidal, she can be sectioned and detained in hospital under the 'Mental Health Act' (as she poses a harm to herself) but still cannot be treated against her wishes (unless there is a court order to do so).
- If she has capacity and is not suicidal, you should provide clear advice on when to return to hospital (after trying your best to ask her to stay).

If the paracetamol level is high, she could be started on oral methionine (if available) and asked to return on the following day for blood tests. It is vital to clearly document all the discussions you have with the patient and the inputs of the psychiatrist and senior most clinician.

OUTCOME

Her blood test results are as follows:

- Full blood count, venous blood glucose, liver function test, serum creatinine and electrolytes and prothrombin time are normal.
- **Paracetamol level is above the treatment line on the nomogram**.
- Salicylate level normal.
- Urine pregnancy test negative.

After counselling, she agrees to stay in hospital and receive NAC. Her stay is uneventful, and she is discharged two days later with appropriate counselling.

It is not surprising that her liver function tests, serum creatinine and prothrombin time were normal, as the blood sample was drawn around two hours after ingestion. Treatment with NAC was clearly indicated based on the results of the serum paracetamol level (*see Figure 38.1*).

NAC is most effective if given within 8 hours from the time of overdose to reduce the risk of liver damage. Some patients may develop skin rashes, flushing, nausea, wheezing or hypotension with NAC. These reactions usually respond to antihistamines and bronchodilators (if wheezing), following which the NAC can be safely restarted at a lower rate. Charcoal is useful only if the patient is seen within one hour of ingestion (but do not give to patients with reduced conscious level, as the emesis may increase the risk of aspiration pneumonia).

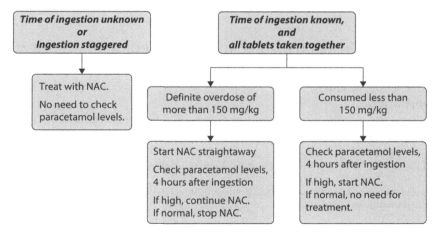

FIGURE 38.1   Flow chart for management of paracetamol overdose with N-acetylcysteine (NAC).

The absolute indication for liver transplantation is arterial pH <7.3 (due to elevated lactate). If pH is >7.3, liver transplant should be considered for patients with (a) encephalopathy, (b) prothrombin time >100 seconds and (c) serum creatinine >300 μmol/L (all three criteria must be met).

The 32-Year-Old Woman with Diarrhoea

Case 39

A 32-year-old woman presents with a three-month history of diarrhoea.
  Her temperature is 36°C, pulse rate 72/minute, BP 116/78 mm Hg, respiratory rate 16/minute and oxygen saturation 98% on room air.

HOW SHOULD THIS PROBLEM BE APPROACHED?

---

*She tells you that her **bowels have been loose** for the last three months. Prior to that, she was opening her bowels once daily, passing solid stools. When the problem first started, she was going to the toilet about two to three times a day. The frequency of bowel movements has since gradually increased, and she is now going **more than a dozen times a day**.*

 Her diarrhoea can be labelled as 'chronic', as it has lasted longer than four weeks. See *Box 39.1* for some common causes of chronic diarrhoea.

> **BOX 39.1   SOME COMMON CAUSES OF CHRONIC DIARRHOEA†**
>
> - Inflammatory bowel disease.
> - Irritable bowel syndrome.
> - Coeliac disease.
> - Infections (e.g. *Giardiasis*, tuberculosis, *Salmonella*, *Cryptosporidium*).
> - Medications (e.g. antibiotics, laxatives, proton pump inhibitors).
> - Hyperthyroidism.
> - Malabsorption (e.g. chronic pancreatitis, lactose intolerance).
>
> † Some rare causes are ischemic colitis, amyloidosis, Zollinger-Ellison syndrome, radiation enteritis, carcinoid syndrome and diabetic autonomic neuropathy.

Further questions to ask:

- Has she noticed ***blood in her stools***?

If there is blood in the stool, ask [a] if the blood is bright red or altered in colour and [b] if the blood is mixed with stools or separate from it.

 DOI: 10.1201/9781003430230-39

Note: Bright red or fresh blood in the toilet paper on wiping is seen in anal disease (like fissure, haemorrhoids or cancer), while altered blood or blood mixed with stool would suggest that the pathology is higher up in the colon.

- Does she *wake up at night to move her bowels*?

Nocturnal diarrhoea would point to organic pathology like inflammatory bowel disease (IBD).

- Ask about *tenesmus*. Does she feel that she hasn't emptied her bowels completely even after going to the toilet because of a sensation of fullness in her rectum?

Tenesmus is a feature of rectal disease (e.g. IBD, rectal cancer).

- Ask about *steatorrhoea*. Are the stools oily, foul smelling and difficult to flush?

Steatorrhea means fat malabsorption. It may be caused by small bowel disease, bile salt deficiency or pancreatic insufficiency.

- Any *abdominal pain*?

Obtain details about the site of pain, radiation, character, aggravating and relieving factors.

- Has she *lost weight*? If so, how much and over how long?
- Ask about *symptoms of hyperthyroidism* (e.g. palpitations, tremors, heat intolerance, lump over the neck).

*She has not noticed blood in her stools. She **wakes up once or twice at night** to move her bowels. She often feels that she hasn't emptied her bowels fully, as there is a **sensation of fullness in her back passage**. The stools do not float in the pan and are not difficult to flush. She gets a generalised **discomfort in her tummy** that feels like a cramp, with no specific aggravating or relieving factors. She has **lost around 6 kg in the last three months**, without trying. She has gone down from around 52 to 46 kg. She has **lost interest in food**. There are no symptoms of hyperthyroidism.*

There are several features in keeping with IBD, including [a] the long duration of diarrhoea (>4 weeks), [b] nocturnal symptoms, [c] tenesmus and [d] unintentional loss of about 10% of her body weight over a short span of time. The abdominal pain is non-specific. The absence of overt lower gastrointestinal bleeding would not exclude IBD.

Irritable bowel syndrome (IBS) should not be entertained in a patient with red flag symptoms, such as nocturnal diarrhoea and weight loss. The relevant blood tests should be requested to rule out hyperthyroidism and coeliac disease although they are somewhat less likely because of tenesmus and abdominal discomfort, and absence of other thyroid symptoms. She is too young to get bowel cancer. Chronic infection and pseudomembranous enterocolitis are still possible, so a *travel history* and history of *prior antibiotic use* would be important to elicit.

She went to Majorca for two weeks, about three months prior to the onset of her symptoms. She has never been outside Europe all her life. She does not take any regular medication. She did not receive antibiotics prior to the onset of her symptoms.

- Ask about *joint pain*, *back pain*, *skin rashes*, previous episodes of *red eyes* (ocular inflammation due to uveitis) and *mouth ulcers* (e.g. Crohn's disease).

IBD may be associated with extra-intestinal symptoms such as arthritis, spondylitis, uveitis and skin rashes (pyoderma gangrenosum and erythema nodosum). Skin rashes are also a feature of coeliac disease (dermatitis herpetiformis).

- Complete the *rest of the history*.

She denies joint pain, back pain and skin rashes. She has never had red eyes or mouth ulcers. Her past medical history is blameless. She has never smoked and seldom drinks alcohol. She has been in a stable relationship with her boyfriend for over seven years and never been pregnant. There is no one in her immediate family with bowel problem. Her menses are regular. She is a manager in a GP practice.

The absence of a history of travel to a tropical country reduces the likelihood of a chronic infection like *Salmonella* or *Giardia*. Pseudomembranous colitis is unlikely, as she did not receive antibiotics prior to the onset of her symptoms.

WHAT SHOULD YOU LOOK FOR ON EXAMINATION?

You should

- Check her *hydration status*.

Signs of dehydration include tachycardia, hypotension, reduced skin turgor and dryness of mucous membranes.

- Perform a *general examination*.

This might help to detect the effects of her illness (e.g. cachexia, malnourished state or pallor) *or* suggest the cause of diarrhoea (e.g. cutaneous signs of IBD or coeliac disease, oral ulcers in Crohn's disease, signs of hyperthyroidism).

- Examine the *abdomen*.

Check for tenderness, rigidity, guarding and rebound tenderness.

*She looks **thin and tired**. She seems well hydrated. There are no skin rashes or oral ulcers. She is clinically euthyroid. Abdominal examination reveals **generalised mild tenderness**.*

HOW SHOULD THIS PATIENT BE INVESTIGATED?

- *Blood tests*, including full blood count, C-reactive protein, liver function tests, serum creatinine and electrolytes.
- The investigation of choice is *colonoscopy with biopsy*.

She should be referred to a gastroenterologist.

Investigations to request in selected patients (depending on the clinical presentation) include:

- *Stool examination*.

Ask for microscopy and culture, and *Clostridium difficile* toxin.

- *Faecal calprotectin* (protein released by neutrophils in the bowel wall) can help to distinguish inflammatory from non-inflammatory bowel disease.
- *Coeliac screen* (anti-endomysial or anti-tissue transglutaminase antibody and serum IgA).

- *Thyroid function tests*.
- *Anti-Saccharomyces cerevisiae antibody* (ASCA) and *perinuclear anti-neutrophil cytoplasmic antibody* (p-ANCA).

These tests may help to distinguish Crohn's disease from ulcerative colitis. The former is more specific for Crohn's disease, while the latter is associated with ulcerative colitis.

WHAT SHOULD YOU TELL THE PATIENT?

You should tell her that

- Her diarrhoea is most likely due to inflammatory bowel disease.

'I suspect your diarrhoea is caused by inflammation of the bowel. We call this inflammatory bowel disease. We do not know what causes this kind of inflammation. Another possible cause is bowel infection, but I think that is less likely'.

- You would like to arrange some investigations, including blood and stool tests.

'I'll first ask for some blood tests. I'll also ask for a stool test to rule out some common infections'.

- You would recommend admission to the hospital for a few days.
- You would ask a gastroenterologist to see her.

'I'll ask a bowel specialist to see you. It is very likely that he will arrange a camera test. The camera test involves passing a thin long tube with a camera at one end through your back passage to look at the inner lining of your bowel and to take a small piece of tissue to be examined under a microscope. This test will help to confirm the inflammation. The bowel specialist will explain this to you'.

- The gastroenterologist will discuss the treatment options.

'The specialist will discuss the treatment options based on the results of your tests'.

- You will update her when the test results are back.

OUTCOME

Her blood tests show

- **Haemoglobin 108 g/L, MCV 84.**
- **White cell count 13.4 × 10⁹/L.**
- Platelet count 480 × 10⁹/L.
- **Erythrocyte sedimentation rate 68 mm/hour.**
- **C-reactive protein 126 mg/L.**
- Thyroid and liver function tests (including serum albumin), serum creatinine and electrolytes are normal.

*She is referred to the gastroenterologist. Colonoscopy shows evidence of **proctitis and distal colitis**, involving the sigmoid and descending colon. Biopsies taken from the rectum are reported as showing features consistent with **ulcerative colitis**. She is commenced on oral prednisolone, steroid enema and mesalazine.*

The 42-Year-Old Woman with Diarrhoea

Case 40

A 42-year-old woman with scleroderma presents with a six-month history of diarrhoea.

HOW SHOULD THIS PROBLEM BE APPROACHED?

---

*She tells you that her **bowels have been loose** for the last six months. She is **moving her bowels about three to four times a day**. She was previously moving her bowels only once daily, passing solid stools.*

 Scleroderma affects multiple parts of the gastrointestinal (GI) tract (*see Box 40.1*). Clinical manifestations arise because of fibrosis of the wall of the GI tract and inefficient forward peristalsis. Her diarrhoea is possibly related to her scleroderma and caused by malabsorption.

BOX 40.1 GASTROINTESTINAL MANIFESTATIONS OF SCLERODERMA

- Dry mouth due to associated Sjögren's syndrome.
- Dysphagia due to oesophageal involvement.
- Gastro-oesophageal reflux disease.
- Vomiting due to gastroparesis.
- Hematemesis or iron deficiency anaemia due to gastric antral vascular ectasia.
- Malabsorption due to small bowel involvement.
- Faecal incontinence due to rectal or anal involvement.

Initial questions to ask:

- Has she noticed **blood in her stools**?
- Are there any features of **steatorrhea** (fat malabsorption)?

This is the key question to ask, given the background history of scleroderma. Fat absorption requires (a) a normal small bowel mucosa, (b) bile salts to emulsify and (c) the pancreatic enzyme lipase to digest the fat. Steatorrhea therefore results from small bowel disease, bile salt deficiency or pancreatic insufficiency. The stools in steatorrhea are pale, oily or greasy and malodorous. They tend to float in the toilet bowl and are difficult to flush away.

DOI: 10.1201/9781003430230-40

- Any *tenesmus* or *urgency*?
- Does she *wake up at night to move her bowels*?
- Any *abdominal pain*?
- Has she *lost weight*? If so, how much and over how long?

*She has not noticed blood in her stools. Her **stools look pale and oily, float in the toilet bowl and are difficult to flush away**. She denies tenesmus or urgency. She does not wake up at night to move her bowels. Her **abdomen feels bloated**, but it is not painful. She has **lost about 2–3 kg in the last six months**.*

The next set of questions should explore her **background history of scleroderma** and features that may suggest **involvement of other parts of the GI tract**.

*She was diagnosed with **scleroderma** more than five years ago, when she presented with **joint pain and Raynaud's phenomenon**. About two years ago, she was told that her **lungs were scarred**, but she does not get breathless on exertion and her breathing tests have been stable. Her annual heart scan, blood pressure and urine tests have been normal so far. She takes amlodipine, omeprazole and fish oil.*

*She used to get **heartburn**, but it has been a lot better since she started taking omeprazole. Her **mouth is always dry**. She denies problems with swallowing, vomiting or faecal incontinence. She has never had a camera test to investigate her bowel.*

Her description is in keeping with steatorrhoea, related to her scleroderma. Omeprazole increases the risk of *Clostridium difficile* infection, but her presentation is not in keeping with this. Apart from the dry mouth (due to possible Sjögren's syndrome) and gastro-oesophageal reflux, she does not seem to have any other GI manifestation of scleroderma.

Scleroderma increases the risk of small intestinal bacterial overgrowth (SIBO). The entire length of the GI tract contains microorganisms, but there are more bacteria in the colon than in the small bowel. In scleroderma, the inefficient forward peristalsis allows colonic bacteria to get to the small bowel, where food is digested and absorbed. The bloated feeling that she is describing is due to the gas produced by bacteria when food is broken down. Weight loss occurs because bacteria compete with the host for nutrients. Malabsorption of other nutrients may cause oedema or muscle wasting (protein), osteoporosis or osteomalacia (calcium) and peripheral neuropathy (vitamin B_{12}).

She denies ankle swelling, or tingling, numbness or weakness in her limbs. She has never broken any bones.

WHAT SHOULD YOU LOOK FOR ON EXAMINATION?

You should focus on the diarrhoea rather than trying to elicit all the signs of scleroderma.

- Ask for her *vital parameters*.
- Check for signs of *dehydration* (dryness of the mucous membrane).
- Examine the *abdomen* to check for tenderness or mass.

*Her vital signs are satisfactory. Her mucous membranes are moist. The abdomen is soft and non-tender. There are signs of scleroderma, including **skin thickening in her face and distal limbs**. **Telangiectasias** are present over her face. There are **fine end-inspiratory crackles** in her lung bases.*

HOW SHOULD SHE BE EVALUATED FURTHER?

You should request

- **Blood tests**, including full blood count, liver function tests, serum creatinine and electrolytes, calcium and phosphate, iron, vitamin B_{12}, folate and vitamin D.

Other tests that may be requested are serum zinc, magnesium and selenium.

- **Faecal fat estimation** is generally not done in practice.

In patients with suspected exocrine pancreatic insufficiency, measurement of **faecal elastase** is useful. Levels would be low in patients with exocrine pancreatic insufficiency. Elastase is preferred, as it is not degraded during transit through the GI tract.

- The **hydrogen breath test** is useful to diagnose SIBO (usually requested by the gastroenterologist).

The patient is given a lactulose drink and exhaled hydrogen is measured. Lactulose is chosen because it is not digested in the small bowel and goes intact to the colon, where it is broken down by colonic bacteria to produce hydrogen. This is seen as a single H+ peak on the breath test. In the presence of SIBO, lactulose is broken down in the small bowel itself, thus causing a double H+ peak ('small bowel' and 'large bowel' peaks).

WHAT SHOULD YOU TELL THE PATIENT?

You should tell her that

- Her diarrhoea is most likely due to malabsorption related to her scleroderma.

'I suspect your bowels are loose because of scleroderma. Scleroderma not only causes thickening of the skin, but also the bowel lining. Thickening of the bowel lining makes it difficult to absorb nutrients, and this leads to diarrhoea'.

- Scleroderma increases the risk of SIBO.

'Our bowel is made of two parts. They are called small bowel and large bowel. The small bowel digests and absorbs all the nutrients from food, while the large bowel turns undigested food into poo and stores it until it can be excreted. We normally have a lot of bacteria in the large bowel. In scleroderma, the forward bowel movement is not so efficient, and this causes bacteria in the large bowel to move backwards into the small bowel. The build-up of these bacteria in the small bowel interferes with the digestion and absorption of nutrients'.

- Her steatorrhoea and bloated feeling are due to fat and carbohydrate malabsorption.

'The fats that are not absorbed appear in the stools and make them oily. You feel bloated because of the gases released by bacteria when they break down the sugars in your food'.

- You will arrange some blood tests to check '*if proteins, vitamins and minerals are being absorbed well*'.
- You will refer her to a gastroenterologist, who might arrange a hydrogen breath test.

'*I'll ask a bowel specialist to see you. He might arrange a breathing test after giving you a sugar drink. This test will tell us if there are too many bacteria in your small bowel. The bacteria will digest the sugars and release some gases, which can be measured in your breath*'.

- You will also refer her to a dietician.
- Once the investigations are done, the gastroenterologist will plan the treatment.

'*The specialist may suggest medications to stimulate the bowel movement, and use antibiotics if the tests show that there are excessive numbers of bacteria in the small bowel*'.

OUTCOME

Her blood test results are as follows:

- **Haemoglobin 114 g/L**.
- Serum ferritin, vitamin B12 and folate normal.
- **Serum vitamin D 18 ng/mL**.
- Liver and renal function, serum calcium, phosphate and electrolytes normal.
- Stool fat estimation not done.
- **Hydrogen breath test results are in keeping with SIBO**.

The gastroenterologist suggests prokinetic agents, probiotics, cyclical antibiotics and vitamin D replacement. The dietician recommends protein, vitamin and mineral supplementation.

The 59-Year-Old Woman with Recent Change in Bowel Habits

Case 41

A 59-year-old woman presents with a three-month history of change in her bowel habits.

HOW SHOULD THIS PROBLEM BE APPROACHED?

- Start with an open-ended question and ask **how her bowel habits have changed** in the last three months.

*She says she **moves her bowels only about once every two to three days**, despite taking laxatives. Until three months ago, she used to move her bowels every day.*

 Constipation is a common complaint, which denotes reduced frequency of bowel movements (≤3/week) *or* passage of hard, pellet-like stools. In most patients, it is due to lack of dietary fibre, inadequate fluid consumption, lack of exercise or ignoring the urge for a bowel movement. In a small number of patients, there may be an organic cause (*see Box 41.1*).

BOX 41.1   ORGANIC CAUSES OF CONSTIPATION

- **Luminal obstruction** (e.g. bowel cancer).
- **Painful defecation** (e.g. anal fissure of thrombosed piles).
- **Reduced peristalsis** (e.g. medications like opioids, iron or calcium channel blockers, hypothyroidism, hypercalcaemia, irritable bowel syndrome).

Further questions to ask:

- Ask if the **constipation alternates with diarrhoea**.
- Ask if **defecation is painful**.
- Ask about the **shape of the stools**.

DOI: 10.1201/9781003430230-41

The stools may become thin or 'pencil-like' in patients with colonic tumour, as the bowel lumen becomes narrow.

■ Ask if she has noticed **blood in her stool**.

The blood may be bright red (if the bleeding is from rectum), altered to maroon colour (if the bleeding is from distal colon) *or* black and tarry (if blood has remained in the gastrointestinal tract for at least 8 hours).

Note: If the patient reports blood in the stool, ask if it is mixed with the stool or separate from it.

Blood separate from the stool or the presence of blood stain on the toilet paper while wiping would suggest anal disease (e.g. haemorrhoids, fissures or cancer), while blood mixed with stool would suggest that the pathology is higher up in the colon.

■ Ask about **tenesmus** (sensation of incomplete evacuation).

Think of rectal cancer in an older patient with recent-onset constipation and tenesmus.

■ Ask if she has **abdominal pain**.

Patients may complain of abdominal pain due to constipation colic, but you should rule out intestinal obstruction if there is associated abdominal distension and vomiting. In patients with bowel cancer, abdominal pain may be due to bowel obstruction or invasion of peritoneum by the cancer.

■ Ask if there is a recent **change in her weight**.

If she has lost weight, ask how much she has lost and over how long, and if this was intentional or unintentional. Also ask about other constitutional symptoms like loss of appetite, fatigue and weakness. If she says she has gained weight, screen for hypothyroid symptoms.

■ Ask about **family history of bowel cancer** (*'Are you aware of anyone in your immediate family with bowel problems?'* is better than directly using the word cancer at this stage).
■ Ask if she has had **colonoscopy** ('camera test') **or stool tests** before.
■ Complete the **rest of the history**.

Ask about her other medical problems, medications taken (check if she takes opioids, iron or calcium channel blockers), smoking habit and alcohol consumption, her concerns and expectations.

*Her constipation does not alternate with diarrhoea, and she does not experience pain while defecating. She says her **poo has become thin**. On a couple of occasions, she has noticed **blood in her poo**, and it was maroon coloured. She thought the bleeding occurred because of straining. She denies abdominal pain or tenesmus. She has **lost about 6 kg in the last three months**. She always used to weigh around 52 kg but only weighs 46 kg now. The **weight loss is unintentional**. Review of systems is unremarkable.*

*She was previously in good health and seldom visited a doctor. She has never had a bowel examination or stool test before. She does not take any medication. She does not smoke or drink. Her **maternal grandfather died of bowel cancer**, but he was 85 at the time of diagnosis. She lives with her husband. She used to be a hairdresser until three years ago.*

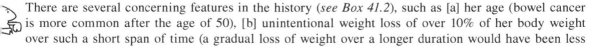

There are several concerning features in the history (*see Box 41.2*), such as [a] her age (bowel cancer is more common after the age of 50), [b] unintentional weight loss of over 10% of her body weight over such a short span of time (a gradual loss of weight over a longer duration would have been less concerning), [c] history of passing blood in her stool, [d] the passage of thin stools and [e] lack of previous screening tests for bowel cancer (either colonoscopy or stool tests). She should be referred to the gastroenterologist urgently.

Colon cancer is the third most common cancer (after prostate and lung in men, and breast and lung in women). The cancer may arise from the large bowel or rectum. They are usually adenocarcinomas that arise from polyps that turn malignant. There are several risk factors for developing colon cancer, such as older age, inflammatory bowel disease, reduced fibre intake, consumption of red meat, smoking and obesity. A family history is relevant because of the increased risk of colon cancer in familial adenomatous polyposis (FAP). The family history of colon cancer at the age of 85 in her maternal grandfather is, however, not relevant and would not merit earlier screening (before the age of 50) of her family members.

BOX 41.2   RED FLAGS IN PATIENTS WITH CONSTIPATION

- Recent onset of constipation in an elderly patient.
- Weight loss.
- Gastrointestinal bleeding (overt or occult).
- Vomiting, abdominal pain and distension.
- Family history of bowel cancer.
- Abdominal mass.
- Unexplained iron deficiency anaemia.

WHAT SHOULD YOU LOOK FOR ON EXAMINATION?

You should

- Perform a *focussed general examination*.

Particularly check for pallor and supraclavicular lymphadenopathy.

- Palpate the *abdomen for a mass* (right-sided tumours may present with a right lower quadrant mass) and *hepatomegaly* (due to liver metastases).

Offer to perform a *digital rectal examination* (rectal tumours may be felt on digital examination).

She looks thin but is not cachectic or emaciated. General examination is unremarkable, with no evidence of pallor or supraclavicular lymphadenopathy. Examination of her abdomen reveals no mass or hepatomegaly.

HOW SHOULD THIS PATIENT BE INVESTIGATED?

You should

- Refer her to a gastroenterologist for *colonoscopy*.
- Ask for *blood tests*, including full blood count, liver function tests, renal function, serum calcium and thyroid function tests.

Do not request **carcinoembryonic antigen** (CEA) to screen asymptomatic patients for colorectal cancer (*see Box 41.3*).

BOX 41.3   CARCINOEMBRYONIC ANTIGEN

- Carcinoembryonic antigen (CEA) was initially thought to be associated with colorectal cancer, but subsequently has been found in other cancers like breast, ovary and thyroid.
- CEA is also found in non-malignant conditions like chronic liver disease and inflammatory bowel disease.
- Not all patients with colon cancer have elevated CEA levels. Hence, CEA should not be used to screen for colon cancer.
- CEA is useful as a prognostic marker (poor prognosis if the levels are high at the time of diagnosis).
- Serial monitoring with CEA is used to assess the response to treatment and predict recurrence.

WHAT SHOULD YOU TELL THE PATIENT AT THIS STAGE?

You should tell her that

- Her recent change in bowel habit should be investigated further.

'Constipation is a common problem. It is usually due to inadequate consumption of fibre, not drinking enough water, lack of exercise or ignoring nature's call. In your case, we should do some tests to find out why you are constipated, as your bowel habits have only changed in the last three months'.

- You are concerned that she has lost weight and is passing blood in her stool.

'I am concerned that you have lost so much weight over such a short span of time and noticed blood in your stool. The weight loss and blood in the stool may be related to the same problem that is causing the constipation'.

- You would refer her to a gastroenterologist (*'bowel specialist'*).
- The gastroenterologist is likely to perform a colonoscopy.

'I am sure the bowel specialist will suggest a camera test. This involves passing a thin long tube with a camera at one end through your back passage to look at the inner lining of your bowel. You will be given an injection to put you to sleep before the camera is passed. The bowel specialist will explain this to you'.

- You will ask for some blood tests in the meantime.
- (If she directly asks if it could be cancer.)

You should address this question sympathetically and tell her that *'A growth in the bowel is one of the possible causes, but it is difficult to be sure about this without doing the camera test to directly look inside. I'll ask the bowel specialist to see you as soon as possible so that we can get the answers quickly'.*

OUTCOME

*Her results show **haemoglobin of 96 g/L**, with **low iron and ferritin**. The white cell and platelet count, serum calcium, liver, renal and thyroid function are normal. The gastroenterologist arranges a colonoscopy, which shows a **growth in her descending colon**. Biopsy is reported as **adenocarcinoma**. CEA is **marginally elevated**. Staging CT scan shows no evidence of lymph node or haematogenous metastases. She is referred to the surgeon to consider left hemicolectomy and the oncologist for chemotherapy.*

 Management of colorectal cancer may include surgery (e.g. right or left hemicolectomy, total or subtotal colectomy, anterior resection of the rectum), chemotherapy (adjuvant, given before surgery, *or* neo-adjuvant, given after surgery), radiotherapy and palliative measures.

Symptomatic bowel cancer is not common, hence the need for regular screening. The aim of screening is to detect cancer early and increase the chance of cure and reduce mortality. In most countries, screening is recommended from the age of 50 (should start earlier for high-risk patients). The gold standard is colonoscopy every ten years if the results are normal each time (as it would take at least ten years for polyps to develop and turn cancerous). For patients who refuse colonoscopy, other screening modalities include CT colonography (but biopsies cannot be taken from polyps or suspicious lesions), air contrast barium enema and flexible sigmoidoscopy (but this can only visualise the left side of the colon and is almost never done these days). An alternative strategy is to perform regular stool tests (for occult blood) and offer endoscopy to patients with positive results.

The 36-Year-Old Woman with Chest Pain

Case 42

A 36-year-old woman presents with a three-month history of intermittent chest pain.

HOW SHOULD THIS PROBLEM BE APPROACHED?

Start with an open-ended question and *explore her main complaint of chest pain*.

*She tells you that she gets **chest pain when she walks her daughters to school**. It is more of a discomfort than pain. This discomfort occurs only when her daughters walk fast, and she must keep pace with them. It usually **resolves in a couple of minutes if she stops walking**. She has never experienced this while walking at a normal pace or during rest. The pain is not related to breathing or eating.*

*The **discomfort is in the central part of the chest**, and it **feels as though someone is squeezing her chest**. The pain does not radiate to arm, neck, jaw or back. This has happened at least a **dozen times in the last three months**.*

Her description is in keeping with stable angina pectoris (*see Box 42.1*). It does not suggest non-cardiac causes, like gastro-oesophageal reflux disease, pleurisy or musculoskeletal chest pain.

BOX 42.1   CHARACTERISTICS OF ANGINA PECTORIS[†]

- Constricting or squeezing discomfort in the central chest.[††]

Patients usually describe it as tightness or discomfort rather than pain. Occasionally, the discomfort may only be felt in the arm or jaw.

- Precipitated by physical exertion.
- Relieved by rest or sub-lingual nitrate within 5 minutes.

[†] If only two out of these three features are present, it is known as *atypical angina*. Presence of none or only one of these three features is known as *non-anginal chest pain*.
[††] It is important to bear in mind that many patients with ischaemic heart disease (particularly elderly patients and those with co-morbidities like diabetes) may not present with typical angina. Conversely, patients with typical angina may not necessarily have coronary artery disease on further evaluation.

DOI: 10.1201/9781003430230-42

The most common cause of angina is atherosclerotic coronary artery disease (CAD). The incidence of CAD rises with advancing age, and it is more common in men than in women. Hence, what is unusual about this story is that she is not in the right age group or sex to develop anginal chest pain. She might as well have traditional cardiovascular risk factors, but the history should aim to elicit the features of conditions that cause non-atherosclerotic CAD (*see Box 42.2*).

BOX 42.2   SOME CAUSES OF ANGINA TO CONSIDER IN A YOUNG PERSON

- Premature atherosclerosis (e.g. *familial hyperlipidaemia*).
- *Valvular heart disease* (e.g. aortic stenosis or regurgitation) and *hypertrophic obstructive cardiomyopathy*.

Angina occurs in aortic stenosis or HOCM because of (a) increased oxygen demand and (b) compression of coronary branches by the hypertrophied left ventricle. In aortic regurgitation, the back-flow of blood from aorta to the left ventricle reduces coronary perfusion.

- Coronary vasculitis due to *Takayasu's arteritis*.
- Coronary vasospasm due to *cocaine*.

- Ask about *risk factors for atherosclerosis*, such as hypertension, diabetes, hyperlipidaemia and smoking habit, and if she has previously suffered a heart attack or stroke.
- Obtain a *family history*.

Ask if any of her immediate family members have suffered a heart attack or stroke at a very young age (<55 years in male and <65 years in female relatives).

- Ask about *other cardiac symptoms*, such as breathlessness, paroxysmal nocturnal dyspnoea, orthopnoea, palpitations, syncope and exertion-induced fatigue.

The presence of these symptoms might suggest left heart failure (e.g. breathlessness, paroxysmal nocturnal dyspnoea, orthopnoea), arrhythmia or volume overload (e.g. palpitation), *or* fixed cardiac output due to ventricular outflow obstruction (e.g. syncope, exercise-induced fatigue).

- Ask about *constitutional symptoms* (e.g. fever, weight loss or joint pain) and *arm claudication* (pain in her arms when she elevates them above the level of her head).

The presence of these features might point to Takayasu's arteritis.

- Ask if she uses *illicit drugs like cocaine*.
- Ask if her *menses are heavy*.

Although anaemia *per se* may not cause angina, it may exacerbate the symptoms of CAD.

*She was very well until three months ago, with no known medical problems. She has never had a heart attack or stroke. Her blood pressure and blood sugar were normal, when last checked during her pregnancies more than eight years ago. Her blood cholesterol has never been checked. Her **father and his brother died of heart attack during their early 40s**. She has an older brother, who is well.*

She denies breathlessness, paroxysmal nocturnal dyspnoea, orthopnoea, palpitations, blackouts, fatigue, fever, joint pain, weight loss or arm claudication. She does not take any medication. She has never smoked or used illicit drugs and always been teetotal. She lives with her husband and two daugh-ters, aged 10 and 8. Her menses are regular and not heavy. She is a housewife.

The premature death of her father and his brother due to heart attack is relevant and possibly due to familial hypercholesterolemia (FH), which is inherited in an autosomal dominant manner. She should be screened for hyperlipidaemia.

WHAT SHOULD YOU LOOK FOR ON EXAMINATION?

You should

- Ask for her **body mass index** and **waist-hip circumference** (if she looks heavy).
- Look for **pallor**.
- Check for **tendon xanthomas** (look at the extensor tendons), **xanthelasma** and **corneal arcus**.
- Ask for her **blood pressure in both arms** (a difference of >10 mm Hg between the two sides may suggest Takayasu's arteritis).
- Examine her cardiovascular system.

Palpate all her **peripheral pulses**, listen to the **carotid and femoral arteries for bruits** and auscultate the **heart for murmurs**.

*Her body mass index is 22. There is no pallor. There are **tendon xanthomas over the extensor aspect of her elbows and Achilles tendons**. There is evidence of **corneal arcus**. Her blood pressure is 124/74 in the right arm and 122/70 in the left arm. Heart sounds are normal and there are no murmurs.*

The tendon xanthomas and corneal arcus point to FH. Corneal arcus generally occurs after the age of 45, so its presence in someone of her age is pathological.

(A detailed examination of the peripheral pulses was omitted, as the tendon xanthomas and corneal arcus have pointed to the cause of her angina.)

FH is an autosomal dominant condition. It can be homozygous (two faulty genes) or heterozygous (one faulty gene). In those with homozygous FH, cardiovascular events usually occur as early as the first or second decade of life. FH is characterised by

- Elevated LDL-cholesterol.
- Premature CAD.
- Family history of elevated LDL-cholesterol *or* premature CAD.
- Tendon xanthomas and arcus senilis (<45 years of age).

LDL-receptors are present on hepatocytes. The presence of more LDL-receptors means that more LDL will be taken from the plasma into cells, thus reducing plasma LDL concentration and *vice versa*. Apo-B is a ligand that helps to bind LDL to the LDL-receptor. PCSK-9 (proprotein convertase subtilisin kexin type 9) degrades LDL-receptors.

FH is caused by mutations of genes that code for LDL-receptor, apo-B or PCSK-9. The result of these mutations is reduced uptake of LDL by liver cells, leading to elevated plasma LDL-cholesterol. The commonest defect is LDL-receptor gene mutation, which prevents LDL-receptors from taking in more LDL from the plasma into hepatocytes. Apo-B gene mutation results in ineffective binding of LDL to its receptor, while PCSK-9 gene mutation results in increased LDL-receptor degradation (it is a 'gain in function' mutation).

HOW SHOULD SHE BE EVALUATED FURTHER?

First-line investigations should include

- **Blood tests**, including haemoglobin, liver and renal function, fasting glucose, HbA_1c and lipid profile.
- A **12-lead ECG**.

The ECG may show evidence of old infarcts, like pathological Q waves or left bundle branch block. In Prinzmetal angina, transient ST segment elevation or depression may be seen during an attack of angina.

- An **echocardiogram** is useful to obtain information about cardiac function and anatomy.

A reduction in left ventricular ejection fraction (LVEF) or regional wall motion abnormalities may point to ischaemic myocardial damage. Echocardiography will also help to rule out other causes of chest pain, like valvular heart disease.

The opinion of a cardiologist should be sought to plan the next line of investigation. She can be referred to a geneticist for **genetic testing** and counselling.

WHAT SHOULD YOU TELL THE PATIENT?

You should tell her that

- Her chest pain is due to angina.

'I suspect you are getting chest pain because of reduced blood flow to the heart muscle. We call this angina. This occurs due to fat deposition on the inner lining of blood vessels that supply the heart muscle, making them narrow. When you exercise, your heart muscle works harder and therefore needs more oxygen, but the narrowed blood vessels are unable to meet this demand'.

- The tendon xanthomas are a sign of high cholesterol.

'The lumps on your elbows and heels suggest that your blood cholesterol level may be high. A high cholesterol level increases the risk of fat deposition in blood vessels'.

- Her hypercholesterolemia is inherited.

'I suspect your high cholesterol is caused by a faulty gene. You probably inherited this from your father'.

- You will arrange a few tests in the first instance.

'I'll arrange some blood tests, a tracing of the heart and a heart scan'.

- You will seek an opinion from a cardiologist.

'I'll ask a heart specialist to see you. He will discuss further tests that you may need and suggest treatments to improve the blood flow to the heart muscle'.

- You would suggest a statin (*'cholesterol-lowering tablet'*) if the tests confirm that her blood cholesterol is high.
- She should eat healthily (*'limit the intake of fats and sugars'*) and increase her physical activity.
- Her immediate family members should be screened for hypercholesterolemia.

'The specialist might suggest a test to check for the faulty gene. If you are found to have the gene, there is a 50% chance that your brother and daughters have got the gene and they too should be tested'.

- You will update her when the test results are back.

OUTCOME

Her results are as follows:

- Full blood count, liver and renal function normal.
- Fasting glucose 5.2 mmol/L and HbA$_1$c 36 mmol/mol.
- **Low-density lipoprotein 5.8 mmol/L** (target <2.7).
- Triglycerides 2.0 mmol/L (target <1.7).
- High-density lipoprotein 1.1 mmol/L (target >1.0).
- Her 12-lead ECG is normal.

Echocardiogram shows no evidence of valvular heart disease, chamber hypertrophy or wall motion abnormalities. Ejection fraction is 65%.

*The cardiologist discusses various options to investigate her chest pain. After a detailed discussion, she opts for invasive coronary angiogram, which shows **significant obstructive disease in the proximal left anterior descending and left circumflex arteries**. She undergoes stenting of these two vessels. She is commenced on a statin, dual anti-platelet therapy and anti-anginal drugs, and given advice on healthy lifestyle measures. She is referred to a geneticist for genetic testing and counselling.*

Management of angina should focus on healthy lifestyle measures, such as cessation of smoking, consuming a healthy diet (high in vegetables, fruits and whole grains, with limited intake of saturated fat, and avoidance of processed foods and sugar-sweetened drinks) and increasing physical activity (at least 30–60 minutes of moderate activity on most days).

Pharmacological management should start with a calcium channel blocker or β-blocker. A long-acting nitrate (e.g. isosorbide mononitrate) should be considered if calcium channel blocker or β-blocker is contraindicated, poorly tolerated or insufficient to control the symptoms. Other options include ivabradine, nicorandil and ranolazine. Anti-platelet therapy should be used for patients with previous myocardial infarction or revascularisation.

Statins are the first-line drugs for FH. If statins fail to reduce the LDL-cholesterol by >50%, other options include ezetimibe (reduces gut absorption of lipids), PCSK-9 inhibitors (prevents LDL-receptor degradation, thus allowing more LDL to get into hepatocytes), bile acid sequestrants (reduce enterohepatic recirculation of bile, which causes more hepatic cholesterol to be converted to bile acids) and niacin. The availability of PCSK-9 inhibitors has greatly reduced the need for LDL apheresis.

The 46-Year-Old Man with Palpitations

Case 43

You are asked to see a 46-year-old man in the medical admissions unit. He had presented earlier that morning with palpitations and his 12-lead ECG at the time showed fast atrial fibrillation with ventricular rate of 140/minute. His symptoms have now resolved, and his ECG shows normal sinus rhythm.

His oxygen saturation is 98% on room air, pulse 76/minute and regular, BP 134/80 mm Hg, respiratory rate 16/minute and temperature 36°C.

HOW SHOULD THIS PROBLEM BE APPROACHED?

Palpitations may be caused by (a) sinus tachycardia, secondary to increased adrenergic activity (e.g. anxiety, panic disorder, alcohol withdrawal, hypoglycaemia, hyperthyroidism, phaeochromocytoma, β-agonist therapy), (b) arrhythmia (e.g. atrial fibrillation [AF], atrial flutter, supraventricular tachycardia, ventricular tachycardia, ectopic beats) *or* (c) volume overload (e.g. aortic regurgitation, dilated cardiomyopathy).

In this patient, palpitations were clearly caused by AF, based on the 12-lead ECG taken at the time. His AF is paroxysmal, as he is back in sinus rhythm now (*see Box 43.1*).

BOX 43.1 CLASSIFICATION OF ATRIAL FIBRILLATION (AF)

- Paroxysmal AF (lasts <7 days).
- Persistent AF (lasts >7 days).
- Long-standing persistent AF (lasts >1 year).
- Permanent AF (if the decision is made to not restore sinus rhythm).

- First, find out **what happened that morning**.

When did the palpitations begin? What was he doing at the time? Were there any associated symptoms, like chest pain, breathlessness or light headedness? How long did the episode last?

Note: In patients in whom the cause of the palpitation is not known, you should ask if the onset was sudden or gradual, and if the palpitations were regular or irregular (ask the patient to tap on the desk and show you).

- Ask if he has had **similar episodes in the past**.

DOI: 10.1201/9781003430230-43

*He says he **suddenly felt his heart racing**, soon after his breakfast. His **heartbeat was fast and irregular**. Soon afterwards, he **felt light headed** and wanted to lie down. He did not develop chest pain or feel breathless. As the palpitations did not subside, his wife drove him to the emergency department. The palpitations **stopped on its own**, without any treatment, a few minutes after the heart tracing was taken in the emergency department. The **whole episode lasted about an hour and a half**.*

*He has had **two similar episodes recently**. The first episode occurred two months ago and lasted ten minutes. The second one occurred a couple of weeks ago and lasted about 15 minutes. On both occasions, the palpitations started suddenly and subsided spontaneously, and he felt light headed. He is unable to recall any specific triggers and not sure what he was doing at the time. He did not seek medical advice, as the episodes were short-lived.*

The two previous episodes were also most likely due to paroxysmal AF, so essentially, he has had three separate episodes of symptomatic AF over a short span of time.

The next step is to determine if there is an underlying cause for his AF, particularly structural heart disease *or* reversible factors, like sepsis, hypoxia, electrolyte derangement or thyroid disease (*see Box 43.2*). If an underlying cause is not found, it should be labelled as 'lone AF'. In patients with paroxysmal AF, it is useful to check what triggered the AF. 'Adrenergic AF' is triggered by physical exertion or emotional stress, while 'vagal AF' occurs at rest or after a heavy meal. This distinction helps to choose the right drug (e.g. β-blockers are useful for adrenergic AF).

BOX 43.2   SOME UNDERLYING CAUSES OF ATRIAL FIBRILLATION

- Ischemic heart disease.
- Hypertensive heart disease.
- Structural heart diseases characterised by atrial enlargement (e.g. mitral valve disease, atrial septal defect, cardiomyopathy).
- Thyrotoxicosis.
- Hypoxia (e.g. pneumonia, pulmonary embolism, obstructive sleep apnoea).
- Electrolyte imbalance (e.g. hypokalaemia, hypomagnesemia).
- Toxins (e.g. alcohol, tricyclic anti-depressants, sympathomimetics).
- Sepsis.

Patients with AF are at risk of developing thromboembolic stroke, which can be predicted using the CHA_2DS_2-VASc score (*see Box 43.3*). It is important to note that patients with paroxysmal AF have the same risk of developing stroke as those with persistent AF.

BOX 43.3 CHA_2DS_2-VASc SCORE

C	Congestive cardiac failure	1
H	Hypertension (blood pressure consistently above 140/90 or treated hypertension on medication)	1
A_2	Age >75	2
D	Diabetes mellitus	1
S_2	Previous or current cardioembolic stroke/TIA	2
V	Vascular disease (coronary artery disease, myocardial infarction, peripheral vascular disease or aortic plaque)	1
A	Age 65–74	1
Sc	Sex category, female gender	1

The next set of questions should explore (a) the components of CHA_2DS_2-VASc score and (b) features that may suggest an underlying cause. You should ask about

- **Recent illnesses** (e.g. pneumonia, sepsis, pulmonary embolism, electrolyte disturbance).

Although this question is less relevant in patients with recurrent episodes of paroxysmal AF, it is important to ensure that reversible factors are not missed.

- **Symptoms of thyroid disease** (e.g. loss of weight, diarrhoea, tremors, heat intolerance).
- **Snoring at night** (obstructive sleep apnoea is an important reversible factor).
- **Symptoms of cardiac failure** (e.g. breathlessness on exertion, paroxysmal nocturnal dyspnoea or orthopnoea, reduced urine output, ankle swelling).
- His **past medical history**, particularly hypertension, diabetes, and history of stroke or transient ischaemic attack, ischaemic heart disease and peripheral arterial disease.
- His **regular medications**, **smoking habit** and **alcohol consumption**.
- **Family history** of sudden death (especially in patients with palpitations in whom the diagnosis of the rhythm disturbance has not been made yet).

*He denies recent illnesses. There are no symptoms of thyroid disease or cardiac failure, and he does not snore at night. His medical history is unremarkable. He is not a known hypertensive or diabetic. He last had his blood sugar checked less than six months ago. He has never had a heart attack or stroke. His legs do not hurt when he walks. He **smokes 10 cigarettes/day** and drinks alcohol only socially. The relevant family history is unremarkable. He is a policeman and lives with his wife.*

 The history has not revealed any features to suggest underlying heart disease or reversible factors. His AF is 'vagal', as it occurred at rest, after a meal. His CHA_2DS_2-VASc score is zero, which means his risk of thromboembolic stroke is very low (the annual risk of stroke progressively increases from 1.3% for CHA_2DS_2-VASc score of 1 point to 15.2% for a score of 9 points). Hence, there is no need to consider anticoagulant treatment unless there is evidence of valvular heart disease (*see later*).

WHAT SHOULD YOU LOOK FOR ON EXAMINATION?

You should

- Check his **pulse rate and rhythm** (to confirm that he is in sinus rhythm).
- Check for **signs of cardiac failure** (elevated jugular venous pressure, ankle oedema and lung crackles).
- Listen to the heart for **murmurs**.
- Check for **signs of hyperthyroidism**.

He appears comfortable at rest. His pulse is 72/minute and regular. His JVP is not elevated and there is no ankle oedema. His lungs are clear and there are no murmurs. He is clinically euthyroid.

HOW SHOULD HE BE EVALUATED FURTHER?

You should request

- **Blood tests**, including full blood count, liver and renal function, thyroid function, serum potassium and magnesium, and troponin.
- **Chest X-ray**.
- **2D echocardiogram** (to look for structural heart disease and assess cardiac function).

WHAT SHOULD YOU TELL THE PATIENT?

You should tell him that

- His palpitations were caused by AF.

'You felt unwell this morning because your heartbeat became fast and irregular for a short-while. We do not know why your heartbeat suddenly became irregular'.

- The two previous episodes were also most likely due to AF.

'From your description, it appears that the two previous episodes were also due to the heartbeat becoming irregular for a short while'.

- This can happen again (very important to warn him.)
- You would arrange further investigations.

'I'll arrange some blood tests, an X-ray of your chest and a heart scan to see if there is an underlying problem that keeps causing your heartbeat to become irregular'.

- You would refer him to a cardiologist (*'heart specialist'*).
- The cardiologist might suggest medications to prevent or treat the paroxysmal arrhythmia.

'The heart specialist might suggest a medication to treat this. It may be a pill that you take every day to prevent further episodes of irregular heartbeat or one that you take only when feel your heart racing so that the episode can be aborted quickly'.

- He should stop smoking.
- You would get in touch with him when the test results are back.

OUTCOME

His blood tests and chest X-ray are normal. His 2D echocardiogram shows no evidence of structural heart disease or regional wall motion abnormalities. His ejection fraction is normal. The cardiologist, after discussing the treatment options, prescribes flecainide to take only when he gets palpitations.

The tests have not revealed any evidence of structural heart disease or reversible factors. There is no evidence of impaired cardiac function either. Hence, flecainide would be a good choice for him (flecainide should not be used in patients with structural heart disease or impaired cardiac function, as it is negatively inotropic). Flecainide can be taken during an attack (*pill in the pocket* approach), or every day, depending on the frequency of episodes and patient choice. Ablation therapy is an alternative, especially for patients who do not respond to pharmacological therapy. The principle of ablation therapy is to burn the area between the pulmonary veins and left atrium using radiofrequency waves, as the triggers for AF usually come from pulmonary veins.

Anticoagulant treatment should be commenced early, ideally within 30 days from the event, in patients in whom it is indicated. In addition to stroke, patients with AF are at risk of dementia (due to multiple small emboli going to the brain). The decision to commence anticoagulant treatment should be based on the CHA_2DS_2-VASc score or presence of valvular heart disease.

- All patients with underlying valvular heart disease should be commenced on an anticoagulant, irrespective of the CHA_2DS_2-VASc score. Warfarin is preferred.
- If the CHA_2DS_2-VASc score is 0 in men or 1 in women, there is no need for anticoagulant treatment.
- If the CHA_2DS_2-VASc score is ≥2 in men or ≥3 in women, anticoagulant treatment is recommended. A novel oral anticoagulant (e.g. apixaban, rivaroxaban, dabigatran) is preferred to warfarin.
- If the CHA_2DS_2-VASc score is 1 in men or 2 in women, the decision to commence anticoagulant treatment is taken on a case-by-case basis.

Anticoagulant treatment is recommended for patients ≥65 years of age, as it is a stronger risk factor for thromboembolism than the other factors conferring one point. For younger patients with only one non-sex risk factor, the decision depends on AF burden, risk of bleeding and patient choice.

- Aspirin is not recommended for patients with low CHA_2DS_2-VASc score unless there is evidence of underlying coronary artery disease.

The 56-Year-Old Woman with Syncope

Case 44

A 56-year-old woman is brought to the medical admissions unit after an episode of blackout that morning.

Her oxygen saturation is 98% on room air, pulse rate 80/minute, BP 112/78 mm Hg, respiratory rate 16/minute and temperature 36.3°C.

HOW SHOULD THIS PROBLEM BE APPROACHED?

The history is the most important tool to make a diagnosis in patients who present with transient loss of consciousness. Ideally, the history should be obtained from an eyewitness if one is available.

The first step is to decide if the loss of consciousness was due to syncope (reduced blood flow to the brain) or seizures (excess electrical discharge by cerebral neurones).

- Ask what happened *before the event*.

What exactly was she doing at the time? Did she experience any chest pain, breathlessness, palpitations, giddiness or aura?

- What happened *during the event*?

Was there actual loss of consciousness? For how long was she unconscious? Was there any limb shaking? Did she bite her tongue or become incontinent?

- Did she sustain *any injuries* because of the fall?
- What happened *after the event*?

Was she able to get up and walk immediately after the event *or* was there a prolonged period of drowsiness, confusion or lethargy?

*She and her husband went to the shopping mall that morning and they had been walking around for over two hours before she **fainted**. She did not experience any chest pain, breathlessness, palpitations, giddiness, nausea or sweating before she fainted.*

*She learnt from her husband later that it **happened suddenly**, and she was **unconscious for a minute or two**. There was no jerking of her limbs, and she did not wet herself. Her tongue was not sore when she regained her consciousness. She felt **exhausted after the episode** but was able to get up and start walking*

DOI: 10.1201/9781003430230-44

a few minutes later. She does not recall being drowsy or confused. She did not sustain any injuries, as her husband was able to support her when she was about to hit the floor. She feels well now.

 His description suggests syncope (*see Box 44.1*), as she rapidly regained consciousness and started walking within a few minutes.

BOX 44.1   FEATURES THAT HELP TO DIFFERENTIATE SEIZURES FROM SYNCOPE

	SEIZURES	*SYNCOPE*
What triggered the event?	Usually sleep deprivation, flashing lights, alcohol intoxication or withdrawal.	Crowded room, warm environment, unpleasant sight or smell, sudden emotional stress [vasovagal syncope]. Assuming the erect posture [postural syncope].
How did the patient feel before the event?	There may be an aura (e.g. odd smell, strange sensation in the stomach).	Nauseous, warm and sweaty (vasovagal syncope). Chest pain, breathlessness, palpitations and dizziness, but often no preceding symptoms (cardiac syncope).
How was the patient during the event?	Rigid, jerking movements, cyanosis, incontinence, tongue biting (*Tongue biting is specific for seizures*)	Pale, cold, sweaty and floppy (convulsive movements and incontinence do not help to differentiate syncope from seizures).
How was the patient after the event?	Slow recovery, with prolonged period of confusion.	Usually rapid recovery within a minute (the *most useful feature to differentiate syncope from seizures*), but there may be prolonged fatigue or nausea after vasovagal syncope.

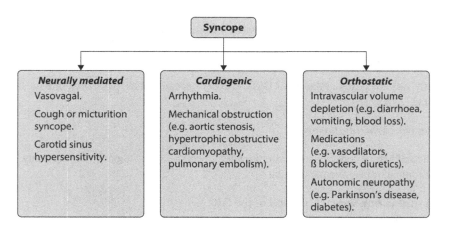

FIGURE 44.1   Mechanisms of syncope.[1]

[1] An underlying cause may not be found in about 30% of patients presenting with syncope.

Having established that her blackout was most likely due to syncope, the next step is to try and find out why it happened (*see Figure 44.1*). Among the three major groups of causes, postural syncope is least likely, as it did not happen when she rose from a supine position. The main differentials are therefore vasovagal and cardiogenic syncope. The former (a) builds up gradually, (b) usually occurs in a crowded or warm environment and is (c) preceded by nausea, light headedness and sweating. Because her syncope was so sudden and occurred without warning, following a period of exertion, cardiogenic syncope should be considered (*see Box 44.2*).

BOX 44.2   SOME HELPFUL POINTERS TO CARDIAC SYNCOPE

- Exertional syncope.†
- Syncope that occurs without warning (*malignant syncope*).
- Syncope in a supine position.
- Cardiac symptoms like chest pain or dyspnoea, murmur or clinical signs of heart failure.
- Family history of sudden cardiac death.

† Systemic vasodilatation occurs during exertion, calling for increased cardiac output to fill the blood vessels. Cerebral hypoperfusion occurs if the cardiac output cannot meet this demand.

Cardiogenic syncope essentially means that the heart is unable to generate enough cardiac output to perfuse the brain. It can be caused by (a) ventricular outflow tract obstruction *or* (b) an arrhythmia (either tachy or bradyarrhythmia). There is inadequate time between two beats to fill the ventricles in tachyarrhythmia, and the heart rate is too slow in bradyarrhythmia.

Further questions to ask:

- Ask if she has *fainted before*.
- Ask about *recent illnesses*, *diarrhoea* or *vomiting*.
- Ask about other *cardiac symptoms*, such as chest pain, breathlessness and palpitations.
- Ask about *features that may suggest pulmonary embolism* (e.g. history of thrombosis, swelling of the calf, recent immobilisation).
- Ask about her *medications* (e.g. drugs that cause bradycardia, hypotension, prolonged QT interval or hypoglycaemia), *alcohol* intake and use of *recreational drugs*.
- Obtain a *family history*. Ask if she is aware of anyone in her immediate family with seizure disorder or history of sudden cardiac death.
- Ask about her *occupation*.
- Ask if she *drives*.

*She **nearly fainted about a month ago** but did not lose consciousness on that occasion. It happened on a particularly busy day, when she was running around, hosting some guests at home.*

*She denies recent illnesses, diarrhoea, vomiting, chest pain, breathlessness, palpitations or leg swelling. Her past medical history is unremarkable. She does not take any medication. She has never smoked or used recreational drugs and seldom drinks alcohol. Her family history is unremarkable. She is not working at present. She **drives her grandchild to school every day**.*

WHAT SHOULD YOU LOOK FOR ON EXAMINATION?

- Check for *external injuries*.
- Look for *pallor*.
- Examine her *cardiovascular system*.

Check for irregular pulse, signs of left ventricular outflow obstruction (e.g. murmur of aortic stenosis, carotid bruit) and signs of heart failure.

- (In patients with suspected postural syncope), ask for *lying and standing blood pressures*.

A significant postural drop is a [a] fall in systolic BP of at least 20 mm Hg *or* [b] a fall in diastolic BP of at least 10 mm Hg *or* [c] a fall in systolic blood pressure to <90 mm Hg, after standing for ~3 minutes.

*There are no external injuries. She is not pale. Her **carotid pulse is slow rising**. Rhythm is regular. Jugular venous pressure is not elevated. Her apex is in the left 5th intercostal space, one cm medial to the mid-clavicular line. It is **heaving**. There is an **ejection systolic murmur over the precordium**, best heard over the aortic area and **radiating to the carotid**. The **second heart sound is soft**. The lungs are clear and there is no pedal oedema.*

The clinical signs are in keeping with aortic stenosis. Although aortic stenosis can cause syncope, it is possible that she had a paroxysmal arrhythmia. Continuous rhythm monitoring (either telemetry *or* outpatient Holter monitoring) should therefore be considered.

The stenosis is likely to be at the valvular level, as the second heart sound is soft. Common causes of aortic stenosis are (a) senile calcific aortic stenosis, (b) congenital bicuspid aortic valve and (c) rheumatic fever. Of these, rheumatic heart disease is least likely, as it usually also affects the mitral valve and seldom the aortic valve in isolation. She should however be asked if she recalls being diagnosed with rheumatic fever during her childhood. You should ask about joint pain, heart problem or abnormal involuntary movements, and if she received penicillin injections for prophylaxis.

The classic triad of symptoms of aortic stenosis includes exertional angina (due to increased oxygen demand by the hypertrophied myocardium), breathlessness and syncope. However, patients with aortic stenosis may be well and asymptomatic for several years, prior to onset of symptoms. Mortality dramatically rises after the onset of symptoms, so patients who are symptomatic should be referred for aortic valve replacement early.

She did not suffer with joint or heart problem during her childhood and did not receive antibiotic injections.

HOW SHOULD SHE BE EVALUATED?

You should request

- ***Blood tests***, including full blood count (to check for anaemia) and glucose.
- A ***12-lead ECG***, ***chest X-ray*** and ***2D echocardiogram***.

The echocardiogram is useful to study the valve anatomy and orifice size, presence of calcification and estimate the pressure gradient across the aortic valve.

Note: Patients with severe aortic stenosis (mean pressure gradient of over 40 mm Hg) should be referred for aortic valve replacement even in the absence of symptoms.

- ***Telemetry*** or ***Holter monitoring*** for prolonged rhythm monitoring.

WHAT SHOULD YOU TELL THE PATIENT?

You should tell her that

- Her syncope was most likely caused by aortic stenosis.

'We have four chambers in the heart. Blood moves from one chamber to another through openings called valves. I suspect you passed out this morning because one of the valves on the left side of your heart is narrow. It is called aortic valve (draw a diagram to illustrate). *Blood that is pumped by the heart normally flows through this valve into a big blood vessel called aorta and then to the rest of the body. Narrowing of this valve can make you pass out because of a sudden drop in blood flow to the brain'.*

- The underlying cause of her aortic stenosis is either congenital bicuspid aortic valve or senile calcific aortic stenosis.

'It is possible that you were born with a narrow aortic valve. Although the narrowing is present from birth, symptoms may not develop until later in life. Another possible cause of narrowing is deposition of calcium on the aortic valve. This usually happens as we get older'.

- An additional possible reason for the syncope is a transient arrhythmia.

'Although the narrowing of aortic valve would explain the fainting, I would like to make sure that there isn't another cause, like a brief episode of irregular heartbeat. We will monitor your heartbeat to see if this happens again'.

- You would ask for *'some blood tests, an X-ray of the chest, tracing of the heart and a heart scan'*.
- You would refer her to a *'heart specialist'*.
- Her syncope may recur, so she should not drive until the evaluation is complete.
- The heart specialist will discuss the treatment plan once she has had the tests.

'If the tests confirm that your aortic valve is narrow, the heart specialist might suggest a procedure to replace this valve. This can be done by passing a thin long tube with the replacement valve through the groin into the big blood vessels, which can then be guided into the heart. He will explain this further'.

OUTCOME

Her 12-lead ECG shows **left ventricular hypertrophy.** *Chest X-ray is normal. Echocardiogram confirms* **aortic stenosis due to bicuspid aortic valve, with pressure gradient of 50 mm Hg.** *Holter monitoring does not pick any arrhythmia. Coronary angiogram is performed to exclude significant coronary artery disease. She is referred for transcatheter aortic valve replacement.*

The 28-Year-Old Woman with Shortness of Breath

Case 45

A 28-year-old Indian woman presents with a six-month history of shortness of breath on exertion.

HOW SHOULD THIS PROBLEM BE APPROACHED?

---

*She tells you that she gets **out of breath when she exerts**. Although she has never really been an active person, her exercise tolerance was previously unlimited. When this problem first began about six months ago, she was getting out of breath only when she walked uphill or climbed one flight of stairs. Her **breathing problem has slowly worsened** during these six months to the extent that she must now stop after less than ten minutes even while walking on level ground at her own pace.*

 She has presented with gradually worsening, chronic shortness of breath on exertion. In patients with chronic shortness of breath, the first step is to ascertain if it is due to cardiac, respiratory or another cause (*see Box 45.1*). This can be done based on (a) associated symptoms and (b) her background medical problems and risk factors (*see below*).

BOX 45.1   CAUSES OF CHRONIC SHORTNESS OF BREATH

- *Cardiac failure*.
- *Respiratory causes* (e.g. chronic obstructive pulmonary disease, interstitial lung disease, chronic pulmonary thromboembolism, pleural effusion, neuromuscular disease affecting the respiratory muscles, thoracic cage problem).
- *Other causes* (e.g. anaemia, chronic kidney disease, thyroid disease, gross obesity, anxiety).

Underlying causes to consider in this young woman are anaemia, cardiac failure, interstitial lung disease, chronic pulmonary thromboembolism and chronic kidney disease. Among the other causes, chronic obstructive pulmonary disease is unlikely in someone of her age (unless caused by the rare α-1 antitrypsin deficiency), as the lung damage that is severe enough to cause breathlessness occurs after several decades of smoking. Neuromuscular and thoracic cage problem often present with other manifestations related to the primary disease rather than with breathlessness alone.

DOI: 10.1201/9781003430230-45

Obtain a further history and check for associated symptoms.

- Ask about *symptoms that may suggest cardiac disease*, like paroxysmal nocturnal dyspnoea, orthopnoea, leg swelling, chest pain, palpitations (*'Do you become aware of your heartbeat from time to time?'*), and exertional fatigue and syncope (*'Have you ever blacked out?'*).
- Ask about *respiratory symptoms*, like cough, expectoration, wheezing (*'noisy breathing'*) and haemoptysis.

Cough, haemoptysis and wheezing are not specific for respiratory disease.

- Ask if her *menses* has been heavy (the commonest cause of anaemia in someone of her age).

*In the last three months, she has **woken in the middle of the night on several occasions**, **gasping for breath**. When this happens, she would get off her bed and open the windows to get some fresh air. Her breathing would then gradually return to normal after about 15–20 minutes. On several nights, she has woken more than once. For the last two weeks, she has been feeling **breathless soon after lying in bed**, which has forced her to sleep propped up on her recliner chair.*

*She denies chest pain, palpitations, blackouts, swelling of her legs, cough, expectoration, wheezing and haemoptysis. She **gets tired very easily after any form of exertion** and has been struggling with her household chores as a result. Her periods are not heavy.*

She describes paroxysmal nocturnal dyspnoea (PND), a symptom that highly suggests left heart failure. In patients with mitral stenosis, PND can occur in the absence of left ventricular dysfunction. PND occurs when increased venous return to the right side of the heart in the supine position is not matched by a corresponding increase in left ventricular output. This leads to increased left atrial pressure, pulmonary venous congestion, interstitial or alveolar oedema and reduced lung compliance. Orthopnoea occurs when the left atrial pressure rises further due to progression of the underlying disease. Orthopnoea is not specific for cardiac disease, as it can also occur in patients with asthma, diaphragmatic weakness, pregnancy or gross ascites. Exercise-induced fatigue is a non-specific symptom, but in the context of cardiac disease, it denotes fixed cardiac output (failure of the heart to appropriately increase its output during exercise).

The absence of cough makes it less likely that her breathlessness is due to chronic lung disease. Pulmonary thromboembolism can be excluded because it would not cause PND or orthopnoea (as the right ventricular output is reduced, and lungs do not get congested). Chronic kidney disease causes breathlessness due to anaemia or fluid overload, and the latter usually presents acutely.

The next step is to try and determine the underlying cause of her left heart failure. Common causes include (a) ischaemic heart disease, (b) hypertension, (c) aortic or mitral valve disease and (d) cardiomyopathy. Of these, ischaemic heart disease and hypertension are less likely in someone of her age. The absence of chest pain and syncope would make aortic stenosis less likely, although not impossible. Aortic stenosis is usually clinically silent for several years or decades because of left ventricular hypertrophy and compensation, but progression is very rapid once symptoms begin. Mitral stenosis, on the other hand, has a short latency phase, as the left atrial pressure rises early, and this is quickly transmitted to the pulmonary veins. Breathlessness occurs on exertion because the duration of diastole gets shortened with increased heart rate, and this results in further reduction in left ventricular inflow and increase in left atrial pressure.

Further questions to ask:

- Ask if she recalls being diagnosed with *rheumatic fever* during childhood.

Note: Rheumatic fever is by far the most common cause of mitral stenosis, but many patients may not be able to recall this. You should ask about joint pain, heart problems or abnormal involuntary movements, and if she received penicillin injections for prophylaxis.

- Complete the **rest of the history**.

Ask about her other medical problems, medications taken, family history, obstetric history or pregnancy plans, and her occupation.

*She **migrated to the UK from India a couple of years ago** after marrying a UK-based banker. She is trained as an accountant but hasn't worked since moving to the UK. She **recalls missing school on several occasions because of joint problems**, when she was around eight to ten years old. She **received penicillin injections every month** but could not continue this for more than a couple of years, as her father, who worked for Indian railways, was regularly getting transferred to different cities.*

*Her medical history is otherwise unremarkable, and she does not take any medication. She has never smoked and always been teetotal. Her family history is unremarkable too. She has never been pregnant, but **she and her husband are keen to try for a baby now**.*

The history of joint problems during her childhood and monthly penicillin injections suggests that her current symptoms are possibly due to rheumatic valvular heart disease. She should be strongly advised to hold her pregnancy plans, pending further evaluation and advice from a cardiologist.

WHAT SHOULD YOU LOOK FOR ON EXAMINATION?

You should

- Ask for her **vital signs**.
- Look for **pallor**.
- Check for **signs of cardiac failure** (e.g. elevated jugular venous pressure, ankle oedema and lung crackles).
- Examine her **heart**.

She is moderately built and comfortable at rest. There is no pallor. Her pulse rate is 84/min and regular in rhythm, respiratory rate 16/minute and BP in her right arm (upright) is 110/70 mm Hg. Her jugular venous pressure is not elevated.

*Her apex is in the left fifth intercostal space, 1 cm medial to the mid-clavicular line, and **tapping in character**. There is no parasternal heave or thrill, and the pulmonary component of the second heart sound (P_2) is not palpable. On auscultation, the **first heart sound is** loud. A **mid-diastolic murmur with pre-systolic accentuation is heard at the apex**. There is no systolic murmur. There are no murmurs over the rest of the precordium and P_2 is normal in intensity. Her lungs are clear.*

The clinical signs are in keeping with mitral stenosis. There are no features of atrial fibrillation or pulmonary hypertension, which are known complications of long-standing mitral stenosis.

The first heart sound becomes loud because of the longer distance that the valve leaflets have to travel (increased left atrial pressure forces the leaflets far apart, so they have to travel a longer distance at the onset of ventricular systole). The tapping apex is due to the loud first heart sound, and pre-systolic accentuation denotes strong atrial contraction (this is lost when atrial fibrillation develops).

HOW SHOULD SHE BE EVALUATED?

You should ask for

- **Blood tests**, including haemoglobin, renal function and thyroid function.

In addition, brain natriuretic peptide (BNP) level is useful in patients with breathlessness in whom the diagnosis of cardiac failure is not certain. If BNP and 12-lead ECG are normal, it would make it extremely unlikely that the breathlessness is due to cardiac failure.

- **Chest X-ray**.

A chest X-ray may reveal (a) enlargement of left atrium (seen as a double contour on the right heart border, also known as 'shadow within shadow'), (b) straight heart border due to enlargement of left atrial appendage and pulmonary arteries, (c) signs of cardiac failure (alveolar oedema, Kerley B lines, cardiomegaly, upper lobe diversion and pleural effusion, easily remembered by the acronym ABCDE) and (d) mitral valve calcification.

- **12-lead ECG**.

ECG findings of mitral stenosis include (a) prolonged P waves due to left atrial enlargement (*P mitrale*), (b) right axis deviation and right ventricular hypertrophy due to pulmonary hypertension and (c) atrial fibrillation.

- **Echocardiogram**.

A 2D echocardiogram is useful to confirm the diagnosis of mitral stenosis. It can provide information on the size of the mitral valve orifice, trans-valvular gradient across the mitral valve, pulmonary artery systolic pressure and presence of mitral regurgitation or associated aortic valve disease. A trans-thoracic echocardiogram should be performed to rule out left atrial thrombus in all patients with atrial fibrillation, *or* prior to planning surgical or interventional treatment.

WHAT SHOULD YOU TELL THE PATIENT?

You should tell her that

- Her breathlessness is due to mitral valve disease.

'We have four chambers in the heart. Blood moves from one chamber to another through openings called valves. You are getting breathless because one of the valves on the left side of your heart is narrow. It is called mitral valve (draw a diagram to illustrate.) *Narrowing of this valve is restricting the flow of blood from the lungs to the left side of the heart. This is causing pressure to build up in the lungs and making you breathless. This is worse at night because more blood returns to the heart when you lie down, which further increases the pressure in the lungs'.*

- The mitral valve disease is due to rheumatic fever.

'I suspect this is related to the joint problem you had during your childhood. It is called rheumatic fever. It is a form of bacterial infection. The immune system, while trying to clear the bacteria, causes inflammation of the joints and heart. The inflammation of the heart leads to narrowing of the valve'.

- You will arrange some investigations.

'I will arrange some blood tests, a tracing of your heart, an X-ray of your chest and a heart scan'.

- She should sleep propped up and restrict her fluid and salt intake.
- You will give her *'a medication to remove the excess fluid'*, which should help to improve her breathing.
- You will refer her to a *'heart specialist'*.
- She should hold off her pregnancy plans, pending the advice of the cardiologist.
- The heart specialist will discuss the treatment plan once she has had the tests.

'If the tests confirm that your mitral valve is narrow, the specialist might suggest a procedure to widen the opening of the valve. This can be done by passing a thin long tube through the groin into the big blood vessels, which can then be guided into the heart. If he thinks this won't be possible, he might suggest an operation to replace this valve. He will explain this further'.

OUTCOME

Her chest X-ray shows **left atrial enlargement**. *The cardiothoracic ratio is normal and there is no evidence of pulmonary congestion. Her 12-lead ECG shows* **P mitrale**. *The 2D echocardiogram confirms the diagnosis of mitral stenosis. Her mitral valve area is 1.3 cm², transvalvular gradient is 9 mm Hg and pulmonary artery systolic pressure is 32 mm Hg, suggesting* **moderate mitral stenosis**. *There is no evidence of mitral regurgitation or other valvular lesions. Ejection fraction is 62%. Her blood tests show Hb 128 g/L and normal liver, renal and thyroid function.*

Medical management of mitral stenosis should include (a) diuretics for heart failure, (b) β-blockers or calcium channel blockers to slow the heart rate and improve diastolic filling of the left ventricle and (c) anticoagulation with warfarin for those with atrial fibrillation, evidence of left atrial thrombus or history of previous stroke (*not* direct oral anticoagulants, which should only be used in those with non-valvular AF). Precipitants of cardiac failure, such as anaemia, thyrotoxicosis, fever, infection, non-steroidal anti-inflammatory drugs and fast atrial fibrillation, should be managed appropriately. Prophylaxis against infective endocarditis prior to invasive procedures is not necessary for those with mitral stenosis and only indicated in those with prosthetic mitral valve.

Patients with moderate to severe mitral stenosis and those who continue to progress despite medical therapy should be considered for interventional or surgical treatment. Percutaneous balloon mitral commissurotomy (PBMC) is the treatment of choice in those with favourable mitral valve morphology. Patients with associated mitral regurgitation, left atrial thrombus or heavy mitral valve calcification are not candidates for PBMC and should be offered mitral valve replacement instead, either with tissue or prosthetic valve. She should be able to try for a baby if PBMC is successful.

The 62-Year-Old Woman with Shortness of Breath

Case 46

A 62-year-old woman with rheumatoid arthritis presents with a six-month history of gradually worsening shortness of breath on exertion.

Her oxygen saturation is 97% on room air, pulse rate 80/minute and regular in rhythm, respiratory rate 16/minute and blood pressure 126/84 mm Hg.

Her recent chest X-ray and blood tests, including full blood count, thyroid panel, liver function tests and serum creatinine, are normal.

HOW SHOULD THIS PROBLEM BE APPROACHED?

*She tells you that she gets **short of breath when she walks**. She is not sure when exactly this problem began, but the distance that she can walk before getting out of breath has gradually shortened over the last several months. She is now unable to walk for more than 10 minutes even at her own pace.*

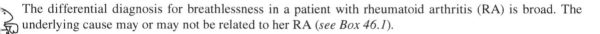 The differential diagnosis for breathlessness in a patient with rheumatoid arthritis (RA) is broad. The underlying cause may or may not be related to her RA (*see Box 46.1*).

**BOX 46.1   CAUSES OF BREATHLESSNESS IN A
PATIENT WITH RHEUMATOID ARTHRITIS**

- Interstitial lung disease related to rheumatoid arthritis.
- Drug-induced pneumonitis (e.g. methotrexate).
- Opportunistic infection due to immunosuppressive therapy (e.g. tuberculosis, pneumocystis jiroveci pneumonia).
- Pleural effusion.
- Bronchiectasis or bronchiolitis obliterans with organising pneumonia.
- Lung cancer.
- Pulmonary hypertension.
- Congestive cardiac failure (secondary to hypertension or ischemic heart disease).
- Anaemia of chronic disease.

DOI: 10.1201/9781003430230-46

The first step is to ascertain if her shortness of breath is due to cardiac, respiratory or another cause.

- Ask about **exacerbating and relieving factors** (e.g. orthopnoea in left heart failure, seasonal variation in chronic obstructive pulmonary disease).
- Check for **associated symptoms**, like chest pain, palpitations, exertional fatigue, syncope, ankle swelling, cough, expectoration, wheezing, haemoptysis and constitutional symptoms like fever and loss of weight.
- Ask about her **background medical problems**.

Ask particularly if she has been diagnosed with heart, lung or kidney disease.

- Ask if she **smokes**.

Smoking increases the risk of both heart and lung disease (e.g. ischaemic heart disease, chronic obstructive pulmonary disease, lung cancer).

*Her shortness of breath is mainly brought on by any form of physical exertion like walking or heavy household chores. She has never woken up at night with breathlessness. She is comfortable lying flat in bed and sleeps with one pillow. There is no seasonal variation in her breathing. She has been **troubled with an irritating cough** for several months. She has never coughed up phlegm or blood. She denies chest pain, palpitations, blackouts, ankle swelling, wheezing, fever and weight loss. Her weight has always been steady around 56 kg. She has never knowingly been in contact with anyone with tuberculosis.*

*She was diagnosed with **high blood pressure** about ten years ago, for which she takes amlodipine. Her blood pressure has been well controlled on amlodipine. She has not been diagnosed with heart, lung or kidney problem. She tried a few cigarettes when she was 18 but never took up the habit.*

 The dry cough, although non-specific, points to a respiratory cause for her breathlessness. Her breathlessness is most likely due to interstitial lung disease (diffuse parenchymal lung disease), related to her RA.

Chronic obstructive pulmonary disease can be excluded based on the negative smoking history, absence of expectoration and lack of seasonal variation. Tuberculosis is unlikely because of the absence of constitutional symptoms and negative contact history. The normal chest X-ray excludes pleural effusion and reduces the likelihood of lung cancer. Hypertension can lead to congestive cardiac failure, but the absence of paroxysmal nocturnal dyspnoea, orthopnoea and ankle oedema combined with the normal chest X-ray would make this less likely. Anaemia, thyroid and renal disease can be excluded because the relevant blood tests are normal. She is not obese. Unlike ankylosing spondylitis, RA does not involve the thoracic cage. There is no weakness, dysphagia or dysarthria to suggest a neuromuscular problem. If she had been anxious, she would have sought medical advice much earlier. Moreover, none of these conditions is associated with a chronic dry cough.

Further questions to ask:

- Ask **about her rheumatoid arthritis**, and how well this is controlled.
- Complete the **rest of the history**, particularly focussing on underlying causes of diffuse parenchymal lung disease (*see Box 46.2*).

Ask about her regular medications, current and previous jobs (to gather evidence of exposure to organic or inorganic dust), pets at home and date of her last mammogram (lymphangitis carcinomatosa due to breast cancer can present with breathlessness).

- Ask **how the breathlessness is affecting her life**.

*She was **diagnosed with rheumatoid arthritis** five years ago. She has been on **methotrexate** from the time of diagnosis, and it has been immensely helpful. She sees her rheumatologist every six months but*

BOX 46.2   UNDERLYING CAUSES OF DIFFUSE PARENCHYMAL LUNG DISEASE

- Autoimmune disease (e.g. rheumatoid arthritis, systemic sclerosis, systemic lupus erythematosus, anti-Jo-1 antibody syndrome, sarcoidosis).
- Drugs (e.g. methotrexate, amiodarone).
- Occupational or environmental exposure to inorganic or organic dust (e.g. asbestosis, coal workers' pneumoconiosis, silicosis, farmer's lung, extrinsic allergic alveolitis).
- Radiotherapy.
- Cancer (e.g. lymphangitis carcinomatosa).

*did not mention about the shortness of breath or cough when she last saw her four months ago, as it was not too bad at the time. She gets a **discomfort in her knees**, which her rheumatologist put down to osteoarthritis. She has otherwise been well. Apart from methotrexate, she takes one folic acid tablet on the day after methotrexate and paracetamol for pain in her knees.*

*She worked as a secretary for a legal firm for more than 30 years before retiring 4 years ago. She has not done any other jobs. She had a mammogram less than a year ago and it was normal. She has never been diagnosed with cancer. She does not keep any pets. She drinks a glass of wine only when she goes out to eat. She went through her menopause in her late 40s. The shortness of breath is increasingly making it **difficult for her to perform household chores or walk long distances**.*

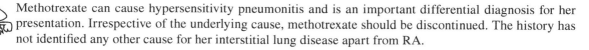

Methotrexate can cause hypersensitivity pneumonitis and is an important differential diagnosis for her presentation. Irrespective of the underlying cause, methotrexate should be discontinued. The history has not identified any other cause for her interstitial lung disease apart from RA.

WHAT SHOULD YOU LOOK FOR ON EXAMINATION?

You should

- Perform a *focussed general examination*.
- Examine the *respiratory and cardiovascular systems*.
- Briefly *examine her joints* to check for active synovitis (keep this brief, as the focus of this consultation is her breathlessness).

*She is comfortable at rest. There is no pallor, cyanosis, ankle oedema or finger clubbing. Jugular venous pressure is not elevated, and cardiac apex is not displaced. Heart sounds are normal. There are **fine end-inspiratory crackles in both lung bases**, which are not altered by coughing. There is bony enlargement and crepitus in both knees. There are no joint deformities or active synovitis.*

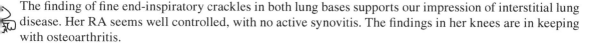

The finding of fine end-inspiratory crackles in both lung bases supports our impression of interstitial lung disease. Her RA seems well controlled, with no active synovitis. The findings in her knees are in keeping with osteoarthritis.

HOW SHOULD THIS PATIENT BE INVESTIGATED FURTHER?

The two key investigations to request are as follows:

- ***High-resolution computed tomography scan of her chest*** (HRCT).

HRCT can help to confirm the diagnosis of interstitial lung disease. It may show lung fibrosis, traction bronchiectasis, honey combing and ground glass opacities (due to alveolar inflammation).

- **Pulmonary function tests**.

Interstitial lung disease leads to a restrictive pattern, which is characterised by reduced FVC (<0.8), normal FEV_1/FVC ratio (>0.7) and reduced gas transfer.

WHAT SHOULD YOU TELL THE PATIENT?

You should tell her that

- Her presentation is suggestive of interstitial lung disease.

'The oxygen that we breathe passes through the breathing tubes and millions of tiny sacs in both lungs before getting into the blood (Draw a diagram to illustrate.) I suspect you are getting breathless because the lining of these sacs is inflamed and thickened, thereby restricting the amount of oxygen that gets into your blood. You feel breathless when you exert yourself because you need extra oxygen at the time and the lungs are unable to provide this'.

- The underlying cause could be the rheumatoid arthritis or methotrexate.

'This is most likely related to your arthritis. In some people with rheumatoid arthritis, the immune system attacks the lungs and causes this kind of inflammation. Another possible cause is methotrexate'.

- Her blood tests and chest X-ray were normal. You will arrange a high-resolution CT scan and pulmonary function tests.

'Your chest X-ray is normal, but we often do not see the changes of lung inflammation on an X-ray, especially in the early stages. I'll therefore ask for a scan of your lungs. Scans are much better at showing lung inflammation than X-rays. I'll also arrange some breathing tests, which will tell us how well your lungs are working'.

- She should stop the methotrexate straightaway.
- You will refer her to a respiratory clinic.

'I'll refer you to a lung specialist, who will explain the results of your scan and breathing tests, and discuss the treatment options'.

- You will also let her rheumatologist know so that she could try an alternative medication for her arthritis.

OUTCOME

*The HRCT scan shows **fibrotic changes in both lungs** in keeping with interstitial lung disease. Pulmonary function tests show FEV_1 64% predicted, **FVC 62% predicted**, FEV_1/FVC ratio 84%, **gas transfer 58% predicted** and **total lung capacity 65% predicted**. An echocardiogram shows normal pulmonary artery systolic pressure.*

She is seen by a respiratory consultant, who commences her on prednisolone and mycophenolate, after discussing with her rheumatologist. He notes that she has already received the flu, pneumococcal and COVID vaccines.

The 22-Year-Old Man with Wheezing   Case 47

A 22-year-old man presents to the clinic with a three-month history of shortness of breath and wheezing.

HOW SHOULD THIS PROBLEM BE APPROACHED?

*He tells you that he developed **shortness of breath**, **wheezing and cough** soon after he moved house three months ago. He used his mum's blue inhalers about two to three times a day and his symptoms gradually improved in a couple of days. He had a further episode of shortness of breath and wheezing a week ago, which lasted a couple of days and again responded to inhalers. He is currently symptom-free.*

The history of brief episodes of shortness of breath, wheezing and cough combined with a good response to bronchodilator therapy points to reversible narrowing of airways, secondary to either bronchial asthma *or* infective bronchitis. Of the two, asthma seems more likely, as his symptoms (a) occurred soon after he moved house, when he was probably exposed to dust and (b) recurred a few weeks later.

In asthma, hyper-responsiveness to innocuous stimuli, such as pollen, dust, feather, hay or drugs (e.g. aspirin, non-steroidal anti-inflammatory drug, β-blocker), leads to inflammation and narrowing of airways. In some patients, it may be triggered by exercise ('exercise-induced asthma') or exposure to cold. Pathological changes in airways include (a) bronchial smooth muscle contraction, (b) inflammatory cell infiltration of airways and (c) increased mucus secretion and mucus plugging. Patients may have associated atopic disorders (e.g. rhinitis, nasal polyps, eczema) and family history of similar illnesses.

Asthma usually starts in childhood, and less often, during adulthood. Childhood asthma may either (a) go away after some years, (b) continue into adulthood *or* (c) go away and return during adulthood. The four typical symptoms of asthma are shortness of breath, wheezing, cough and chest tightness. Patients may present with any combination of these symptoms, with varying degrees of severity, and it is important to bear in mind that not everyone with asthma will present with wheeze. Diurnal variation is characteristic, with symptoms often being worse at night or early in the morning. Unlike in chronic obstructive pulmonary disease (COPD), the airway inflammation in asthma is reversible.

Further questions to ask:

- Has he been completely well, apart from the two recent episodes?
- Does he get **breathless on exertion**?
- Does he get **nocturnal symptoms**, and if so, how often?

- Did he suffer from *asthma during his childhood*?
- Apart from his mother, is there *any other family member with asthma or other atopic disorders*?
- Does he have *other atopic problems*, like rhinitis, nasal polyps or eczema?
- Check for *exposure to possible triggers*.

What is his occupation? Does it involve exposure to dust or smoke? Does he or anyone else around him smoke? Does he keep any pets at home? Does he live in a house with a garden?

- Does he get *heartburn*? Does he *snore at night*?

Patients with asthma may have associated gastro-oesophageal reflux disease or obstructive sleep apnoea.

*He has been completely asymptomatic apart from the two episodes. He does not get breathless on exertion. He has never had nocturnal symptoms. He learnt from his mother that **he had asthma as a child** but is not sure if this was confirmed with tests. He **grew out of asthma during his early teenage years** and did not have any problems until three months ago. His **mother has asthma**. Apart from her, there is no one else in his immediate family with asthma or other atopic disorders. He has a younger brother, who is well.*

*He **gets hay fever during the spring and summer months** but has never had polyps in his nose, sinus problems or eczema. His medical history is otherwise unremarkable, and he does not take any regular medication. His job is office-based. He has never smoked. His **father is a heavy smoker** though he tends not to smoke around him or his mother. He does not keep any pets. He denies heartburn, and no one has told him that he snores at night. He is single and lives alone in a flat.*

The salient features are (a) the history of childhood asthma, (b) family history of asthma in his mother, (c) his tendency to develop hay fever during summer and spring months and (d) possible passive smoking. The history has not identified any other triggers for asthma.

WHAT SHOULD YOU LOOK FOR ON EXAMINATION?

You should

- Ask for his *vital signs*.

In patients with acute exacerbation of asthma, it is important to record the oxygen saturation, respiratory rate, pulse rate, blood pressure, temperature, conscious level, ability to speak in full sentences, use of accessory muscles of respiration and presence of cyanosis.

- Examine the *respiratory system*.

Examination may be normal when the patient is well. Rhonchi are heard only during an exacerbation. The wheeze in asthma is typically *polyphonic* (many different tones are heard simultaneously), as the airway obstruction is dynamic, and sounds originate from oscillation of airways at many sites. By contrast, *monophonic wheeze* is a single tone and arises due to fixed obstruction of a large airway (e.g. tumour, foreign body).

His vital signs are normal. There are no rhonchi or other abnormal findings on examination of his respiratory system.

HOW SHOULD THIS PATIENT BE EVALUATED FURTHER?

The preferred diagnostic test is *spirometry*, which will help to demonstrate reversible airway obstruction (*see Box 47.1*). Spirometry is often normal in asthma, especially if it is performed when the patient is well and asymptomatic.

Alternative tests (less accurate than spirometry) are (a) *serial peak flow measurements* for two to four weeks to demonstrate diurnal variation due to variable airway obstruction *and* (b) *provocative testing* with methacholine or histamine to check for airway hyper-responsiveness. In practice, (c) a *trial of therapy* is often given to patients with high likelihood of asthma. If the patient responds to therapy, treatment is continued, and the diagnosis confirmed with objective testing later.

BOX 47.1   FVC, FEV$_1$ AND PEFR EXPLAINED

Spirometry measures the amount of air that the patient can forcefully breathe out from the lungs after maximal inspiration ('Take a deep breath and take in as much as you can. Then blow out as hard and fast as you can until no more air comes out').

There are two basic measures that are tested during spirometry: *forced vital capacity* (FVC) and *forced expiratory volume in the first second* (FEV$_1$). The total volume of air that is forcefully breathed out in *one breath* is called FVC, while the volume that is breathed out in the *first second* is FEV$_1$. Both FVC and FEV$_1$ are measured in litres and expressed as a percentage of a predicted value (the predicted 'normal' value is based on age, sex, ethnicity and height). During health, more than 70% of the predicted volume of air is blown out in the first second (FEV$_1$), and more than 80% over the entire duration of expiration (FVC).

The FVC and FEV$_1$ can help to differentiate obstructive from restrictive lung disease.

- In obstructive lung disease, air flows out of the lungs more slowly than it should (just like how it takes longer for traffic to get past a stretch of a dual carriageway when one lane is blocked). Hence, FEV$_1$ is reduced, FVC is normal and FEV$_1$/FVC ratio is reduced (<0.7).
- In restrictive lung disease, the total amount of air that can be inhaled into the 'smaller lungs' is reduced. Hence, FVC is reduced (and therefore FEV$_1$ as well) and FEV$_1$/FVC ratio is normal (>0.7).

If asthma is suspected, spirometry should be repeated after administering a bronchodilator, like salbutamol. Asthma is characterised by 'reversibility' (improvement in FEV$_1$ or FVC by >12% and >200 mL, following administration of the bronchodilator).

Peak expiratory flow rate (PEFR) measures the *maximum speed of expiration* as opposed to how much air is blown out in one breath or in the first second. The patient is asked to take a deep breath and blow out as fast as possible into the peak flow meter (just like 'blowing out a candle'). Unlike in spirometry, there is no need to try and empty the lungs. The normal value ranges from 400 to 700 L/minute. Peak flow can be done at home, thus allowing patients to maintain a peak flow diary. Serial peak flow measurements over two to four weeks are particularly helpful in patients with normal spirometry. A diurnal variation in peak flow of more than 20% *or* an improvement of at least 20% after inhaling a rapidly acting bronchodilator would support a diagnosis of asthma.

Patients should measure the baseline peak flow when they are well so that they know what their 'normal values' are. When they feel unwell, they can measure the peak flow and compare with their baseline value. This will help to monitor their progress at home. Peak flow is also useful to diagnose occupational asthma. The peak flow should be performed several times a day for two weeks, while the patient is working, and then for a similar period when the patient is away from work. A lower PEFR during the working weeks would establish the diagnosis of occupational asthma.

- There is no need for a *chest X-ray* to diagnose asthma.

Chest X-ray is only indicated in patients with atypical symptoms *or* those who do not respond to treatment.

- In some patients, full blood count might show evidence of *eosinophilia* (an indicator of atopic tendency).
- *Skin prick tests* and *allergen-specific serum IgE* may help to identify specific allergens once the diagnosis of asthma has been confirmed with objective testing.

WHAT SHOULD YOU TELL THE PATIENT?

You should tell him that

- His symptoms are due to bronchial asthma.

'I suspect your asthma has come back. In asthma, the airways become narrow because of inflammation and tightening of the muscles around the breathing tubes. An attack of asthma is usually triggered by external particles like dust, pollen or feather'.

- You would arrange spirometry.

'I'll arrange some breathing tests to confirm this. There is no need for an X-ray or blood tests. Once we confirm the diagnosis of asthma, I'll arrange some tests to find out what exactly you are reacting to'.

- You would suggest a regular low-dose corticosteroid inhaler.

'I'll prescribe a steroid inhaler to use every day. This will reduce the inflammation in airways and help to prevent the attacks of asthma. Sometimes, steroid inhalers can cause thrush in the mouth, which is a white patch caused by a fungus. To reduce the risk of thrush, you should rinse your mouth and spit out the water each time you use the inhaler so that the medicine is cleared from the mouth'.

- He should use the salbutamol inhaler as and when needed.

'The blue inhaler opens the airways and should be used when you develop breathing difficulty, wheezing or chest tightness. If your symptoms don't respond to the blue inhaler, you should seek medical advice'.

- You would ask the asthma nurse to check his inhaler technique.
- He should try and avoid the triggers as much as possible.

'You should try and avoid potential triggers as much as possible. You should avoid smoky environments and exposure to dust and pollen. Keep your windows closed during the pollen season and make sure your pillows, mattresses and bedding have covers. Do not take anti-inflammatory tablets like ibuprofen, as they can trigger an attack of asthma'.

- You would refer him to a respiratory clinic (*'lung specialist'*) if symptoms are difficult to control with the above measures.

OUTCOME

*Spirometry reveals **normal FEV₁ and FVC** (he is asymptomatic at the time of the test). The respiratory physician advises him to check his peak flows at home, at least three to four times a day for two weeks and maintain a peak flow diary. The diary shows a **dip of more than 20% in the evenings** in keeping with asthma. He is seen by the asthma nurse, who advises him to avoid potential triggers. He is commenced on low-dose inhaled corticosteroid along with a β-agonist inhaler to be used as and when necessary.*

The normal spirometry results are not surprising. The diurnal variation noted on serial peak flow measurements combined with his clinical presentation supports the diagnosis of asthma, although it would be good to repeat the spirometry at a later date to confirm the diagnosis.

The treatments used for asthma target the three main pathological changes in airways: (a) short- and long-acting β-agonists (e.g. salbutamol, salmeterol) dilate the bronchi by relaxing the bronchial smooth muscle, while (b) corticosteroids (either inhaled, oral or intravenous) reduce airway inflammation and (c) anti-cholinergics (e.g. ipratropium) reduce airway secretions. The most recent addition to the therapeutic armamentarium is omalizumab, which is an anti-IgE antibody.

The 63-Year-Old Man with Breathlessness

Case 48

A 63-year-old man presents with a 2-year history of gradually worsening shortness of breath. He is afebrile. His oxygen saturation is 94% on room air, pulse rate 72/minute, respiratory rate 18/minute and blood pressure 136/88 mm Hg.

HOW SHOULD THIS PROBLEM BE APPROACHED?

---

*He tells you that he gets **breathless on exertion**. His breathing has gradually worsened over the last two to three years. He was previously able to walk a fair distance but is now unable to keep pace with his wife or friends and must stop after walking a few hundred yards to catch his breath.*

 This patient describes gradually worsening chronic breathlessness. Possible causes are congestive cardiac failure, chronic obstructive pulmonary disease (COPD), interstitial lung disease, chronic kidney disease (CKD) and anaemia.

Questions to ask:

- Ask about **cardiac symptoms**, like paroxysmal nocturnal dyspnoea, orthopnoea, leg swelling, reduced urine output, chest pain, palpitations, exertional fatigue and syncope.

Note: Orthopnoea, leg swelling and reduced urine output are symptoms of fluid overload, which may be secondary to cardiac or renal disease.

- Check for **features that may suggest a respiratory cause**, like cough, expectoration, haemoptysis, wheeze, seasonal variation in symptoms, and constitutional symptoms like loss of weight and fever.

Note: Cough, haemoptysis and wheeze are not specific to respiratory disease.

- Complete a **review of systems**.

Ask particularly about symptoms that may suggest an autoimmune connective tissue disease (e.g. joint pain, skin rashes).

- Complete the **rest of the history**.

 DOI: 10.1201/9781003430230-48

Ask about his other medical problems (particularly a previous diagnosis of heart, lung or kidney disease), regular medications, current and previous occupations, pets at home and smoking habits.

*He has been troubled with a **long-standing cough**. He coughs up a small amount of phlegm nearly every day, which normally looks white or grey. He has had a **couple of chest infections in the last year**, which responded promptly to antibiotics. On both occasions, he became more breathless and the phlegm turned yellow. He has never been admitted to a hospital for this problem. He has never coughed up blood or lost weight. His symptoms are **usually worse during winter**. He sleeps with one pillow and has never woken in the middle of the night with breathlessness. He denies leg swelling, reduced urine output, chest pain, palpitations, exertional fatigue or blackouts.*

*He had a **heart attack five years ago**, following which stents were placed in two of his blood vessels around the heart. He takes aspirin, atenolol, valsartan and atorvastatin. He started smoking at the age of 20 and used to smoke 20 cigarettes/day but cut this down to **10 cigarettes/day** after the heart attack. He has been unable to cut down any further. He drinks a glass of wine with his dinner nearly every day. He worked in a printing press for nearly 30 years until 5 years ago. Prior to that, he did some office-based jobs in his early 20s. He does not keep any pets and has no hobbies. He lives with his wife.*

There are several features that favour COPD, including (a) the gradually worsening chronic breathlessness, (b) chronic productive cough, (c) seasonal variation in symptoms (worse during winter months), (d) his heavy smoking habit (about 40-pack years) and (e) intermittent worsening of breathlessness due to chest infection. COPD encompasses the clinical term chronic bronchitis (sputum production for at least three months in a year for ≥2 consecutive years) and the pathological term emphysema (destruction of alveolar walls).

Based on the Medical Research Council (MRC) dyspnoea scale (*see Box 48.1*), he is between grades 2 and 3.

BOX 48.1   MRC GRADING OF DYSPNOEA IN COPD

- *Grade 0* Gets breathless with strenuous exertion.
- *Grade 1* Gets breathless while hurrying on level ground or walking uphill.
- *Grade 2* Walks slower than people of same age because of breathlessness.
- *Grade 3* Gets breathless after 100 m or a few minutes of walking on level ground.
- *Grade 4* Too breathless to leave the house or gets breathless even while dressing or undressing.

The background history of ischaemic heart disease increases his risk of developing cardiac failure, but the absence of orthopnoea, paroxysmal nocturnal dyspnoea and leg swelling does not suggest this. Interstitial lung disease is unlikely, as it usually presents with dry cough. His haemoglobin and kidney function should be checked but his overall presentation does not support a diagnosis of CKD or anaemia.

There are no clinical features of *cor pulmonale* (pulmonary hypertension and right ventricular failure), like fatigue, exertional syncope or ankle swelling, but it can indeed be clinically silent in the early stages. His smoking habit increases his risk of developing lung cancer but there are no suggestive features, like weight loss or haemoptysis.

WHAT SHOULD YOU LOOK FOR ON EXAMINATION?

You should

- Perform a *focussed general examination*.

Check for nicotine staining of his fingers, clubbing, cervical lymphadenopathy, elevated jugular venous pressure (JVP) and leg oedema.

- Examine the *respiratory system* and particularly check for signs that may suggest COPD.
- *Auscultate the pulmonary area* of the heart for loud P_2.

*He is comfortable at rest, with no signs of respiratory distress. There is **nicotine staining of his fingers**. There is no clubbing, lymphadenopathy or leg oedema. The calves are supple. His JVP is not elevated.*

*His **chest is barrel shaped**, with increased anteroposterior diameter. The **cricoid-sternal distance is reduced** to two fingerbreadths. The chest is **hyperresonant on percussion**, with **loss of hepatic and cardiac dullness**. Air entry is equal on both sides, but **breath sounds are generally quiet** with **prolonged expiratory phase**. Heart sounds are normal.*

Physical signs are in keeping with COPD. The narrowing of airways, destruction of alveolar walls, air trapping and hyperinflation cause the barrel shape of the chest, reduced cricoid-sternal distance (normally three to four fingerbreadths), reduced chest expansion, hyperresonant percussion note and quiet breath sounds. There are no pointers to lung cancer, like clubbing or lymphadenopathy. There are no signs of cardiac failure or cor pulmonale either.

HOW SHOULD HE BE EVALUATED?

You should request

- A *chest X-ray*.

Chest X-ray findings in COPD include reduced cardiothoracic ratio, hyperinflated lungs and flat diaphragm. The chest X-ray may also help to reveal consolidation, lung mass, pneumothorax or features of heart failure.

- A *12-lead electrocardiogram*.

The ECG may reveal signs of old ischemic heart disease, atrial fibrillation and evidence of right ventricular strain (increased height of P waves and right ventricular hypertrophy).

- *Blood tests*, including full blood count and renal function.

Patients with COPD may be polycythaemic due to chronic hypoxia and smoking habit. In younger patients with COPD, especially those who have never smoked, *serum α-1 antitrypsin* should be checked.

- *Pulmonary function tests* (spirometry with gas transfer).

COPD is characterised by reduced FEV_1 and FEV_1/FVC ratio (<0.7), with reduced gas transfer (because of destruction of alveolar walls). The airway obstruction in COPD is not reversible with bronchodilators, unlike asthma.

WHAT SHOULD YOU TELL THE PATIENT?

You should tell him that

- His breathlessness is due to COPD.

'You are getting breathless because your airways have become narrow. We call this chronic obstructive pulmonary disease or COPD for short. Chronic means long-standing. It is called obstructive because there is obstruction to the flow of air into the lungs. The word pulmonary refers to the lungs'.

- COPD is caused by cigarette smoking and air pollution.

'This is most often caused by smoking or air pollution. The lining of the airways gets damaged by the harmful substances that are present in cigarettes or air pollutants'.

- You would arrange some investigations.

'I'll ask for some blood tests, an X-ray of your chest and breathing tests. These tests will help to confirm the narrowing of airways'.

- He should stop smoking.

'I would strongly advise you to stop smoking. If you stop smoking, we can reduce the risk of further damage to the lungs'.

- You would prescribe a short-acting bronchodilator inhaler and refer him to a respiratory physician.

'I'll prescribe an inhaler medication, which will help to open your airways when you feel breathless. I'll refer you to a lung specialist, who will suggest other types of inhalers that you can use in the long-term. His team will teach you some exercises to improve your breathing and make it easier for you to perform your day-to-day activities'.

- COPD increases the risk of chest infection. You will arrange for him to receive flu and pneumococcal vaccines.

'Narrowing of the airways increases your risk of getting lung infections. When you get an infection, your breathing may suddenly get worse. You may start coughing up more phlegm or the phlegm may turn yellow or green. You should see a doctor when that happens. I'll arrange for you to receive flu and pneumonia vaccines to reduce your risk of catching an infection'.

- You would give him an information booklet about COPD (or suggest useful websites).

OUTCOME

*His chest X-ray shows **reduced cardiothoracic ratio, hyperinflated lungs and low flat diaphragm** in keeping with COPD. The 12-lead ECG shows **Q waves** in keeping with old myocardial infarction and **P pulmonale**. His full blood count shows **Hb of 158 g/L**. Renal function is normal. Pulmonary function tests show **FEV$_1$ of 45%, FVC 78% and gas transfer 56%** in keeping with obstructive airway disease. Reversibility is not tested.*

 The results are in keeping with COPD. Cessation of smoking is the most important aspect of management. All patients should be given rescue short-acting bronchodilator (e.g. salbutamol). Long-term options include long-acting β-agonist or LABA (e.g. salmeterol), long-acting muscarinic antagonist or LAMA (e.g. tiotropium) and inhaled corticosteroids. All patients should receive influenza and pneumococcal vaccines. He should be referred for pulmonary rehabilitation to increase his exercise capacity. Pulmonary rehabilitation includes exercise therapy, disease education, and psychological and social interventions.

Infective exacerbation of COPD is usually due to *Streptococcus pneumoniae, Haemophilus influenzae, Moraxella catarrhalis* or rhinoviruses. Management of an exacerbation should include oxygen, bronchodilator nebulisers, corticosteroids and antibiotics.

Long-term home oxygen therapy should be considered (provided the patient has quit smoking) if (a) the PaO$_2$ is <7.3 kPa *or* (b) the PaO$_2$ is between 7.3 and 8 kPa, in the presence of pulmonary hypertension, peripheral oedema or polycythaemia. Selected patients may benefit from lung volume reduction surgery.

The 56-Year-Old Man with Haemoptysis

Case 49

A 56-year-old Caucasian man presents to the emergency unit with haemoptysis.
His oxygen saturation is 96% on room air, pulse rate 76/minute, BP 128/76 mm Hg, respiratory rate 16/minute and temperature 37°C.

HOW SHOULD THIS PROBLEM BE APPROACHED?

Having ensured that oxygen saturation and hemodynamic parameters are satisfactory, start with an open-ended question and obtain a focussed history.

*He tells you that he **coughed up a small amount of blood** earlier that morning and it happened again a few hours later. He is unable to precisely quantify the amount but says it was probably **one to two teaspoonfuls on each occasion**. The blood was not mixed with phlegm. He has never coughed blood before.*

- First, ***confirm that he is describing haemoptysis*** and not haematemesis.

Preceding nausea or associated melena and abdominal pain, dark or coffee ground appearance (due to formation of acid haematin), presence of food particles in the expelled contents and background history of gastrointestinal or liver disease (e.g. peptic ulcer, liver cirrhosis) would favour haematemesis, while preceding cough, bright red or pink and frothy appearance (as it is mixed with air) and background history of lung disease (e.g. tuberculosis, bronchiectasis, lung cancer) would favour haemoptysis. Occasionally, haemoptysis may be confused with bleeding from the nose or gums.

*He is quite certain that he coughed up the blood. The blood **looked bright red**. He denies nausea, vomiting, abdominal pain, melena or bleeding from the nose or gums.*

Massive haemoptysis carries a high mortality. There is no consensus on the definition of massive haemoptysis, as the literature describes a wide range from >100 mL/24 hours to >1000 mL/24 hours. What is more relevant is probably whether it is life-threatening, as the rate of bleeding and underlying lung disease also determine the outcome and not just the amount of blood expectorated. In this patient, the haemoptysis could be categorised as 'non-life-threatening' on the basis that his vital parameters are currently satisfactory.

Haemoptysis may be the presenting symptom of several diseases (*see Box 49.1*).

BOX 49.1   SOME UNDERLYING CAUSES OF NON-TRAUMATIC HAEMOPTYSIS IN ADULTS[†]

Airways

- Bronchitis.
- Bronchiectasis.
- Cancer (e.g. bronchogenic carcinoma, carcinoid, lung metastases).

Lung parenchyma

- Necrotising pneumonia or lung abscess.
- Tuberculosis.
- *Paragonimus westermani* infection (also known as lung fluke).[††]
- Mycetoma.

Blood vessels

- Pulmonary embolism.
- Diffuse alveolar haemorrhage due to pulmonary capillaritis (e.g. ANCA-associated vasculitis, systemic lupus erythematosus, Goodpasture's syndrome).
- Left heart failure or mitral stenosis due to elevated pulmonary capillary pressure.
- Ruptured arterio-venous malformation (e.g. hereditary haemorrhagic telangiectasia).

[†] Bronchitis, bronchiectasis and tuberculosis are the most common causes of haemoptysis. An underlying cause may *not* be found in about 10% of patients.

[††] *Paragonimus westermani* infection is endemic in many parts of Eastern Asia, Africa and South America, and is a common cause of haemoptysis in these regions.

Further questions should explore the features that may suggest an underlying cause. You should ask about:

- Associated **respiratory symptoms**, like cough, expectoration, breathlessness, wheezing and pleuritic chest pain.
- **Constitutional symptoms**, like fever, night sweats and weight loss.

If constitutional symptoms are present, ask about possible **contact with tuberculosis** and obtain a **sexual history** (as HIV infection increases the risk of tuberculosis disease or reactivation of latent infection).

- **Features of pulmonary embolism**, like unilateral calf swelling or recent immobilisation (e.g. long-distance travel, recent hospitalisation).
- **Joint pain**, **skin rashes**, **reduced urine output** or **change in colour of the urine** (may suggest systemic vasculitis, systemic lupus erythematosus or Goodpasture's syndrome).
- His **background medical problems**, particularly chronic lung disease (e.g. bronchiectasis, tuberculosis), cancer, diabetes and autoimmune connective tissue disease.
- **Regular medications** (ask particularly if he takes anticoagulant or immunosuppressive medications).

- *Smoking habit.*
- *Occupational history* (current as well as past).
- Ask about possible *exposure to asbestos.*

*He has had a **dry cough for the last three to four months**. He was coughing for a few weeks after COVID-19 infection two years ago but has not had a cough at any other time. He denies breathlessness, orthopnoea, wheezing, chest pain and ankle swelling. He says he has **lost about 4–5 kg** in the last few months without trying but denies fever or night sweats. He also denies calf swelling, recent immobilisation, joint pain, skin rashes, reduced urine output or change in colour of the urine.*

*He takes amlodipine for **hypertension**. His medical history is otherwise unremarkable and he does not take any other medication or 'over-the-counter' preparation. His blood sugar and cholesterol were found to be normal when last tested about six months ago. He has not knowingly been in contact with anyone with tuberculosis. He has **smoked about 20 cigarettes/day since the age of 18**. He drinks a can of beer two to three times a week. He works as a security officer for a private firm. He has not done any other jobs in the past. He lives with his wife, who has been his only sexual partner ever.*

We can rule out certain conditions based on the history. The absence of fever, productive cough, breathlessness, wheezing and pleuritic chest pain combined with the normal vital signs would rule out acute bronchitis or pneumonia. Diffuse alveolar haemorrhage is unlikely, as he is not breathless and his oxygen saturation is normal. Also, there are no features of an underlying autoimmune connective tissue disease. His presentation does not suggest left heart failure or mitral stenosis, as he denies breathlessness or orthopnoea. There are no pointers to pulmonary embolism, like breathlessness, pleuritic chest pain, calf swelling, recent immobilisation, low oxygen saturation, tachycardia or tachypnoea. The absence of long-standing productive cough makes chronic bronchitis or bronchiectasis unlikely.

So the two possible diagnoses to consider are lung cancer and tuberculosis. Both can present with persistent cough, weight loss and haemoptysis. Of the two, tuberculosis seems somewhat less likely, as he is Caucasian, with no tuberculosis contact history or other constitutional symptoms like fever or night sweats. His heavy smoking habit (38 pack-years) indeed places him at a higher risk for developing lung cancer.

- Ask a few more focused questions to check for *other features of lung cancer* (*see Box 49.2*).

BOX 49.2   MANIFESTATIONS OF LUNG CANCER

- The tumour may be silent and *detected on a routine chest X-ray*, cause bronchial occlusion leading to *collapse* or *recurrent pneumonia* or spread to the pleura and cause *pleural effusion*.
- *Spread of cancer to the surrounding tissues* can result in compression of the oesophagus (dysphagia), trachea (stridor), left recurrent laryngeal nerve (hoarseness of voice), phrenic nerve (diaphragmatic weakness), sympathetic chain (Horner's syndrome), brachial plexus (pain, weakness and numbness in the arm) or superior vena cava (swelling of the face).
- *Lymphatic spread* causes hilar lymphadenopathy and mediastinal widening.
- *Haematogenous spread* occurs to the liver, brain, bones and adrenal gland.
- *Non-metastatic paraneoplastic manifestations* include finger clubbing, hyponatraemia, hypercalcaemia, Cushing's syndrome, Eaton-Lambert syndrome, neuropathy and cerebellar degeneration.

He denies problems with swallowing, noisy breathing, change in his voice, pain in the arm, swollen lymph glands or weakness of his limbs.

WHAT SHOULD YOU LOOK FOR ON EXAMINATION?

Examination should be focused and aimed at checking for features that may suggest lung cancer or tuberculosis (rather than trying to look for signs of all possible conditions that can cause haemoptysis). You should

- Examine the ***respiratory system***.

Particularly check for clubbing, supraclavicular nodes, air entry on both sides (e.g. collapse and pleural effusion can reduce air entry) and crepitations (e.g. pneumonia).

- Examine the abdomen for ***palpable liver***.

Rare signs include those of Horner's syndrome (miosis, ptosis and enophthalmos), swelling of the face and distended veins due to superior vena cava obstruction, and wasting of the small muscles of the hand due to compression of brachial plexus.

*He is moderately built and looks comfortable at rest. Examination reveals **clubbing** and **nicotine staining of his fingers**. His lungs are clear and air entry is equal. There is no hepatomegaly. The rest of the examination is unremarkable.*

HOW SHOULD THIS PATIENT BE INVESTIGATED?

You should request

- A ***chest X-ray*** (this can be omitted if CT scan can be performed soon, but it is readily available and will help to rapidly check for lung mass).

Note: The chest X-ray may be completely normal in patients with early lung cancer, bronchitis, endobronchial tuberculosis or pulmonary embolism.

- ***CT scan of the chest and upper abdomen*** (to include the adrenals).
- ***Blood tests***, including full blood count, liver function tests, serum creatinine and electrolytes, calcium, coagulation screen, and group and cross match.

If the test results clearly point to lung cancer, ***sputum for acid fast bacilli***, ***polymerase chain reaction and TB culture*** can probably be omitted.

If CT findings are suspicious for cancer, subsequent steps in the evaluation will include (a) confirmation of the diagnosis by ***biopsy*** (bronchoscopy for centrally placed tumours and CT-guided biopsy for peripherally placed tumours) and (b) ***staging scans***. Treatment depends on the histological type and stage of cancer.

WHAT SHOULD YOU TELL THE PATIENT AT THIS STAGE?

You should tell him that

- You would recommend admission to hospital.

'I would recommend that you get admitted to hospital because you could cough up blood again'.

- His vital signs are stable at the moment.

'When you cough up a lot of blood, the blood pressure and oxygen level in the blood can go down. Your blood pressure and oxygen level are normal but we should continue to monitor this closely'.

- You would ask for a chest X-ray and some blood tests.
- You would prescribe codeine to suppress the cough, and tranexamic acid to reduce bleeding.

'I'll prescribe a cough mixture to suppress your cough and another medication to try and reduce the bleeding'.

- You will refer him to a respiratory physician.

'I'll come back and talk to you once you have had the X-ray. I'll be asking a lung specialist to see you. He might suggest further tests depending on what the X-ray shows'.

OUTCOME

*His chest X-ray shows a **lung mass in the left mid-zone**. His full blood count, liver function tests, serum creatinine, sodium and calcium are normal. An urgent CT scan of the chest and upper abdomen is arranged. This shows a **spiculated mass in the left middle lobe**.*

*The respiratory physician arranges bronchoscopy and biopsy, as the lesion is central. Biopsy is reported as **squamous cell carcinoma**. Tests for tuberculosis are negative. Further evaluation with positron emission tomography (PET)-CT scan and MRI of the brain shows no evidence of metastases. Following discussion in a multi-disciplinary meeting, he is referred to a cardiothoracic surgeon to consider lobectomy, as the cancer is localised.*

Note: Spiculated lesion is more likely to be due to cancer. The spicules denote the extension of cancer cells into the surrounding lung parenchyma.

The 54-Year-Old Man Who Snores at Night

Case 50

A 54-year-old overweight man is referred to the medical clinic, as his wife has been complaining that he snores loudly at night.

HOW SHOULD THIS PROBLEM BE APPROACHED?

Snoring occurs because of narrowing of the upper airways. Apart from causing annoyance to the bed partner, simple snoring does not affect the quality of sleep or result in any clinical sequelae. However, in some patients, the narrowing of upper airways may be severe enough to cause repetitive episodes of reduction *or* cessation of airflow (hypopnoea or apnoea). This is known as obstructive sleep apnoea (OSA). The resulting hypoxia stimulates an increase in inspiratory effort and awakens the person several times at night, leading to sleep fragmentation, daytime sleepiness and tiredness (*see Figure 50.1*).

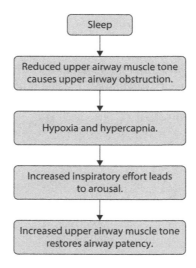

FIGURE 50.1 Mechanism of apnoea or hypopnoea in obstructive sleep apnoea.

DOI: 10.1201/9781003430230-50

- After the open-ended question, ask *whether he feels sleepy during the day* (not just tired).

*He tells you that his **wife has been complaining about his snoring** for a long time. Of late, she has been sleeping in a separate room because of his snoring. He admits that he **wakes up feeling unrefreshed** and **feels sleepy during the daytime**.*

The daytime sleepiness indicates that he might have OSA and not just simple snoring. The effects of daytime sleepiness may range from impaired performance at work *to* potentially fatal motor vehicle accidents. Patients may also report morning headaches, low mood, cognitive decline and reduced libido. OSA leads to increased risk of hypertension, insulin resistance, ischaemic heart disease and stroke, arrhythmias (e.g. atrial fibrillation), pulmonary hypertension and congestive heart failure.

Risk factors for OSA include male sex, older age (>50 years), obesity, large neck circumference (>17 inches in men and >16 inches in women) and orofacial anatomical abnormalities (e.g. acromegaly, retrognathia, large tongue, enlarged tonsils or adenoids, low-lying soft palate).

Further questions to ask:

- Ask if his wife has ever told him that he *stops breathing in the middle of the night*.
- Ask about his *occupation*, and if the daytime sleepiness affects his performance at work.
- Ask *how the sleepiness affects his day-to-day life*.
- Ask *if he drives*, and if he has ever dozed off behind the wheel.
- Ask about his *weight gain*.

If the weight gain is recent, screen for thyroid and adrenal disease.

- Obtain details of his *medical problems*, *regular medications*, *smoking habit* and *alcohol consumption*.
- Ask if he has previously been evaluated for the sleep problem or snoring.

*His wife has never told him that he stops breathing during sleep. He works as a supervisor in a garment factory. He **drives a car**, but only to the supermarket or shops, as his company bus takes him to work every day. He **gets tired very easily**, so he is no longer able to help his wife with household chores like how he used to. He **tries to catch a wink whenever he gets an opportunity** at home or during lunch time at work. He usually **falls asleep in the company bus**, **while watching television or whenever he is idle**. He denies problems with mood or memory. He has not consulted anyone about this problem.*

*His medical problems include **hypertension**, **impaired glucose tolerance**, **hyperlipidaemia and stage 3 chronic kidney disease**. He has never had a heart attack or stroke. He says he has gradually piled on the pounds over many years. He takes amlodipine 5 mg/day, lisinopril 10 mg/day, atorvastatin 20 mg/day and metformin 500 mg twice daily. He says his **blood pressure control hasn't been too good** although he has been compliant with his medications. He **smokes 5 cigarettes/day**. He cut down from 20 cigarettes/ day about five years ago but hasn't been able to quit the habit. He **drinks 1–2 cans of beer most evenings**.*

The daytime sleepiness is clearly affecting his ability to perform his daily tasks, and probably his performance at work as well. He should be screened using the *Epworth Sleepiness Scale* (ESS), which is a self-administered questionnaire designed to assess daytime sleepiness. Patients are asked to rate on a 4-point scale, their chance of dozing off or falling asleep while engaged in eight different activities.

OSA cannot be ruled out on the basis that his wife has not witnessed apnoeic episodes. His poor blood pressure control is probably due to OSA, and he has other cardiovascular risk factors as well, which could be exacerbated by OSA. He should be advised to quit smoking and cut down his alcohol intake (alcohol can exacerbate OSA by reducing the tone of upper airway muscles). He is driving a car, which is concerning. It could prove dangerous if he were to doze off while driving, so he should be asked to immediately stop driving and inform the driving vehicle licensing agency pending further evaluation.

WHAT SHOULD YOU LOOK FOR ON EXAMINATION?

You should

- Ask for his *body mass index* and *measure his neck circumference*.
- Ask for his *blood pressure*.
- Examine his *neck and orofacial region* (e.g. acromegaly, goitre, retrognathia, large tongue, enlarged tonsils, low-lying soft palate).
- *Listen to the lungs* (OSA often co-exists with chronic obstructive pulmonary disease) and *pulmonary area of the heart* for loud P_2 (pulmonary hypertension).
- Check for *leg oedema* (*cor pulmonale*).

His body mass index is 32 kg/m² and neck circumference is 19 inches. His blood pressure is 168/102 mm Hg. His neck looks large, but there are no specific anatomical abnormalities. His lungs are clear, and the second heart sound is normal in intensity. There is no leg oedema.

HOW SHOULD HE BE EVALUATED FURTHER?

- He should be *referred to a sleep clinic*.

The sleep specialist is likely to arrange sleep studies. The sleep study can be conducted at home unless more detailed information is required, in which case, the study would be conducted in the sleep lab in hospital. The aim of the sleep study is to measure the apnoea-hypopnoea index (AHI), which is the total number of episodes of apnoea (complete cessation of breathing for ≥10 seconds) or hypopnoea (reduction in ventilation by >50% for ≥10 seconds) per hour (*see Box 50.1*).

**BOX 50.1 SEVERITY OF OBSTRUCTIVE SLEEP APNOEA
BASED ON THE APNOEA-HYPOPNOEA INDEX (AHI)**

- AHI <5 normal
- AHI 5–14 mild sleep apnoea
- AHI 15–29 moderate sleep apnoea
- AHI ≥ 30 severe sleep apnoea

In the home sleep study, only basic measures such as airflow and oxygen saturation are monitored at night to determine the AHI. The sleep study in hospital is more detailed and includes recording of electrical activities of the brain, eyes, muscles and heart along with airflow, chest and abdominal movements, and oxygen saturation.

WHAT SHOULD YOU TELL THE PATIENT?

You should tell him that

- He is snoring because of narrowing of the upper airways.

'Snoring occurs when the airway around the throat becomes narrow during sleep'.

- His daytime sleepiness is most likely due to OSA.

'Sometimes the airways become too narrow or close completely for a few seconds. When this happens, it'll stop your breathing for a few seconds and cause the blood oxygen level to go down. The brain will sense this and wake you up so that you can take some extra breaths to get more oxygen. You will then instantly go back to sleep and not even realise that you woke up. The problem is that this can happen repeatedly throughout the night and reduce the quality of sleep. We call this obstructive sleep apnoea or OSA for short, as the obstruction of the airway during sleep leads to apnoea. Apnoea is the medical term for brief cessation of breathing. I wonder if this is the reason why you feel so sleepy during the daytime'.

- The daytime sleepiness not only affects performance of day-to-day tasks but also leads to increased cardiovascular morbidity.

'Poor quality of sleep will not only reduce your ability to perform day-to-day tasks, but also increase the risk of developing high blood pressure, diabetes, heart attack and stroke'.

- You will give him a questionnaire to complete and refer him to a sleep clinic.

'The sleep specialist will assess your problem and arrange some tests to check your breathing during sleep. If these tests confirm that you do have OSA, he might suggest using a breathing machine at night to keep your airway open. The specialist will explain this to you'.

- His quality of sleep can be significantly improved with treatment (it is important to stress this.)
- He should stop driving in the meantime.

'You should temporarily stop driving, as there is a chance that you could fall asleep behind the wheel. You may be able to resume driving once the problem is treated by the sleep specialist'.

- He should *'start exercising and eat healthily to lose weight, stop smoking and cut down the alcohol'.*
- You would suggest increasing the dosage of his anti-hypertensive medication.
- He may be able to reduce the dosage once the sleep problem is addressed.

OUTCOME

*His **Epworth Sleepiness Score is 18/24, indicating severe daytime sleepiness.** The sleep specialist arranges a home sleep study, which shows **AHI of 20 per hour.** Following counselling, he is commenced on treatment with continuous positive airway pressure (CPAP). His daytime sleepiness improves remarkably with CPAP, and repeat sleep study shows that his AHI is down to 2 per hour. His blood pressure control improves and he is able to reduce the dosages of his anti-hypertensive medications.*

The treatment of choice for patients with moderate or severe OSA (AHI ≥ 15) is continuous positive airway pressure (CPAP). CPAP is also considered for patients with mild OSA (AHI 5–14) in the presence of symptoms *or* cardiovascular co-morbidity. The aim of CPAP is to maintain airway patency by delivering continuous positive pressure, thus eliminating nocturnal apnoeic or hypopnoeic episodes. Mask designs have considerably improved in recent years, and patients can roll over in bed, wear glasses to read a book or even travel! CPAP improves not only symptoms and quality of sleep, but also cardiovascular morbidity. It is usually a life-long treatment and patients must remain compliant.

For patients who refuse CPAP or those with mild OSA (AHI <5), mandibular devices to retain the mandible in a forward position *or* positional therapy (avoiding sleeping on the back so that the tongue doesn't fall backwards) can be tried. Surgery (uvulopalatopharyngoplasty) is only a last resort option.

The 25-Year-Old Man with Marfanoid Habitus

Case 51

A 25-year-old man presents to A and E with right-sided chest pain. Chest X-ray shows a small pneumothorax. The A and E doctor does not feel that aspiration or chest drain is warranted, as the visible peripheral rim of air is less than 2 cm. She asks for your opinion, as she feels that he has Marfanoid habitus.

His oxygen saturation is 96% on room air, pulse rate 68/minute, respiratory rate 18/minute and blood pressure 124/68 mm Hg.

HOW SHOULD THIS PROBLEM BE APPROACHED?

After introducing yourself, ask him if he feels well. Has the chest pain resolved? Does he feel breathless? What have the doctors told him?

*You note that **he looks tall and slim**. He says he developed pain on the right side of his chest earlier that day, but it has gone now. He denies breathlessness. He is aware that he has a pneumothorax, which is a collection of air around his lungs. The A and E doctor told him that there is no need to remove the air, as the collection is small. He is waiting to see a lung specialist.*

Tell him why you have come to see him.

> *'I am the medical registrar. The A and E doctor has asked for my opinion because she wonders if you have an underlying medical condition that may have caused the pneumothorax. I'll ask you a few questions and examine you, and I'll then tell you what I feel'.*

 Not everyone who is tall and slim will have Marfanoid habitus. Marfanoid habitus includes a constellation of features, such as tall stature, long limbs, arachnodactyly, joint hypermobility, kyphoscoliosis, pectus carinatum or excavatum, hind-foot deformity and high-arched palate. It may suggest a heritable connective tissue disorder, like Marfan syndrome, Ehlers-Danlos syndrome (EDS), Loeys-Dietz syndrome (LDS) or homocystinuria. These conditions are caused by mutations of genes that code for various proteins in connective tissues. If your examination confirms that he has Marfanoid habitus, it is likely that he has one of these conditions, as they all can present with pneumothorax. Of these, Marfan's syndrome and the hypermobile variant of EDS are the most common, each with incidence of around 1:5000. Diagnosis of a heritable connective tissue disease is important because of its implications for genetic counselling, monitoring of complications and obtaining insurance.

DOI: 10.1201/9781003430230-51

Marfan syndrome is caused by a mutation of FBN1 gene on chromosome 15, which codes for fibrillin 1, an extra-cellular matrix protein that provides elasticity to connective tissues (easily remembered as the 3Fs: FBN1, Fibrillin and chromosome Fifteen). As fibrillin is a structural protein, Marfan syndrome is inherited in an autosomal dominant manner. The phenotype is characterised by skeletal, ocular and cardiovascular manifestations (*see Box 51.1*).

BOX 51.1   CLINICAL MANIFESTATIONS OF MARFAN SYNDROME

- Hypermobility of joints, kyphoscoliosis, pectus excavatum or carinatum, hindfoot deformity (pes planus ± valgus), arachnodactyly, increased arm span (arm span to height >1.05), reduced upper to lower segment ratio (<0.85).
- Ectopia lentis (subluxation of lens), Myopia of >3 dioptres.
- Aortic root dilatation, aortic dissection, mitral valve prolapse and regurgitation, aortic valve regurgitation.
- Spontaneous pneumothorax, apical blebs and bullae.
- Dolichocephaly (longer head), enophthalmos, malar hypoplasia, high-arched palate.

EDS is an umbrella term that is used for 13 clinically and genetically heterogeneous conditions. It is due to defective synthesis and processing of collagen. All subtypes are characterised by (a) abnormalities of skin (e.g. skin hyperextensibility, easy bruising, atrophic scarring, poor wound healing), (b) joint hypermobility and (c) tissue fragility, which in extreme cases can cause rupture of blood vessels or organs (e.g. gravid uterus, intestine).

LDS is caused by mutations of genes that code for transforming growth factor-β (TGF-β). It is characterised by (a) more severe cardiovascular manifestations, such as widespread aortic (not just the root as in Marfan syndrome) and arterial aneurysms and tortuosity, (b) hypertelorism (widely spaced eyes) and (c) bifid uvula and cleft palate. Ectopia lentis is typically absent (this is a key distinguishing feature from Marfan's syndrome). Homocystinuria is least likely, as it usually presents early in life, and clinical features include mental retardation, seizures, thrombosis and osteoporosis. Interestingly, the direction of lens dislocation is downwards and inwards in homocystinuria, whereas it is upwards and outwards in Marfan syndrome.

Further questions to ask:

- Obtain a *family history*.
- Ask if he has *previously had pneumothorax*.
- Ask about *cardiac symptoms* like shortness of breath, palpitations, dizziness on standing up or syncope.

Note: These symptoms may be caused by valvular heart disease. Some patients may have postural orthostatic tachycardia syndrome (POTS), which causes postural dizziness or syncope due to the inability of blood vessels to constrict upon standing up.

- Ask if he has *joint pain*. Is he *double-jointed* or do the *joints get easily dislocated*?
- Ask if his *skin* stretches easily. Does he bruise easily or do the wounds heal poorly?
- Ask if he is *short-sighted*.
- Complete the *rest of the history*.

Ask about his other medical problems, regular medications, smoking habit, occupation and hobbies (e.g. diving).

*His **father is tall**, but he is healthy and not known to have any medical conditions. His father has one sister, who is well. He has no siblings. His medical history is blameless, and he has never had a pneumothorax before. He denies chest pain, breathlessness, palpitations, dizziness or syncope. He is **double-jointed** but his joints have never been painful. His skin is normal. He is **short-sighted**, and his power is 2 dioptres on both sides. He does not take any medication. He has never smoked. He has just graduated in engineering. He has no hobbies.*

WHAT SHOULD YOU LOOK FOR ON EXAMINATION?

You should

- Look for '**Marfanoid' features**. Ask for his arm span and height, and upper to lower segment ratio.

Examine the (a) hands and wrists for thumb sign and wrist sign (*see below*), (b) sternum for pectus carinatum or excavatum, (c) spine for kyphoscoliosis and (d) legs for hind-foot valgus deformity.

Notes:

1. Positive wrist sign and thumb sign would suggest arachnodactyly (means 'spider-like' long and slender fingers). Wrist sign is positive if the tip of the thumb overlaps the entire fingernail of the fifth finger when wrapped around the contralateral wrist. Thumb sign is positive when the entire distal phalanx of the adducted thumb extends beyond the ulnar border of the palm.
2. In people with Marfanoid habitus, the arm span to height ratio is more than 1.05, and the upper to lower segment ratio is reduced to less than 0.85 because of long legs (upper segment is head to symphysis pubis, and lower segment is symphysis pubis to the sole).

- *Inspect the face*, *eyes and mouth*.

Certain facial features may offer a clue (e.g. dolichocephaly in Marfan syndrome, hypertelorism in LDS). Look at the eyes for iridodonesis (tremulousness of the iris during eye movement due to subluxation of lens), and mouth for high-arched palate, cleft palate and bifid uvula.

- Check for *joint hypermobility* (*see Box 51.2*).

BOX 51.2   BEIGHTON SCORE TO ASSESS JOINT HYPERMOBILITY[†]

- Passive hyperextension of the fifth metacarpophalangeal joint beyond 90 degrees.
- Passive apposition of the thumb to the flexor aspect of the forearm.
- Passive hyperextension of the elbow beyond 10 degrees.
- Passive hyperextension of the knee beyond 10 degrees.
- Ability to flex the spine with the knees fully extended so that the palms of the hands rest flat on the ground.

[†] Maximum score is 9 (the first four elements are given two points each, as they are checked on both sides). A score of ≥4 indicates joint hypermobility due to ligamentous laxity.

■ *Examine the skin* for hyperextensibility, atrophic scars and striae.

Gently pull the skin at the hairless volar aspect of the wrist or forearm until resistance is met. If the skin can be stretched >1.5 cm, it indicates hyperextensibility. In EDS, the scars widen over time, giving rise to the characteristic 'cigarette paper scars'.

■ *Auscultate the heart*.

Auscultate over the mitral area for mid-systolic click and late systolic murmur, and aortic area for regurgitant murmur.

*He is 182 cm tall. His **arm span is 1.06 and upper to lower segment ratio is 0.82**. Wrist sign is positive but thumb sign is negative. He has **pectus excavatum**. There is no kyphoscoliosis or hind-foot defor-mity. There are no characteristic facial features, or iridodonesis. He has a **high-arched palate**. There is evidence of joint hypermobility, with **Beighton score of 6/9**. His skin looks normal, with no evidence of hyperextensibility. Heart sounds are normal, with no added sounds or murmurs.*

Examination has confirmed that he has Marfanoid habitus. EDS is unlikely because of the absence of skin hyperextensibility, and he does not seem to have any phenotypic features of LDS.

It is likely that he has Marfan syndrome but this cannot be diagnosed yet. *In patients with a positive family history* (the family member should also satisfy the criteria for diagnosis), Marfan syndrome can be diagnosed if any of the following is present:

■ Aortic root dilatation (Z-score ≥ 2).
■ Ectopia lentis.
■ Systemic score ≥7 (the systemic score is calculated based on skeletal manifestations, pneumo-thorax, myopia, skin striae and facial features).

In the absence of a family history, the patient should satisfy one of the following criteria:

■ Aortic root dilatation *plus* ectopia lentis.
■ Aortic root dilatation *plus* systemic score ≥7.
■ Aortic root dilatation *plus* FBN1 mutation.
■ Ectopia lentis *plus* FBN1 mutation with previous aortic involvement.

His family history cannot be considered relevant unless his father is clinically assessed and found to satisfy the diagnostic criteria for Marfan syndrome. The patient should be referred for an echocardiogram to check for aortic root dilatation, and slit lamp examination to check for ectopia lentis. His systemic score is 5 (one point each for positive wrist sign, pectus excavatum and long limbs, and two points for pneumothorax). A systemic score of 7 will be useful to make a diagnosis if (a) he has no evidence of aortic root dilatation or ectopia lentis, but his father satisfies the diagnostic criteria for Marfan syndrome, *or* (b) he has aortic root dil-atation, but no ectopia lentis or positive family history. An X-ray of the pelvis can then be requested to check for protrusio acetabuli (2 points), and if this is normal, MRI of pelvis to check for dural ectasia (2 points).

WHAT SHOULD YOU TELL THE PATIENT?

You should tell him that

■ You suspect he has Marfan syndrome.

'I wonder if you have a condition called Marfan syndrome. It is one of the conditions that can cause pneumothorax. In our body, we have connective tissues that connect different parts together. In Marfan

syndrome, the connective tissues become weak and stretchy because of a faulty gene. This may be the reason why you are double-jointed and your breast bone is sunken into your chest'.

▪ You would refer him for an echocardiogram and slit lamp examination of the eyes.

'I need more information from a couple of tests before I can say for sure that you have Marfan syndrome. One is a scan of your heart to see if the aorta, the big blood vessel that leaves the heart, is enlarged. The second is an eye test to check if the lens in your eye has moved out of its normal place. If these tests show that your aorta is enlarged and the lens has moved out of its place, it'll confirm that you have Marfan syndrome. If not, we'll have to do a blood test to check if you have the faulty gene'.

▪ It is important to diagnose Marfan syndrome so that he can be monitored for complications.

'It is important to know if you have Marfan syndrome so that we can monitor you for possible complications. People with this condition need regular heart scans, as the aorta could progressively widen and increase the risk of developing a tear on its inner lining. Medications are available to slow down the widening of the aorta, which I will discuss after you have had the heart scan'.

▪ There is a risk of recurrence of pneumothorax. The respiratory physician will discuss measures to reduce this risk.

'You are at risk of developing pneumothorax again. The lung specialist will discuss measures to reduce this risk'.

▪ You will refer him to a geneticist, if the diagnosis is confirmed. His father and aunt should be assessed as well.

'If you do have Marfan syndrome, there is a 50% chance that your children will inherit this from you. If we confirm the diagnosis, I will refer you to a genetic specialist who will discuss this with you. Your father and aunt should be assessed as well'.

▪ You will book an appointment to see him in clinic to discuss the test results.

OUTCOME

---

*He is discharged later that day. His 2D echocardiogram reveals **aortic root dilatation**, **with a Z score of 2.74**. There is no mitral valve prolapse or aortic regurgitation. Slit lamp examination shows **upward and outward subluxation of the lens on both sides**. He is commenced on a β-blocker and losartan in an attempt to slow the progression of aortic root enlargement. CT scan of the lungs shows **apical blebs**. The respiratory physician arranges pleurodesis. He is referred to the geneticist and advised to get his father and aunt assessed for Marfan syndrome.*

Marfan syndrome can be diagnosed in this patient based on the presence of both aortic root dilatation and ectopia lentis, irrespective of the family history. The presence of ectopia lentis rules out LDS, and the upward subluxation is not in keeping with homocystinuria. Aortic dissection and rupture are the most feared complications of Marfan syndrome, hence the need to do regular echocardiograms and monitor his blood pressure. Preventive aortic root surgery is usually offered when the measurement reaches 5 cm.

In Marfan syndrome, the FBN1 mutation results in excessive TGF-β signalling, which is mediated by angiotensin-II. Losartan, the angiotensin receptor blocker, has been shown to slow the progression of aortic root enlargement and is used in combination with a β-blocker. The presence of apical blebs and background history of Marfan syndrome increases his risk of recurrence of pneumothorax, hence the decision to perform pleurodesis.

The 62-Year-Old Man with Transient Right-Sided Weakness

Case 52

A 62-year-old man presents to the emergency department after a brief episode of weakness in his right upper and lower limb earlier that morning. He has fully recovered now.

His temperature is normal, pulse rate 76/minute, blood pressure is 164/102 mm Hg, respiratory rate 16/minute and oxygen saturation 98% on room air. Capillary blood glucose is 6 mmol/L.

HOW SHOULD THIS PROBLEM BE APPROACHED?

- Start with an open-ended question and find out ***what exactly happened***.

*He tells you that he was at home earlier that morning, talking to his daughter over the phone. He suddenly dropped the handset because his **right handgrip became weak and the whole of his right arm felt heavy**. His **speech became slurred** at the same time. He called his wife, and she disconnected the phone call after telling the daughter that they will call later. The wife started rubbing the arm but the heaviness was still there. After a minute or so, he stood up and tried to walk to the bedroom but **had to drag his right leg**, **as it felt heavy and weak**.*

*His wife straightaway got him into the car and drove to the hospital. When he got off the car just outside the A and E, he realised that the weakness had completely resolved and he was able to speak normally. The **whole episode probably lasted about 40 minutes**.*

Say some reassuring words before proceeding further with the history. *'That must have been really frightening for you both, but I am glad that you have fully recovered now. Please allow me to ask you a few questions and I will then try to explain what might have happened'.*

- Establish the ***extent of neurological dysfunction***.

Ask about facial weakness (*'Did you notice that your mouth was drooped on one side?'*), sensory symptoms in his limbs and face, and visual loss.

- Ask if he experienced a ***headache*** at the time.

It is pointless to ask about seizures or loss of consciousness, as he has given a very good description of the sequence of events from start to finish.

He is not sure if there was drooping of the mouth or numbness in his limbs and face. There was no headache or loss of vision.

 It is clear that he experienced an episode of transient focal neurological dysfunction that [a] started suddenly and [b] resolved quickly. The differential diagnosis is broad (*see Box 52.1*), but the most likely cause in someone of his age is a transient ischemic attack (TIA). A TIA is defined as a 'transient episode of neurological dysfunction caused by central nervous system ischaemia *without* infarction'.

BOX 52.1   CAUSES OF TRANSIENT NEUROLOGICAL DYSFUNCTION

- Transient ischaemic attack.
- Post-ictal paralysis after generalised tonic-clonic seizures.
- Hemiplegic migraine.
- Hypoglycaemia.
- Hypertensive encephalopathy.
- Multiple sclerosis.
- Chronic subdural haematoma.
- Functional.

Among the other causes, postictal paralysis can be ruled out, as his consciousness was preserved throughout. Hemiplegic migraine need not be considered in the absence of headache, and it is also unlikely to present for the first time at the age of 62. Hypoglycaemia can present with hemiplegia without other neuroglycopenic symptoms like mental obtundation or seizures, but complete recovery without receiving glucose is not possible. Although his blood pressure is elevated, hypertensive encephalopathy is unlikely, as it usually presents with altered mental state and symptoms will not resolve without anti-hypertensive treatment. A functional disorder is a diagnosis of exclusion and should not be entertained at this stage.

Further questions to ask:

- Ask if he has experienced *similar episodes in the past*.

You should not only ask about limb weakness or numbness but also loss of vision, diplopia, speech disturbance, vertigo and unsteadiness of gait (*see Box 52.2*).

- Ask about *vascular risk factors*, such as hypertension, diabetes and hyperlipidaemia.
- Ask if he *smokes*.
- Ask about *cardiac symptoms*, like chest pain, breathlessness or palpitations, and if he has previously been diagnosed with *heart problem* (source of embolism.)

*There is no history of previous episodes of neurological dysfunction. He was diagnosed with **hypertension** about ten years ago, for which he was prescribed amlodipine to take once daily. He admits that he **takes the amlodipine only when he remembers**, maybe about two to three times a week. He was last screened for diabetes and hyperlipidaemia just over a year ago and told that his 'glucose was normal and **cholesterol was high**'. He was advised to take a medication for high cholesterol, but he was not keen. He has **smoked about 10 cigarettes a day since the age of 20**. He has no cardiac symptoms. He has never been diagnosed with a heart problem.*

BOX 52.2   CLINICAL MANIFESTATIONS OF A TRANSIENT ISCHEMIC ATTACK

An *anterior circulation TIA* (also known as carotid TIA) involves the carotid and anterior or middle cerebral artery. Patients may present with:

- Contralateral limb weakness and numbness.
- Dysphasia (if the dominant hemisphere is involved).
- Homonymous hemianopia.
- Transient ipsilateral monocular blindness (*amaurosis fugax*).

A *posterior circulation TIA* (also known as vertebrobasilar TIA) involves the vertebral, basilar or posterior cerebral arteries and their branches. They supply the occipital and medial temporal lobes, brain stem, cerebellum and thalamus. Patients may present with:

- Dizziness and vertigo, diplopia, dysarthria, dysphagia and dysmetria (the 5Ds).
- Macular sparing homonymous hemianopia *or* cortical blindness due to involvement of the occipital pole (the macula is spared, as it is supplied by middle cerebral artery).
- Crossed paralysis (ipsilateral cranial nerve palsies with contralateral hemiparesis due to brain stem involvement).

- Complete the *rest of the history*.

Ask about his other medical problems (particularly, a history of peptic ulcer disease, before starting aspirin), regular medications, alcohol consumption, use of recreational drugs (e.g. cocaine), occupation and drug allergies.

He developed gastritis after an alcoholic binge at the age of 18 but has since not had any problems with his stomach. He does not take any medication apart from amlodipine. He drinks a glass of wine with his dinner nearly every day. He has never taken recreational drugs. He has no drug allergies. He is a retired secondary school teacher.

The presence of vascular risk factors, such as smoking habit, hypertension and hyperlipidaemia, strengthens our clinical impression of a TIA. It is quite possible that he has got undiagnosed diabetes mellitus or impaired glucose tolerance as well. The distribution of his neurological symptoms points to an anterior circulation TIA due to transient occlusion of the left middle cerebral artery. In anterior circulation TIA, thrombus usually forms in the carotid and travels to anterior or middle cerebral artery. The [a] complete resolution of symptoms within a short span of time, [b] preservation of consciousness and [c] absence of headache would rule out a haemorrhagic stroke.

WHAT SHOULD YOU LOOK FOR ON EXAMINATION?

You should

- Briefly examine the *nervous system* to check for (residual) focal neurological deficits.
- Perform a focussed examination of the cardiovascular system.

Check for *irregular rhythm*, *carotid bruits* and *heart murmurs*.

*He is moderately built, **with central obesity**. A quick neurological examination reveals normal power and sensation in the limbs. There is no facial asymmetry. His speech is normal. His pulse is regular, and there are no carotid bruits or heart murmurs.*

HOW SHOULD THIS PATIENT BE INVESTIGATED?

You should ask for

- ■ ***Non-contrast computed tomography (CT) scan or magnetic resonance imaging (MRI) of the brain*** (within 24 hours of symptom onset).

The imaging modality of choice depends on local availability. CT scan of the brain is often requested in the emergency setting because of its ready availability and ability to rule out haemorrhage. An infarct can be missed on CT scan, so MRI scan should be requested if the CT scan is normal.

- ■ ***Blood tests***, including full blood count, liver function tests, serum creatinine, fasting blood glucose and lipid panel.

Note: All patients with TIA or ischemic stroke should be commenced on statin anyway, but knowledge of the lipid panel results is useful to optimise the dosage and lower the low-density lipoprotein to target.

- ■ ***12-lead electrocardiogram*** may reveal arrhythmia.

Further investigations may include

- ■ ***Telemetry*** in the inpatient setting or ***Holter monitoring*** in the outpatient setting to detect occult atrial fibrillation.
- ■ ***2D Echocardiography*** (to look for a cardiac source of embolism, like patent foramen ovale, valvular heart disease or thrombus in the heart).
- ■ ***Imaging of the carotids and cerebral circulation*** (e.g. CT angiogram, MR angiogram, carotid Doppler).

WHAT SHOULD YOU TELL THE PATIENT?

You should tell him that

- ■ His symptoms were most likely caused by a transient ischaemic attack.

'I suspect your arm and leg became weak this morning because of a temporary reduction in the blood flow to a part of your brain. We call this a mini stroke'.

- ■ A TIA results from thrombotic occlusion of a cerebral blood vessel.

'A mini stroke occurs when a blood clot blocks the blood vessel in the brain. The weakness spontaneously improves after a while because the blood clot breaks down and blood flow is restored. Blood clots like this can develop when there is fat deposition in blood vessels'.

- ■ You would arrange a CT scan, blood tests and 12-lead ECG.

'I'll ask for a brain scan, some blood tests and a tracing of your heart'.

- ■ There is a risk of further TIAs or stroke but several measures can help to reduce this risk.

'There is a risk of further mini strokes or even a full blown stroke but several measures can help to reduce this risk' (very important point).

- You would like to start him on aspirin (*'blood thinning medication'*) if the scan rules out bleeding, and a statin (*'cholesterol-lowering medication'*).
- He should take his blood pressure medications regularly.

'Taking amlodipine regularly will keep your blood pressure under control and reduce the risk of heart attack or stroke in the future'.

- He should stop smoking.

(You should impress upon him that controlling the blood pressure, stopping smoking and taking aspirin and statin would reduce the risk of further TIAs or stroke.)

- He should not drive for at least a month (in the UK).
- You will refer him to the neurologist (*'brain specialist'*).

OUTCOME

CT scan of his brain is reported as normal. His full blood count, liver function tests and serum creatinine are normal. Fasting glucose is 5.2 mmol/L. **Low-density lipoprotein is elevated at 4.2 mmol/L.** *MRI and MRA are normal, with no evidence of infarction. Carotid Doppler shows* **62% stenosis in the right carotid and 80% stenosis in the left carotid artery.** *His ABCD$_2$ score is calculated as 5 (see Box 52.3), thus placing him at a higher risk of recurrence.*

He is commenced on aspirin, clopidogrel and atorvastatin and encouraged to take amlodipine regularly. He is strongly advised to quit smoking, eat healthily and exercise regularly. His 2D echocardiogram and Holter are normal. The neurologist refers him for left carotid endarterectomy.

BOX 52.3   THE ABCD$_2$ SCORE[†]

Age	≥60 years (1)
	<60 years (0)
Blood pressure	Systolic ≥140 or diastolic ≥90 (1)
	Normotensive (0)
Clinical syndrome	Unilateral weakness (2)
	Speech disturbance (1)
	Neither (0)
Duration of symptoms	≥60 minutes (2)
	10–59 minutes (1)
	<10 minutes (0)
Diabetes	Yes (1)
	No (0)

[†] Patients with ABCD$_2$ score of ≥4 are at higher risk of developing recurrent TIA or stroke within the next 90 days. For patients with ABCD$_2$ score of ≥4, dual anti-platelet therapy with aspirin and clopidogrel is recommended for 21 days, followed by single anti-platelet therapy.

The 27-Year-Old Woman with Seizures

Case 53

You are asked to see a 27-year-old woman, who was admitted to the medical admissions unit earlier that day after an episode of seizures at home. She has been well since admission, with no further seizures.

She is alert and oriented. Her temperature is normal, pulse rate 72/minute, BP 122/68 mm Hg, oxygen saturation 96% on room air and respiratory rate 16/minute. Capillary blood glucose is 6 mmol/L.

HOW SHOULD THIS PROBLEM BE APPROACHED?

- You should obtain a detailed account of **what happened before**, **during and after the episode**. (Ideally, you should speak to someone who witnessed the episode.)

The history is crucial to clarify if the episode was due to seizures or syncope, as limb jerking can occur in both.

*She is **unable to recall much** and only found out from her husband later about what happened. She remembers going to the kitchen that morning but nothing after that. The next thing she remembers is waking in the ambulance. Her **tongue was sore** at the time.*

*She says her husband told her that he came running to the kitchen when he heard a noise. He found her on the floor, **shaking all four limbs**. She was **stiff all over**, her **eyes were rolled up**, there was **froth at the mouth** and **she had wet herself**. The whole **episode lasted less than a couple of minutes**. He called for an ambulance straightaway and the paramedics arrived within 10 minutes but she had already stopped shaking by then. She was **drowsy and confused for about 15–20 minutes** according to him.*

Her description fits with seizures. The features that point to seizures are (a) the soreness of her tongue (possibly because she bit her tongue), (b) prolonged postictal drowsiness and confusion and (c) her inability to recall anything about the incident.

Tongue biting is not common but it is fairly specific for seizures. Patients with seizures bite their tongue because of stiffness and rhythmic jerking of the jaw muscles, combined with lack of awareness. This does not happen in patients with syncope, as their muscle tone is reduced during the episode. Postictal drowsiness or confusion occurs because of the time it takes for the brain to be reset after the period of excessive neuronal discharge. Patients with syncope usually regain consciousness within 1–2 minutes because the blood flow to the brain is restored as soon as the supine position is assumed.

DOI: 10.1201/9781003430230-53

In patients with suspected seizures, there are three key questions to ask:

Question 1: *What type of seizure is this?*

Knowing the type of seizure will help to choose an appropriate drug (*see Figure 53.1*). Seizures are classified based on the following:

- Onset of seizure activity in the brain.

Focal seizures begin on one side of the brain, whereas *generalised seizures* begin on both sides simultaneously. If the seizure activity begins on one side and then spreads to the other, it is known as *focal to bilateral seizure*. If the onset is not known, it falls into the *unknown onset category*.

- Level of awareness during a seizure.

Focal seizures may or may not affect awareness and are accordingly classified as *focal aware* (previously known as simple partial seizures) or *focal impaired awareness* (previously known as complex partial seizures). Generalised seizures, on the other hand, always affect awareness.

- Presence or absence of motor symptoms.

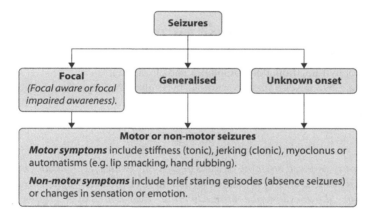

FIGURE 53.1   Simple classification of seizures.

Based on this classification, it appears that this woman had generalised tonic-clonic seizures. The seizure activity could have begun on both sides of the brain simultaneously (generalised) *or* begun on one side and then spread to the other (focal to bilateral). Patients with generalised seizures may report 'aura', which is essentially a focal aware seizure. The aura may be an unusual smell or taste, strange sensation in the stomach, sudden intense feeling of joy or fear, the sensation that one leg or arm is bigger or smaller than the other one *or* visual hallucinations.

She says she was well before the episode and did not experience anything unusual.

Question 2: *What is the risk of recurrence of the seizures?*

This is probably the most important question from the patient's perspective. Epilepsy is the tendency to develop seizures, or the occurrence of more than one seizure, at least 24 hours apart. Anti-epileptic drug therapy is indicated in patients at higher risk of recurrent seizures. The following questions will help to decide the risk of recurrence:

- Ask *if she has had similar episodes before* (would point to epilepsy).

The first seizure may not be the first! It is important to not only ask about previous generalised tonic-clonic seizures but also about absence seizures, myoclonic jerks or episodes of *deja-vu* (only family members or friends may be able to provide this information).

- Obtain a *family history.*

Ask if any of her immediate family members have been diagnosed with epilepsy or seizure disorder (there is a higher risk of developing epilepsy if there is a strong family history).

- Ask relevant questions to **check if the seizures were provoked** (*see Box 53.1*).

Ask about headache, focal neurological symptoms (may be caused by structural brain lesion), recent head trauma, fever, infective symptoms, recent illnesses and history of tuberculosis.

- Obtain a **detailed drug history** (including prescription medications, 'over-the-counter' preparations and illicit drugs), and ask about her **alcohol intake**.

Note: A first seizure that is provoked by an acute brain insult (e.g. toxins, metabolic derangements, infection) is less likely to recur, whereas unprovoked seizures and seizures due to structural brain lesion (e.g. tumour, tuberculoma, scar) have a higher chance of recurrence.

BOX 53.1   PROVOKING FACTORS FOR SEIZURES

- **Toxic** (e.g. alcohol or drug withdrawal, use of illicit drugs and pro-convulsant medications, such as theophylline, tramadol, quinolones and clozapine).
- **Metabolic** (e.g. hypoglycaemia, hyperosmolar hyperglycaemia, hyponatremia, hypocalcaemia).
- **Infection** or **inflammation** (e.g. meningoencephalitis).
- **Structural brain lesion** (e.g. tumour, abscess, tuberculoma, cerebral infarct or haemorrhage).

She says she has never experienced anything like this before. She denies fever, headache and focal neurological symptoms. Her past medical history is blameless, and there is no history of head trauma, recent illnesses or previous tuberculosis. She does not take any medication, 'over-the-counter' preparations or illicit drugs. She does not smoke or drink. There is no one in her immediate family with epilepsy as far as she is aware.

Question 3: What is the risk for her in case the seizures were to recur?

- Ask about her **occupation** and **hobbies**.

Some occupations (e.g. working with machinery) or hobbies (e.g. rock climbing, scuba diving) may pose a risk to the patient in case the seizures were to recur.

- Ask if she is **pregnant or planning to get pregnant** or takes the **oral contraceptive pill**.

Some anti-epileptic drugs are teratogenic (e.g. sodium valproate, phenytoin, carbamazepine) *or* may interfere with the efficacy of the oral contraceptive pill (e.g. lamotrigine).

- Ask if she **drives** (an important question to ask in all patients with seizures.)

*She is a human resources officer in a finance company. She **drives to work** every day. She plays the flute and likes to bake but does not have any hobbies that would be considered dangerous. She is not pregnant and not planning to have a child for at least another two years. Her husband uses condoms. She does not take the oral contraceptive pill. Her last menstrual period was a week ago.*

Based on the history, it appears that her seizures were unprovoked but the relevant blood tests should be requested to rule out metabolic derangements. Her occupation or hobbies would not pose a threat to her safety in case the seizures were to recur. She should be advised to temporarily stop driving (should be seizure-free for 12 months in the UK for non-commercial vehicles but this rule may be different in other countries).

WHAT SHOULD YOU LOOK FOR ON EXAMINATION?

You should

- Perform a *general examination*.
- Check for any *injuries* that she may have sustained when she fell. Inspect her *tongue*.
- Check for signs of *meningism* and perform a quick screen for *focal neurological deficits*.

Offer to *examine the fundus* to check for papilledema.

General examination is unremarkable. There are no obvious injuries. There is no evidence of bite mark on the tongue. There are no signs of meningism. The fundus could not be examined properly, as the pupils are not dilated. There are no focal neurological deficits.

HOW SHOULD THIS PATIENT BE INVESTIGATED?

You should request

- *Blood tests*, including full blood count, glucose, liver function tests, serum creatinine and electrolytes, serum calcium, phosphate and magnesium.

These tests may identify provoking factors (although the yield is generally very low) *or* serve as a baseline before anti-epileptic drug therapy is commenced.

- A *12-lead electrocardiogram*, as cardiac syncope can cause hypoxic seizures.
- An *electro-encephalogram* (EEG).

The EEG should ideally be performed within 24 hours (the yield is lower if it is delayed). Epileptiform discharges can help to predict recurrence. EEG is also useful to differentiate idiopathic generalised and focal seizures. If the EEG is normal and the diagnosis is in doubt, a sleep-deprived EEG (usually requested by the neurologist) is useful, as it may pick abnormalities that are not detected on a standard EEG.

- *Brain imaging* (preferably, magnetic resonance imaging (MRI), *or* computed tomography scan if MRI is not available).

Brain imaging is useful to look for structural lesions, like tumour, abscess, tuberculoma, old infarct or haemorrhage. The goal of imaging is to identify a lesion that can explain the seizure. It is especially indicated in patients with focal, focal to bilateral or unknown onset seizures and those with focal neurological deficits. It can be omitted in patients with clinical and EEG evidence of idiopathic generalised seizures.

- *Lumbar puncture* is indicated in patients with suspected meningoencephalitis or sub-arachnoid haemorrhage but should only be done if CT scan of the brain is normal.
- *Toxicology screen* (if drug toxicity is suspected).

WHAT SHOULD YOU TELL THE PATIENT?

You should tell her that

- Her presentation is due to seizures.

'I would like to speak to your husband to get a corroborative account but based on what you have told me, I suspect you had fits this morning. Fits occur because of excessive discharge of signals from the brain'.

- Seizures may be secondary to a variety of medical conditions.

'In most people with fits, we do not know why they happen. In some people, there may be an underlying cause like brain infection, stroke, alcohol or low glucose'.

- You would like to arrange some investigations.

'I'll ask for a brain scan and some blood tests to check if there is an underlying medical problem that may have caused the fits. I'll also ask for an electrical tracing of the brain, as it can tell us what type of fits you had and if they are likely to happen again'.

- You will ask a neurologist (*'brain specialist'*) to see her.
- You would like to keep her in hospital overnight. If there are no further seizures, she should be able to go home on the following morning.
- She should not drive pending further advice from the neurologist.

'Because the fits could happen again, you should temporarily stop driving. It would be disastrous if you get fits while driving'.

- She should restrict recreational activities that would pose a risk to herself.

'You should not do anything that would pose a risk to yourself in case the fits were to happen again, like swimming alone, for example'.

- You will talk to her again when the test results are back.

OUTCOME

*The husband arrives later and a corroborative history is obtained. His account of events is consistent with what she described. On further questioning, he recalls that **she sometimes stares blankly**. He did not make much of those episodes, as they usually lasted less than 20 seconds and she would become normal thereafter. This has happened about six to seven times in the last two years that he has known her. He has never observed any limb jerking, head turning or lip smacking during those episodes.*

*All her blood test results are normal. The **EEG shows generalised epileptiform discharges**. The CT scan of the brain is reported as normal. MRI scan is not done. The neurologist commences her on lamotrigine after detailed counselling. She is discharged home on the following morning.*

The blank staring episodes were most likely focal impaired awareness seizures, which suggests that this is not her first seizure. The MRI scan was omitted because of the history of possible absence seizures and generalised epileptiform discharges on the EEG. She is at higher risk of recurrence, hence the decision to commence an anti-epileptic drug (lamotrigine).

The 35-Year-Old Woman with Headache   Case 54

A 35-year-old woman is referred to the medical clinic with a three-month history of headache.

HOW SHOULD THIS PROBLEM BE APPROACHED?

---

*She tells you that she has been troubled with this **headache for the last three months**. It is there most of the time and seems to be gradually **getting worse**. She has never suffered with headaches before.*

Headaches are broadly classified into primary and secondary depending on whether or not there is an underlying organic cause. Primary headaches like migraine and tension headache account for the vast majority (>90%) that are seen in primary care or outpatient setting. In this patient, it is important to look for a secondary cause (*see Box 54.1*), as she presents with a short history of gradually worsening headache.

The pathophysiology of headache involves (a) traction or distension of intracranial pain-sensitive structures like dura mater, large blood vessels and venous sinuses, (b) spasm of the muscles around the head and neck *or* (c) inflammation of the mucous membranes of paranasal sinuses. There are no pain receptors in the pia or arachnoid mater, brain parenchyma and skull.

BOX 54.1   UNDERLYING CAUSES OF HEADACHE ('SECONDARY HEADACHE')

Intracranial

- Head trauma (resulting in intracranial haemorrhage).
- Meningeal inflammation (e.g. bacterial or tuberculous meningitis, subarachnoid haemorrhage).
- Raised ICP (e.g. tumour, abscess, haematoma, obstructive hydrocephalus, cerebral venous sinus thrombosis, *IIH*).

Extra-cranial

- Giant cell arteritis (in patients >50 years of age).
- Acute narrow angle glaucoma.
- Sinusitis.
- Dental problem.
- Cervical spondylosis.
- Medications that cause vasodilatation (e.g. calcium channel blockers, nitrates).

DOI: 10.1201/9781003430230-54

- *Ask further about the headache.*

Ask about the location and whether it radiates, character of the pain, severity (grades 1–10), aggravating and relieving factors and associated symptoms.

Note: You should specifically ask if the headache is worse when she bends forward, coughs or lies in bed.

- Screen for *focal neurological symptoms* (*see Box 54.2*).
- Ask if she has ever *blacked out or had seizures*.

BOX 54.2   FOCAL NEUROLOGICAL SYMPTOMS

- Limb and/or facial weakness and numbness.
- Unsteadiness of gait or clumsiness.
- Loss of vision and diplopia.
- Hearing loss and vertigo.
- Problems with speech, swallowing, and bladder and bowel control.

---

*She feels the pain **over her forehead** on both sides. It does not radiate anywhere. It is a **dull discomfort**, usually around grades 4–5/10. The headache is **worse when she coughs or bends forward**. The pain sometimes **disturbs her sleep** but it gradually improves after she sits up. She occasionally **feels sick with the pain** but has not vomited. She denies focal neurological symptoms. She has never blacked out or had fits.*

The aggravation of headache with coughing, bending forward and recumbency is concerning and suggests that her headache may be due to raised intracranial pressure (ICP).

The skull is a rigid structure that encloses the brain, cerebrospinal fluid (CSF) and blood. An increase in the volume of any of these components will increase the ICP: (a) increased brain volume (e.g. benign and primary or secondary malignant tumours, cerebral abscess, haematoma, large tuberculoma), (b) increased CSF volume (e.g. obstructive hydrocephalus from tumours or meningeal inflammation, idiopathic intracranial hypertension [IIH]) *or* (c) increased blood volume (e.g. cerebral venous sinus thrombosis).

Cerebral oedema due to a variety of acute insults (e.g. traumatic brain injury, infection, stroke, malignant hypertension, hepatic or uraemic encephalopathy, hyponatremia, hypercapnia) can also raise the ICP but need not be considered in this patient because of the longer duration of symptoms.

Further questions should explore the features that may suggest an underlying cause for raised ICP. You should ask about

- *Trauma to the head*, prior to the onset of her headache.
- *Fever*, *night sweats*, *weight loss* and *history of tuberculosis*.
- *Symptoms that may suggest cancer* (e.g. haemoptysis, breast lump, change in bowel habit).
- Her other medical problems, particularly a *previous diagnosis of cancer or thrombosis*.
- *Medications* taken.
- Ask what *analgesics* she takes for her headache and how often.

Note: Analgesic overuse may be associated with headache ('medication overuse headache').

- *Stressors* at home or work.
- Her *concerns and expectations*.

*There was no trauma to her head prior to the onset of headache. She denies fever or sweats. She has always been **overweight since her teenage years**, and her weight has not changed recently. Her only medical problem is **acne**, for which she has been taking **minocycline** for the last six months. This was* *suggested by her dermatologist, as topical treatments were not helpful and she did not want to try isotret-inoin. Review of systems is unremarkable. She was previously healthy, and there is no history of tuber-culosis, cancer or blood clots.*

*She tried paracetamol for her headache but stopped it after a while because it was not so helpful. She does not smoke or drink. She has four children, aged between 14 and 5. She has been sterilised, and her last menstrual period was ten days ago. She does office work and her job is not particularly stressful. She is concerned about her headache, as **her aunt, who had similar symptoms, was eventually diag-nosed with a brain tumour**.*

The recent initiation of minocycline for acne and her increased body weight are relevant and point to IIH. IIH occurs due to impaired CSF absorption from the sub-arachnoid space across the arachnoid villi into dural sinuses. More than 90% of patients with IIH are overweight women in their third or fourth decade of life. Apart from minocycline, several other drugs such as isotretinoin, human growth hormone and vita-min A are known to cause IIH. This condition was previously known as benign intracranial hypertension but this term is no longer used, as it is not really benign and can potentially lead to permanent visual loss. IIH is diagnosed on the basis of elevated CSF pressure after excluding other causes of raised ICP, such as brain tumour, hydrocephalus and venous sinus thrombosis.

She is understandably anxious because of the diagnosis of brain tumour in her aunt, who had similar symptoms. This should be addressed sympathetically.

WHAT SHOULD YOU LOOK FOR ON EXAMINATION?

You should

- Examine her *fundus* to check for papilledema, *eye movements* for evidence of third or sixth nerve palsy and *visual fields* for evidence of hemianopia.
- Perform a quick *neurological examination* to check for focal neurological deficits.
- Ask for her *blood pressure*.
- Offer to perform a thorough *general examination* to detect evidence of malignancy (e.g. breast mass, hepatomegaly, lymphadenopathy).

*There is evidence of **bilateral papilledema**. Her near visual acuity and eye movements are normal. There is no evidence of hemianopia, or weakness or numbness in her limbs or face. Her blood pressure is 132/84 mm Hg. The rest of the examination is unremarkable.*

HOW SHOULD THIS PATIENT BE INVESTIGATED?

- The investigation of choice is *magnetic resonance imaging (MRI) of her brain* with *magnetic resonance venogram (MRV)* (MRI plus MRV).

The MRV should be requested to rule out cerebral venous sinus thrombosis.

- If MRI scan cannot be obtained soon, ask for an urgent *computed tomography (CT) scan of her brain* (with contrast).
- (If the MRI or CT scan do not show any evidence of tumour) perform a *lumbar puncture* to measure the opening pressure and analyse the CSF.

WHAT SHOULD YOU TELL THE PATIENT?

You should tell her that

- Her headache is due to raised ICP.

'I suspect your headache is caused by increased pressure in the brain. This is the reason why your head-ache is worse when you cough, bend forward or lie down. I found some swelling of the nerve at the back of your eye on both sides, which is also in keeping with this'.

- This is possibly due to IIH.

'I wonder if this is due to the antibiotic pill that you are taking for acne. Being overweight can also contribute to the problem or make it worse'.

- You would arrange an urgent brain scan to exclude a brain tumour.

'I'd however like to arrange an urgent brain scan to be absolutely sure that the raised pressure is not due to a growth in the brain. I'll ask for the scan to be done urgently so that we can get the answers quickly and put your mind to rest'.

- The scan will also help to rule out cerebral venous sinus thrombosis (*'blood clots in the brain'*).
- She should stop taking the minocycline (key advice.)
- You will refer her to a neurologist (*'brain specialist'*.)
- If the scan is normal, the neurologist might suggest a lumbar puncture.

'If the brain scan is normal, the specialist may suggest a minor procedure called lumbar puncture. A needle will be inserted into the lower end of your backbone to collect some fluid that surrounds the spinal cord. This test will help to confirm the increased pressure in the brain'.

She should be advised to lose weight but it is best to discuss this after she has had the brain scan.

OUTCOME

*The MRI and MRV are normal, with no evidence of tumour or venous sinus thrombosis. She is referred to a neurologist, who arranges a lumbar puncture. Her **CSF pressure is 32 cm H₂O** (normal 8–20 cm H₂O). CSF examination is normal. She is diagnosed with IIH.*

She is advised to stop the minocycline and lose weight. She is commenced on acetazolamide. She manages to lose 12 kg over the next six months. Her headache gradually improves, and she eventually stops the acetazolamide.

IIH was diagnosed in this patient based on the normal MRI scan and elevated CSF pressure. Management includes (a) weight loss and (b) discontinuation of the offending drug. Other options include (c) acetazol-amide (carbonic anhydrase inhibitor), (d) repeated lumbar punctures (to reduce CSF pressure), (e) optic nerve sheath fenestration (to reduce the pressure of CSF around the optic nerve) and (f) ventriculoperito-neal or lumboperitoneal shunt (to divert CSF into the peritoneal cavity).

The 26-Year-Old Woman with Headache   **Case 55**

A 26-year-old woman presents with a 2-year history of headache.

HOW SHOULD THIS PROBLEM BE APPROACHED?

---

*She says she has been getting a **headache** for the last two years. It comes roughly every two to three months and lasts about two to three days each time. She is asymptomatic between the episodes.*

The long history of recurrent brief episodes is in keeping with primary headache (e.g. migraine, tension headache). A secondary cause (e.g. tumour, infection, bleeding, cerebral venous sinus thrombosis, idiopathic intracranial hypertension) is unlikely, as she is asymptomatic between episodes. However, she should be asked to clarify if the headache is always there and gets worse every few months *or* she is truly asymptomatic except during times when she has the headache.

- *Ask further about her headache.*

Ask about the location and whether it radiates, character of the pain, severity (grades 1–10), aggravating and relieving factors and associated symptoms (e.g. nausea, photophobia, phonophobia).

- Ask what *triggers* these headaches.

Common triggers for migraine are foods like cheese, chocolate or wine, sleep deprivation, irregular meals, dehydration and menstruation.

- Ask if she experiences any *aura or prodromal symptoms* (e.g. temporary visual changes, irritability, food cravings, strange smell, tingling).

Note: Migraine that is preceded by aura is called classical migraine (some patients may just experience aura without the headache), and migraine without aura is called common migraine.

*She confirms that she is asymptomatic between the brief episodes of headache. The pain usually occurs either on the **right or left side of the head**, and never on both sides at the same time. It is **throbbing** in nature and can get to about **grades 8–9/10**. She **feels sick** with the headache and usually **switches off the lights** at the time. She is not sure what triggers these headaches. She does not get prodromal symptoms. The headache is not related to her menstrual cycle.*

DOI: 10.1201/9781003430230-55

Further questions to ask:

- Check for features that may suggest **raised intracranial pressure** (e.g. headache worse with bending forward, coughing or lying in bed) and **focal neurological symptoms**.
- Ask about symptoms of **sinusitis** ('pain over the cheeks, blocked nose, cough and cold'), **tooth ache** and **neck pain**.

Note: Dental problem can cause headache by stimulating the trigeminal nerve.

- Ask about her **other medical problems**.
- Ask what **medications** she takes, including those for the headache.
- Is there any suggestion of **medication overuse**? Does she take the **oral contraceptive pill**?
- Ask if **anyone in her immediate family suffers from headache**.
- Ask about her occupation. Are there any **stressors at home or work**?

Her headache is not worse when she bends forward, coughs or lies in bed. She denies focal neurological symptoms, symptoms of sinusitis, tooth ache and neck pain.

*Her medical history is otherwise blameless. She does not take the oral contraceptive pill or any other medication. She **takes paracetamol only when she gets the headache**, and it helps to a certain extent. She does not smoke and drinks alcohol only socially. Her last menstrual period was three weeks ago. Her **aunt suffers from migraine**. She works in a day nursery as a childminder. She is single and shares a flat with a work colleague. She denies any stresses at home or work.*

 Her history is in keeping with migraine (*see Box 55.1*) as the pain is (a) unilateral, (b) throbbing in nature, (c) associated with nausea and photophobia and (d) it lasts less than three days each time. There are no features to suggest a secondary cause. Tension headache can also present with episodic headache but the pain is felt as a band around the head on both sides, and it is usually brought on by tension, anxiety or stress.

BOX 55.1   FEATURES OF MIGRAINE

- Commonly affects young or middle-aged women.
- Usually triggered by certain foods, sleep deprivation, menstruation ('*menstrual migraine*'), irregular meals or dehydration.
- May or may not be preceded by aura.
- Unilateral headache (the term 'migraine' is derived from hemi-cranium).

(However, in up to a third of the patients, migraine may be bilateral.)

- Throbbing or pulsating in nature.
- Associated with nausea, vomiting, photophobia and phonophobia.
- Usually lasts 4 hours to three days.

WHAT SHOULD YOU LOOK FOR ON EXAMINATION?

You should

- Perform a **focussed neurological examination**.

Examine her visual acuity, look at the fundus for evidence of papilledema and check her eye movements.

- Ask for her **blood pressure**.

Examination is completely normal. There is no evidence of papilledema, and her visual acuity and eye movements are normal. Her blood pressure is 124/76 mm Hg.

WHAT SHOULD YOU TELL THE PATIENT?

You should tell her that

- Her headache is due to migraine.

'I suspect your headache is due to migraine. Migraine can be distressing but it is not serious. I do not feel that your headache is caused by a problem in the brain like tumour, infection or bleeding'.

- The cause of migraine is not known.

'We do not know what causes migraine. It may be due to a problem in the nerves that carry pain signals to the brain'.

- There is *'no need for a brain scan or blood tests'*.
- It is possible to reduce the recurrence of headache by identifying the triggers and avoiding them.

'Migraine tends to recur, and it is often triggered by certain foods. I would suggest that you keep a diary to see if you can relate it to some food. Not getting enough sleep at night, not eating regularly and not consuming enough fluids can also trigger migraine attacks. You should make sure you get enough sleep at night, eat regularly and keep yourself hydrated'.

- You would recommend a simple analgesic or non-steroidal anti-inflammatory medication along with an anti-emetic for the headache and nausea.

'You can either continue to take paracetamol or try an anti-inflammatory medication for the headache, but you should take it as soon as the headache begins. I will prescribe a sickness pill to take along with the painkiller'.

- If the headaches increase in frequency, prophylactic medications can be tried.

'If your headaches keep coming on more often, we can try medications to prevent them. These medications should be taken every day and not just when the pain occurs'.

- You will see her again in a few months to see how she is getting on.

OUTCOME

She accepts the explanation, and the decision to not investigate further with a brain scan. She maintains a diary and notes that sleep deprivation or eating too much chocolate triggers her headaches. She improves her sleep and cuts down her intake of chocolate, and the headaches reduce in frequency.

The 71-Year-Old Man with Dizziness   **Case 56**

A 71-year-old man presents to the emergency department with a two-day history of dizziness. His temperature is normal, pulse rate 76/minute, blood pressure 152/98 mm Hg, respiratory rate 16/minute and oxygen saturation 96% on room air.

HOW SHOULD THIS PROBLEM BE APPROACHED?

Patients may use the term dizziness to describe light headedness or pre-syncope, disequilibrium (loss of balance) *or* vertigo.

- It is therefore important to *first ask him to clarify what he means by dizziness*.

The key question to ask is *whether the room spins around him*. This will help to decide if the dizziness is vertiginous or non-vertiginous.

He says the room spins around him.

- Having established that his dizziness is due to vertigo, ask if it is *episodic or continuous*.

If it is episodic, *how long does each episode last*? Are they brief episodes, lasting less than a minute each time, *or* longer episodes? What *triggers* the dizziness?

- Ask if he has suffered from *vertigo in the past*.

The dizziness started suddenly two days ago. It is there more or less all the time. It becomes worse when he moves his head. He has never experienced this before.

 Vertigo results from a problem in the inner ear, vestibular nerve, vestibular nucleus in the brain stem *or* cerebellum. Vertigo is labelled as either *peripheral* or *central*, based on the anatomical structure that is involved ('peripheral' if it is inner ear or vestibular nerve, and 'central' if it is brain stem or cerebellum).

The three most common causes of recent onset vertigo are (a) benign paroxysmal positional vertigo (BPPV), (b) vestibular neuritis and (c) posterior circulation stroke (*see Figure 56.1*). BPPV is characterised by brief episodes of vertigo that are triggered by a change in head position (e.g. rolling over in bed, bending forward, looking up). All forms of vertigo will be made worse by head movement, but in BPPV, the patient is asymptomatic when the head is still, and the episodes are *triggered* by a change in head position. The vertigo lasts less than a minute each time (although the associated nausea may last longer), and

    DOI: 10.1201/9781003430230-56

nystagmus is typically *absent*. In this patient, the presentation does not suggest BPPV, as his symptoms are more or less continuous.

Both vestibular neuritis and posterior circulation stroke can present with continuous vertigo. Vestibular neuritis usually follows an upper respiratory tract infection. Although it can be incapacitating and sometimes take several weeks to months to resolve, it is self-limiting. Posterior circulation stroke, on the other hand, can lead to permanent disability or even death, and it is *the diagnosis not to miss*. Stroke should certainly be ruled out in this patient, given (a) his age, (b) the sudden onset of symptoms, (c) absence of previous episodes of vertigo and (d) high blood pressure. Posterior circulation includes the vertebrobasilar territory, which supplies the brain stem, cerebellum, occipital lobe and thalamus. The mechanism of stroke is usually vertebrobasilar atherosclerosis or embolism from the heart.

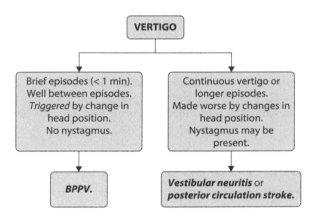

FIGURE 56.1   Simple approach to the three most common causes of vertigo.

Further questions to ask:

- Screen for **neurological symptoms**.

Ask about weakness, numbness or paraesthesia, the 5Ds (dizziness, diplopia, dysphagia, dysarthria and dysmetria), unsteadiness of gait, headache and hiccoughs.

- Check if he has **risk factors for vascular disease**, such as hypertension, diabetes, hyperlipidaemia and smoking habit, and ask if he has previously had a **stroke or heart attack**.
- Ask about **cardiac symptoms** (e.g. chest pain, breathlessness, palpitations, syncope).

Is he known to have an **irregular heartbeat**?

- Ask if he has (or recently had) **symptoms of respiratory tract infection** (e.g. fever, cough, rhinorrhoea, sore throat, breathlessness).
- Ask if he has **hearing loss, tinnitus, nausea or vomiting**.

Note: Hearing loss occurs in Meniere's disease or labyrinthitis but it is not specific for peripheral vertigo and will not help to rule out a stroke.

- What **medications** does he take?

Several medications, such as sedatives, hypnotics, anti-psychotics, anti-hypertensives, anti-diabetics, anti-epileptics and aminoglycosides can cause dizziness or vertigo.

- Does he **drive a vehicle**?

He denies weakness or numbness in his face and limbs, problems with vision, swallowing or speech, headache and hiccoughs. He has not become clumsy. He is able to stand unaided but he has not attempted to walk since his symptoms began. He denies current or recent symptoms of respiratory illness, hearing loss, tinnitus, nausea or vomiting.

*His medical problems include **hypertension and hyperlipidaemia**. He is not a known diabetic. He takes **nifedipine and atorvastatin** daily. He does not take any other medication or 'over-the-counter' preparation. He has never had a stroke or heart attack. He is not known to have an irregular heartbeat. He **has smoked 10 cigarettes/day for the last 50 years**. He drinks a glass of wine about two to three times a week. He is a retired chemical engineer. He lives with his wife, who is well. He **drives a car** but only to the supermarket or to visit friends.*

Posterior circulation stroke should be considered, given the presence of risk factors such as hypertension, hyperlipidaemia and smoking habit. The absence of other neurological symptoms would not rule out a stroke, as vertigo could be the sole manifestation.

There are several less common causes of vertigo, such as Meniere's disease, vestibular migraine, multiple sclerosis and acoustic neuroma. Meniere's disease can be excluded because of the absence of previous episodes of vertigo. He is not in the right age group to develop migraine or multiple sclerosis. Acoustic neuroma usually presents with sensorineural hearing loss, and only less commonly with vertigo.

WHAT SHOULD YOU LOOK FOR ON EXAMINATION?

You should

- Perform a focussed **neurological examination**.

Check for cerebellar signs (*see Box 56.1*). Also, check the pupils and test the sensation in the face and limbs, as posterior circulation stroke can manifest with other signs (e.g. ipsilateral Horner's syndrome, hiccoughs, and loss of pain and temperature in the ipsilateral face and contralateral trunk and limbs in lateral medullary infarction due to occlusion of the posterior inferior cerebellar artery).

BOX 56.1   CEREBELLAR SIGNS

- Gaze-evoked nystagmus.
- Dysarthria ('scanning speech').
- Intention tremor.
- Dysmetria, resulting in past-pointing during the finger-nose test.
- Dysdiadochokinesia.
- Heel-shin incoordination.
- Broad-based and ataxic gait (swaying towards the side of the lesion) or truncal ataxia.

Truncal ataxia is a sign of midline cerebellar lesions.

- Hypotonia and pendular knee jerk.

- Examine the **cardiovascular system** (e.g. atrial fibrillation, heart murmur).
- The **HINTS** test (head impulse test, nystagmus and test of skew) is only indicated in patients with continuous vertigo *and* nystagmus, especially if there are no other obvious neurological symptoms or signs that suggest stroke (*see Box 56.2*).

BOX 56.2   HINTS TEST[†, ††]

- *Head impulse*

Ask the patient to fix his eyes on your nose. Move the head slowly to the right for about 20 degrees and then abruptly bring back to the centre. Repeat on the left side. Look for the presence of saccadic eye movements.

- *Nystagmus*

Ask the patient to gaze to the right and then to the left. Observe if the nystagmus is unidirectional (fast component of the nystagmus is only towards one direction, irrespective of whether the patient looks to the right or left) *or* bi-directional.

- *Test of skew*

Ask the patient to look straight ahead and then cover and uncover each eye in turn. Vertical deviation of the eye after uncovering is abnormal.

[†] Presence of *all three* of the following would suggest a peripheral cause: abnormal head impulse (occurrence of saccadic eye movements), unidirectional nystagmus and normal test of skew.
[††] Presence of *any one of the following* would suggest a central cause: normal head impulse, bi-directional nystagmus or abnormal test of skew.

- The ***Dix-Hallpike's manoeuvre*** should only be performed in patients with suspected BPPV (brief episodes of vertigo, without nystagmus).

Note: The Dix-Hallpike and HINTS should never be performed in the same patient!

*Neurological examination reveals **dysdiadochokinesia and dysmetria in the right arm**. There is no nystagmus, intention tremor or dysarthria. He is unable to walk because of vertigo but there is no heel-shin incoordination. His pupils are normal. A quick sensory examination reveals no sensory loss. His pulse is regular, and there are no heart murmurs.*

The dysdiadochokinesia and dysmetria in the right arm point to posterior circulation stroke, possibly in the right cerebellum (as cerebellar signs occur ipsilateral to the lesion).

HOW SHOULD THIS PATIENT BE INVESTIGATED?

- ***Magnetic resonance imaging*** (MRI) of the brain is more sensitive than computed tomography (CT) for all forms of ischemic stroke (especially so for posterior circulation strokes) but this may not be readily available in the acute setting.

In practice, ***CT with or without CT angiogram*** is often done initially. CT scan can help to rule out haemorrhage.

- ***Blood tests***, including full blood count, liver function tests, serum creatinine, blood glucose and lipid profile.
- ***Cardiac investigations*** to identify a source of embolism, including 12-lead ECG, 2D echocardiogram and cardiac rhythm monitoring with telemetry or Holter.

WHAT SHOULD YOU TELL THE PATIENT?

You should tell him that

- His dizziness is most likely due to stroke.

'I am concerned that your dizziness may be due to stroke. Stroke occurs when a blood clot blocks the blood vessels supplying a part of the brain. Stroke commonly causes weakness or numbness in the limbs and face but when it affects the rear end of the brain, dizziness may be the only symptom'.

- You would admit him to hospital.
- You would like to organise *'an urgent scan of the brain and some blood tests'*.
- You would refer him to the neurologist (*'brain specialist'*).
- If the scan does not show a bleed, you would like to start him on aspirin (*'blood thinning medication'*).
- If the scan confirms a stroke, he would need some cardiac investigations.

'Stroke affecting the rear end of the brain may be caused by a blood clot in the heart that travels to the brain. If the brain scan confirms the stroke, we'll arrange a heart scan to check for blood clots in your heart, and monitor the tracing of your heart'.

- You will update him once the results of the tests are available.

He should also be advised to *stop smoking* but it is best to convey this after he has had the scan, and when he is more stable. If the scan confirms the stroke, he should be advised to *temporarily stop driving*.

OUTCOME

*The CT scan rules out a haemorrhage. MRI and MR-angiogram reveal a **right cerebellar infarct**. His blood tests show fasting glucose of 5.4 mmol/L and **low-density lipoprotein of 3.6 mmol/L**. Cardiac investigations, including 12-lead ECG, 2D echocardiogram and telemetry, are unremarkable.*

He is not considered for thrombolysis or endovascular intervention, as he is past the time window. He is commenced on aspirin and advised to increase the dosages of amlodipine and atorvastatin. He is also advised to stop smoking. His vertigo gradually improves with symptomatic treatment and vestibular physiotherapy.

The 43-Year-Old Man with Facial Weakness

Case 57

A 43-year-old man presents to the casualty complaining that his face looks twisted since that morning.

HOW SHOULD THIS PROBLEM BE APPROACHED?

---

*When you greet him, you note that he is **unable to close the right eye fully**. There is **absence of wrinkles on the right half of the forehead**, **the right nasolabial fold is flattened** and the **angle of the mouth is pulled to the left**.*

*He tells you that he was alarmed when he looked in the mirror that morning, as his **face looked twisted**. His right eye was wide open and the mouth was pulled to one side.*

His description and physical signs are in keeping with right facial palsy. The facial nerve supplies all the muscles of the face (the muscles on the right half of the face are supplied by the right facial nerve, and those on the left half of the face by the left facial nerve). This would explain his inability to raise the eyebrow (occipitofrontalis) or close the eye (orbicularis oculi), and drooping of the mouth (zygomaticus major).

Once you recognise facial palsy, you should establish if it is due to upper or lower motor neurone lesion. This distinction is important because the two most common causes of acute facial weakness are ischemic stroke (upper motor neurone lesion) and Bell's palsy (lower motor neurone lesion), of which the former is a time-sensitive condition that should be treated without delay. At his age, it could be either! An upper motor neurone lesion results in weakness of only the *lower half of the face on the side opposite to the lesion*, as the upper half of the face receives innervation from both cerebral hemispheres. A lower motor lesion, on the other hand, causes *ipsilateral weakness of the entire half of the face*. In this patient, weakness of the upper half of the face (absence of forehead wrinkles and inability to close the eye) suggests a lower motor neurone lesion.

The next step is to check for associated features to further localise the lesion. The facial nerve, soon after arising from the facial nucleus in the lower pons, loops around the abducens nucleus. It then passes through the posterior fossa in company with the fifth and eighth cranial nerves, before entering the internal acoustic meatus. In the facial canal of the temporal bone, it gives rise to (a) parasympathetic fibres that supply the lacrimal and salivary glands (except parotid), (b) nerve to stapedius and (c) chorda tympani, which supplies taste sensation to the ipsilateral anterior two-thirds of the tongue. After exiting the skull, the facial nerve passes through the parotid before giving rise to branches that supply the muscles of facial expression. Hence,

- A lesion at the level of the pons (e.g. stroke) would cause contralateral hemiplegia and ipsilateral sixth and seventh nerve palsies.
- A lesion at the cerebellopontine angle (e.g. acoustic neuroma) would present with associated fifth and eighth cranial palsies.

Acoustic neuromas are slow-growing tumours that present with insidious onset of hearing loss, tinnitus and vertigo. Involvement of the seventh nerve occurs only when the tumour enlarges.

- An intracranial lesion would result in reduced tear production, hyperacusis (intolerance to sound) and loss of taste in the ipsilateral anterior two-thirds of the tongue.
- An extra-cranial lesion (e.g. parotid tumour) would only affect the muscles of facial expression. It will not result in hyperacusis or loss of taste.

Initial questions to ask:

- Ask *how rapidly the symptoms began* and at *what time he was last well*.

The onset of ischemic stroke is acute, with focal neurological deficits developing within seconds to minutes, whereas in Bell's palsy, the deficits develop over several hours.

- Screen for other *neurological symptoms*.

Ask about limb weakness and numbness, visual loss, double vision, facial numbness, hearing loss, tinnitus, vertigo, speech disturbance and dysphagia.

- Ask if he has *pain in or around the ear*.

Pain in or around the ear may be caused by herpes zoster of the geniculate ganglion (also known as Ramsay-Hunt syndrome), otitis or Bell's palsy.

- Ask if he has *lost his taste*, and if the *sounds are louder* on the affected side.

Loss of taste in the anterior 2/3rd of the tongue and hyperacusis would suggest an intracranial lesion.

- Ask if he has noticed any *lumps in the neck or face* (parotid enlargement).

*He first noticed that his face was twisted only that morning. He was **fine when he went to bed the night before**. He denies weakness or numbness in his limbs, loss of vision or double vision, hearing loss, tinnitus, vertigo or speech disturbance. He is able to swallow but the **food tends to collect between the gum and cheek on the right side**, and **saliva is drooling from the corner of his mouth**. He has been **tearing a lot from the right eye**. There is no pain in or around the ear, loss of taste or sensitivity to sounds. He has not noticed any lumps in the neck or face.*

 There are no features of a brain stem problem, like limb weakness, speech disturbance, diplopia or dysphagia. Acoustic neuroma need not be considered, as it usually presents with insidious onset of hearing loss, tinnitus and vertigo, and not with isolated facial palsy. Guillain-Barre syndrome is also unlikely, as it begins with sudden onset of flaccid weakness in the distal limbs, and facial palsy only occurs later, as the weakness ascends. Middle ear infection and cholesteatoma can be ruled out, as he has no hearing loss or ear pain.

BOX 57.1   CAUSES OF LOWER MOTOR NEURONE FACIAL PALSY[†]

- Bell's palsy (the most common cause).
- Brain stem stroke, tumour or demyelination.
- Cerebellopontine angle tumour (e.g. acoustic neuroma).
- Ramsay-Hunt syndrome (herpes zoster of the geniculate ganglion).
- Middle ear infection or cholesteatoma.
- Lyme disease.
- Sarcoidosis.
- Guillain-Barre syndrome.
- Parotid tumour or parotidectomy.

[†] In patients with bilateral facial palsy, think of Guillain-Barre syndrome, sarcoidosis or Lyme disease.

Further questions to ask (*see Box 57.1*):

- Ask if he has *cough*, *breathlessness*, *joint pain or skin rashes* (sarcoidosis).
- Ask about *recent travel or tick bites* (Lyme disease).
- Complete the *rest of the history*. Ask about his other medical problems, previous surgeries (e.g. parotidectomy), medications taken, smoking habit, alcohol consumption and occupation.

Ask particularly about hypertension and diabetes, as they are risk factors for stroke, and Bell's palsy is more common among diabetics.

- Explore his *concerns*.

The disfigurement of the face can push patients into social isolation. It is important to be aware of this and be empathetic and reassuring.

*He denies cough, breathlessness, joint pain or skin rashes. He did not travel anywhere recently and cannot recall being bitten by ticks. His medical and surgical histories are unremarkable, and he does not take any medication. He says he was tested for diabetes about a year ago and told that the result was normal. He has never smoked and drinks alcohol socially. He is a sales assistant in a home appliance shop. He is **quite upset that his face looks different**.*

WHAT SHOULD YOU LOOK FOR ON EXAMINATION?

Having already inspected the face, you should

- Complete the *examination of the seventh cranial nerve*.

Ask the patient to (a) raise the eyebrows and wrinkle the forehead, (b) shut the eyelids as tightly as he can, (c) blow the cheeks and (d) smile.

- Examine the other cranial nerves, particularly his *eye movements* (for VI nerve involvement) and *cranial nerves V and VIII*.

Note: Testing the corneal reflex is only necessary in patients with suspected acoustic neuroma (afferent for corneal reflex is V nerve and efferent is VII nerve).

- Briefly **examine the limbs** to test the strength (e.g. crossed paralysis from brain stem stroke).
- Check for **parotid enlargement**.
- Ask for his **blood pressure** (in case you wish to start him on corticosteroid).

Patients with ear pain should be referred for ENT examination to check for vesicles of herpes zoster.

*He is **unable to raise the right eyebrow, shut the right eye**, **blow the cheeks or smile**. His eye movements are full. There is no sensory loss over the face, and his hearing is normal. There is normal power in the limbs. There is no parotid enlargement. His blood pressure is 118/76 mm Hg.*

His presentation is in keeping with Bell's palsy, as there are no features of any of the known causes of facial palsy. The pathogenesis of Bell's palsy is not known but it is believed to be caused by reactivation of herpes simplex virus.

HOW SHOULD THIS PATIENT BE INVESTIGATED?

There are no specific tests to diagnose Bell's palsy.

- **Blood glucose** should be requested, as diabetes increases the risk of developing Bell's palsy. It is also a good idea to check the glucose if treatment with corticosteroid is contemplated.
- **Magnetic resonance imaging** of the brain or internal acoustic meatus is only needed in patients with other focal neurological deficits that may suggest a tumour.
- **Electromyography and nerve conduction studies** are mainly used to provide prognostic information and predict the outcome in patients with severe Bell's palsy.
- **Other investigations** to request in selected patients may include Lyme serology, tests for sarcoidosis (e.g. chest X-ray, angiotensin-converting enzyme, serum calcium, biopsy of lymph node) and audiometry in patients with hearing loss.

WHAT SHOULD YOU TELL THE PATIENT?

You should tell him that

- His face is weak because of facial nerve palsy.

'You are not able to close your right eye and the mouth is pulled to one side because of a problem with a nerve that supplies the muscles in the face. This nerve is called facial nerve'.

Note: Do not say 'your face looks twisted', although the patient described it that way.

- The most likely cause is Bell's palsy.

'We call this Bell's palsy. We do not know what causes it. It may due to a virus but no one knows for sure. There are some medical conditions that can affect the facial nerve but I haven't found any evidence of those in you'.

- There is no need for investigations apart from blood glucose.

'There is no need for X-rays or scans. I would just recommend checking your blood sugar because Bell's palsy occurs more commonly in those who have diabetes'.

- Spontaneous recovery occurs in a majority of patients (>70%) but it can take some months.

'The weakness generally improves completely without any treatment in most patients but it can take several months'.

- You would recommend a short course of corticosteroid, as it can increase the chance of recovery.

'I would recommend steroid pills for ten days as they can increase your chance of recovery. The sooner we start the steroid, the better. Steroids can make you put on weight, and increase the blood pressure and blood sugar but these side effects generally occur in those who take them for a longer period of time'.

- You would suggest an eye patch to protect the eye and lubricating eye drops.

'Your right eye is at risk of becoming dry as you are unable to close it fully. This can cause irritation and damage to the surface of the eye. I would recommend using artificial tears during the day and an ointment at night to keep it moist. I would also suggest wearing sunglasses during the day and using an eye patch at night to protect your eye'.

- You would refer him to a specialist (plastic surgeon) if there is no improvement.

'If the weakness does not improve as expected, I will refer you to a specialist'.

- You will see him again in a couple of weeks.

OUTCOME

His blood glucose is normal. He is commenced on 60 mg of prednisolone/day to take for five days and advised to taper the dose by 10 mg every day for the next five days. Four weeks later, he starts to notice an improvement in his facial weakness, and over the following two months, he recovers completely.

A majority of patients with Bell's palsy will experience a complete or near-complete recovery. A small number of patients may be left with permanent residual deficits. Patients who do not notice any improvement by six to eight weeks should be referred to a plastic surgeon. In some patients, aberrant regeneration occurs, resulting in regenerating motor neurones innervating inappropriate muscles. For example, the fibres that are intended for salivary glands may innervate the lacrimal glands, causing lacrimation while eating ('crocodile tears'). Recurrence is possible, but fortunately, rare.

It is important to start the steroid early, ideally within 72 hours from the time of onset. It is unlikely to be effective if started after seven days. The inability to close the eye can lead to eye irritation and corneal dryness, which can potentially lead to blindness. Eye protection and lubrication are therefore vital. Some patients may have to be referred to the ophthalmologist to consider tarsorrhaphy (procedure to join the upper and lower eyelids).

The 54-Year-Old Man with Tremor

Case 58

A 54-year-old man is referred to the medical clinic with a one-year history of tremor in his hands.

HOW SHOULD THIS PROBLEM BE APPROACHED?

Common causes of pathological tremor are (a) essential tremor (ET), (b) Parkinson's disease (PD), (c) hyperthyroidism and (d) cerebellar disease. There are two initial questions to ask:

- *Which parts of the body are affected?*

Tremor can involve not only the hands but also the legs, head and voice. ET usually starts in both hands at the same time. In some patients, there may be involvement of the head ('Yes-Yes' or 'No-No' tremors) or voice tremor, but the legs are never affected in isolation. PD, on the other hand, typically starts in one hand and then moves proximally before progressing to the other side. PD can also cause tremor of the legs, but not head or voice tremor.

- *Is the tremor present at rest or only when he tries to do something* (e.g. reading a newspaper, reaching out for an object)?

Tremor is broadly classified into resting and action tremor, and the latter is further sub-classified into postural and kinetic tremor (*see Figure 58.1*). Postural tremor occurs while maintaining a position against gravity (e.g. reading a newspaper), and kinetic tremor during voluntary movement (e.g. reaching out for an object).

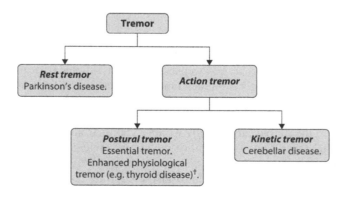

FIGURE 58.1 Classification of the causes of tremor.

† Other causes of enhanced physiological tremor include high-adrenaline states like anxiety, hypoglycaemia and alcohol withdrawal.

DOI: 10.1201/9781003430230-58

The commonest cause of rest tremor is PD, which is classically described as 'pill rolling' (as if the patient is trying to roll a pill between the forefinger and thumb). The tremor becomes less prominent during voluntary activity (patients may be able to drink from a glass of water without spilling) and worsens when the patient is distracted. The tremor of ET is absent at rest and only present when the patient stretches his hands (postural) or tries to reach for an object (kinetic).

*He tells you that the **shaking is present in both hands**. This problem **started about a year ago** in **both hands at the same time**. There is no shaking of the head or leg, or trembling of the voice. To begin with, his **hands were shaky only when he was holding the newspaper** but he is now **shaking even when he tries to pick something**. This is increasingly making it **difficult for him to perform even simple daily tasks**, like drinking from a glass of water, holding the knife and fork, brushing his teeth, shaving or putting on his clothes.*

His description is in keeping with ET, as (a) the tremors started in both hands at the same time, (b) they are postural and kinetic and (c) they are not present at rest. ET typically worsens during voluntary activity, explaining the functional difficulties that he is experiencing. Unlike Parkinson's disease (PD), tremor is the *only* abnormality in ET, and there are no other neurological symptoms or signs.

Among the other differentials, hyperthyroidism is unlikely, as patients usually present with a constellation of 'thyroid symptoms', and the tremor is never bad enough to affect the activities of daily living to this extent. Cerebellar disease also seems unlikely, as patients usually present with incoordination and unsteadiness of gait, and tremor mainly occurs while approaching a target.

Further questions to ask:

- Check for *features of Parkinsonism*.

Does he feel stiff? Has he become slower? Does he take a longer time to finish his meal or cover a certain distance while walking? Has he fallen because of loss of balance?

Note: Features of PD include (a) rigidity (cog-wheel or lead-pipe), (b) bradykinesia (reduced arm swing while walking, expressionless facies, reduced blinking, monotonous voice and small handwriting), (c) postural instability (poor balance, with risk of falls) and (d) shuffling gait. Patients with atypical Parkinsonism may have other features such as dementia, visual hallucinations, autonomic dysfunction and supranuclear palsy.

- Ask about symptoms of *thyroid disease* (e.g. diarrhoea, palpitations, weight loss, heat intolerance, neck swelling).
- Obtain a detailed *medication history*.

Dopamine antagonists like anti-psychotics and anti-emetics can cause Parkinsonism and should always be ruled out before diagnosing idiopathic PD. Other drug-induced causes of tremor include sympathomimetic drugs like β-agonists, amphetamine, cyclosporine, valproate, lithium and theophylline.

- Obtain a *family history* and ask if any other member is affected by tremor.

The family history is important because more than half of the cases of ET are familial, with an autosomal dominant inheritance.

- Complete the *rest of the history*. Ask about his other medical problems, occupation, smoking habit and alcohol consumption.

Ask specifically about the *effect of alcohol on the tremor*, as the tremor of ET may be temporarily suppressed by a small amount of alcohol.

*He does not feel that he has become stiff, slow or unsteady. There are no symptoms of thyroid disease. He takes **amlodipine for hypertension**. His medical history is otherwise unremarkable. He does not take any other medication or 'over-the-counter' preparation. He does not smoke. He drinks a glass of red wine about three to four times a week. The **tremor is indeed slightly better after a drink**. He recalls his **grandfather having similar shaking** in his hands.*

The family history of similar tremor in his grandfather and the suppression of tremors by alcohol are further pointers in favour of ET. Medication-induced tremor can be ruled out. There are no features of PD or thyroid disease.

WHAT SHOULD YOU LOOK FOR ON EXAMINATION?

- **Observe the patient at rest**, and look carefully at the hands, legs and head. Also note if there is a voice tremor.

Ask the patient to count backwards from 20 to distract him (this will make the tremor of PD more obvious).

- Ask the patient to stretch out the arms and hands to **check for a postural tremor**.
- Ask him to **drink from a glass of water**, and **check his handwriting**.

The tremor of ET worsens during voluntary activity (hence, they spill the water), while that of PD improves (they can drink without spilling). The handwriting of patients with PD is smaller, while that of those with ET is large and tremulous.

- Check for **cerebellar signs** (e.g. finger-nose test for intention tremor and past-pointing, dysdiadochokinesia, nystagmus, dysarthria, ataxic gait, heel-shin incoordination).
- In patients with rest tremor, **Check for signs of PD** (e.g. rigidity, bradykinesia, paucity of facial expression, lack of arm swing while walking, shuffling gait).
- Look for **signs of thyroid disease**.

*There are no tremors at rest even with distraction. There are no features of Parkinsonism. The **tremor is brought on by stretching the arms and hands**. It is **present on both sides**. There is no head or voice tremor. He is **unable to drink from a glass of water without spilling**. His **handwriting is large and tremulous**. There are no cerebellar signs. He is clinically euthyroid.*

HOW SHOULD THIS PATIENT BE INVESTIGATED?

ET is a clinical diagnosis. There are no specific tests to confirm the diagnosis.

- **Functional imaging** (Dopamine transporter scan).

This might be useful in difficult cases to distinguish PD from other causes of tremor (PD is characterised by depletion of dopamine).

Note: A good response to Levo-dopa is also useful to make a diagnosis of PD.

- **Thyroid function tests**, for completion.
- In patients under 40 years of age, Wilson's disease should be excluded.

WHAT SHOULD YOU TELL THE PATIENT?

You should tell him that

- You suspect this is essential tremor.

'Your hands are shaking because of a problem in the parts of the brain that control the movements. We call this essential tremor. We do not know why this occurs'.

- Essential tremor is often familial.

'This is probably the same type of shaking that your grandfather had'.

- The tremor is not due to Parkinson's disease.

'This kind of shaking also occurs in a condition called Parkinson's disease. In Parkinson's disease, there is damage in the brain, which progressively gets worse and makes the person stiff, slow and prone to falling. I do not feel that your shaking is due to Parkinson's disease'.

- You would request thyroid function tests.

'Thyroid problem can also cause shaking. Although I do not feel that your shaking is due to thyroid problem, I will ask for a blood test to rule this out'.

- You would seek an opinion from a *'brain specialist'*.
- Medications are available to suppress the tremor.

'Medications are available to reduce the shaking. Although they are not effective in everyone, it is worth a try'.

- You would refer her to an occupational therapist.

'An occupational therapist will teach you some techniques and provide advice on devices that can make it easier for you to perform your day-to-day activities'.

- If the shaking does not respond to medications, the neurologist might try *'other types of treatment'.*

OUTCOME

His thyroid function tests are normal. He is commenced on propranolol. The neurologist decides to monitor his response to propranolol and consider further treatments depending on his response. He is also referred to occupational therapist.

There is no cure for ET, so treatment only aims to manage the symptoms. The drugs of first choice are β-blockers. Primidone is tried in patients who do not respond well to β-blockers. For patients who are resistant to medications, other treatment options that may be tried in specialist centres include focussed ultrasound (delivering ultrasound to create a lesion in the thalamus), deep brain stimulation (using surgically implanted electrodes to deliver high-frequency signals to the thalamus) and radiofrequency or surgical thalamotomy.

The 32-Year-Old Woman with Double Vision

Case 59

A 32-year-old woman presents with a three-month history of double vision.

HOW SHOULD THIS PROBLEM BE APPROACHED?

She tells you that she is seeing double. This problem started roughly about three months ago.

- First, ask *what she means by 'double vision'*.

Is she seeing two images of the same object?

- Establish if it is *monocular or binocular diplopia*.

In monocular diplopia, the double vision resolves when the affected eye is covered. In binocular diplopia, the double vision resolves when either eye is covered. Monocular diplopia is usually due to ophthalmic conditions (e.g. cornea, lens or retina), while binocular diplopia indicates a neurological problem (*see Box 59.1*).

> ### BOX 59.1   CAUSES OF BINOCULAR DIPLOPIA
>
> - *Brain stem* (e.g. stroke, demyelination, tumour).
> - *Cranial nerves III, IV and VI* (e.g. cavernous sinus thrombosis, Miller-Fisher syndrome, Wernicke's encephalopathy, third nerve palsy due to diabetes or posterior communicating artery aneurysm).
> - *Neuromuscular junction* (e.g. myasthenia gravis).
> - *Ocular muscles* (e.g. Graves' disease, giant cell arteritis).

- (In patients with binocular diplopia), ask if the *two images are separated horizontally or vertically*.

A lesion in the sixth nerve causes horizontal diplopia because of lateral rectus weakness, while a lesion in the fourth nerve causes vertical diplopia because of superior oblique weakness. The image

DOI: 10.1201/9781003430230-59

separation is usually greatest in one direction (e.g. maximum separation on looking to the right with right lateral rectus palsy or diplopia on coming down the stairs with superior oblique palsy). A lesion in the third nerve, myasthenia gravis (MG) and thyroid eye disease will cause both horizontal and vertical diplopia.

- Ask about the ***onset and progression of symptoms*** (continuous or variable). If the symptoms are variable, ask if the diplopia is ***worse towards the end of the day***.

*She confirms that she is **seeing two images of the same object**. It **resolves when she covers either eye**. The two images **can be side by side or one above the other**. She always wakes up feeling fine, and the **double vision mainly occurs towards the end of the day**.*

Her diplopia is clearly binocular. Among the differentials, giant cell arteritis can be excluded because of her young age. Acute stroke, cavernous sinus thrombosis and Miller-Fisher syndrome need not be considered because of the longer duration of symptoms. The presence of both horizontal as well as vertical diplopia would exclude an isolated fourth or sixth nerve lesion. The differentials to consider are therefore thyroid disease, third nerve palsy and MG. Of these, MG is the most likely diagnosis because of the fatiguability (occurrence of diplopia towards the end of the day).

MG usually affects younger women in their 20s or 30s, and older men in their 60s or 70s (a strange bi-modal distribution). Motor neurones release acetylcholine (Ach), which binds to receptors on the muscle cell membrane, resulting in muscle contraction. In MG, the autoimmune response blocks the Ach receptors. Weakness becomes more pronounced with repetitive muscle contraction because of the gradual depletion of Ach. Ocular MG affects extra-ocular muscles and eyelids, while generalised MG also involves the limb, bulbar and respiratory muscles. Ocular MG progresses to generalised MG in about 80% of the patients.

- Ask about ***drooping of her eyelids***, ***problems with eyesight*** and ***pain in her eyes or headache***.
- Ask about ***features that may suggest generalised MG*** (e.g. breathlessness, problems with swallowing or choking while eating, problems with speech or voice, difficulty in raising the arms or rising from the seated position, performing repetitive movements or walking long distances).
- Screen for ***thyroid disease*** (e.g. diarrhoea, weight loss, palpitations, heat intolerance, neck swelling).
- Ask if she ***drives a car***.
- Complete the ***rest of the history***.

Ask about her other medical problems, regular medications (e.g. penicillamine can cause myasthenia gravis), family history, occupation, smoking habit, alcohol intake and obstetric and menstrual history.

*She says her **eyelids drop down**, especially when she is tired and towards the end of the day. She denies problems with her eyesight, pain in the eye, headache or problems with eating, swallowing or speech. She has no trouble raising her arms or rising from a seated position. She denies thyroid symptoms.*

*She is an event organiser and **drives to work every day**. Her past medical history is unremarkable except for appendicectomy at the age of 19. She does not take any medication. Her mother suffers from rheumatoid arthritis. She has never smoked and drinks alcohol only socially. She lives with her husband and two young children. She is not planning to have any more children.*

The presence of ptosis ('eyelids dropping down') narrows down the differential diagnosis to oculomotor nerve palsy or MG. Of these, the latter is more likely, as the symptoms are worse in the evening. There don't seem to be any features of bulbar, respiratory or limb muscle weakness. She should be advised to stop driving until the diplopia is controlled with appropriate treatments.

WHAT SHOULD YOU LOOK FOR ON EXAMINATION?

You should

- Examine her *eye movements*.

This will help to detect evidence of cranial nerve palsy. In MG, the eye movements would be expected to be normal.

- Examine her *visual acuity and pupils*.

Note: In patients with third nerve palsy, the size of the pupils can help to distinguish ischemic (e.g. diabetic infarction of the central fibres of the nerve) from compressive lesion (e.g. posterior communicating aneurysm compressing the nerve). Because pupillary fibres are present on the peripheral parts of the nerve, the pupils are spared in diabetic infarction but affected in those with aneurysmal compression. An urgent brain scan should therefore be arranged in those with painful third nerve palsy and dilated pupil.

- Check for *fatiguability*.
  a. Ask the patient to look up for a sustained period (this might bring on the ptosis).
  b. Ask the patient to count up to 50 to check for voice fatiguability.
  c. Test the shoulder abduction before and after repetitive arm movement (move the arm up and down about 20 times).

*Her eye movements are full. Visual acuity and pupils are normal. The **ptosis is brought on by sustained upward gaze**. There is no fatiguability in her voice or limb muscle power.*

HOW SHOULD THIS PATIENT BE INVESTIGATED?

- *Acetylcholine receptor antibody* is present in about 90% of patients with generalised MG, and in about 50% of those with ocular MG.

The muscle-specific tyrosine kinase antibody (MUSK) antibody, which targets a protein in muscle cells, is present in about half of those with negative Ach receptor antibody.

- *Thyroid function tests*.
- *Neurophysiologic tests* in patients with negative Ach receptor and MUSK antibody.

Repetitive nerve stimulation causes decremental response in patients with MG because of gradual depletion of Ach.

- The *tensilon (edrophonium) test* in patients with equivocal neurophysiological studies.

A short-acting anti-cholinesterase like edrophonium is administered (Ach is broken down by the enzyme cholinesterase). An improvement in muscle strength would suggest MG. This test is seldom done these days because of the risk of life-threatening bradycardia.

- *CT scan of the thorax* should be requested in all patients with MG, as about 10% of them have a thymoma.
- *Forced vital capacity* in patients with suspected respiratory muscle weakness.

WHAT SHOULD YOU TELL THE PATIENT?

You should tell her that

- You suspect her diplopia and ptosis are due to myasthenia gravis.

'Our muscles are supplied by nerves. There is a gap between the nerve and muscle. A protein that is present in this gap helps the muscles to work normally. I suspect you are seeing double and your eyelids are dropping down because your immune system is mistakenly attacking the muscles around your eyes, and stopping this protein from working normally. We call this myasthenia gravis'.

- You will request some blood tests.

'I'll ask for a few blood tests, which will help to confirm whether your immune system is attacking the muscles'.

- You will refer her to a neurologist (*'muscle specialist'*).
- The neurologist might arrange further tests depending on the results of the blood tests.
- She should stop driving until the double vision improves.
- She would be commenced on appropriate treatments once the diagnosis is confirmed.

'The muscle specialist is likely to start you on a medication to prevent the protein in the gap between the nerve and muscle from getting depleted, and steroid pills to stop the immune system from attacking your muscles'.

- You will update her once the results of the tests are available.

OUTCOME

*Her results show normal full blood count, glucose and thyroid function tests. Hepatitis B screen is negative. **Acetylcholine receptor antibody is positive**. CT scan of the chest is normal, with no evidence of thymoma. The neurologist explains the diagnosis to her and starts treatment with pyridostigmine, prednisolone and azathioprine, following which her symptoms markedly improve.*

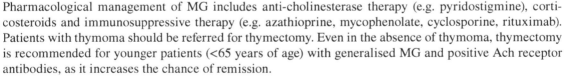

Pharmacological management of MG includes anti-cholinesterase therapy (e.g. pyridostigmine), corticosteroids and immunosuppressive therapy (e.g. azathioprine, mycophenolate, cyclosporine, rituximab). Patients with thymoma should be referred for thymectomy. Even in the absence of thymoma, thymectomy is recommended for younger patients (<65 years of age) with generalised MG and positive Ach receptor antibodies, as it increases the chance of remission.

Some patients may develop life-threatening respiratory muscle weakness (*myasthenic crisis*). It may be difficult to distinguish this from *cholinergic crisis*, which occurs because of excess acetylcholine in patients on anti-cholinesterase treatment. The tensilon test is useful in this situation, as the weakness improves after edrophonium in myasthenic crisis and worsens in cholinergic crisis. Patients with myasthenic crises are managed aggressively with mechanical ventilation, high dose corticosteroids, plasmapheresis and intravenous immunoglobulin.

A closely related entity is Lambert-Eaton myasthenic syndrome, which predominantly affects proximal limb muscles. It is associated with small cell lung cancer and is caused by antibodies to pre-synaptic voltage-gated calcium channels (calcium influx is necessary to release Ach into the synapse). It is characterised by incremental response on repetitive nerve stimulation (as repetitive stimulation releases Ach without the need for calcium).

The 62-Year-Old Woman with Weakness

Case 60

A 62-year-old woman presents with a three-month history of weakness in her limbs.

HOW SHOULD THIS PROBLEM BE APPROACHED?

---

*She tells you that she feels weak. She **finds it difficult to raise her arms** to wash or comb her hair, and reach out for objects above the level of her head. She also **struggles to rise from a chair or get off her bed in the mornings**. This problem began about three months ago, prior to which she was well. The weakness is **gradually worsening**.*

You should establish the distribution of weakness and check for other neurological symptoms in order to bracket the anatomical level of the lesion in the nervous system. (*Where is the lesion?*)

- Does she find it **difficult to turn the tap or key** (weakness of hands)? Does she **slap her feet while walking** (weakness of distal leg muscles)?
- Any **double vision** or **drooping of eyelids** (weakness of ocular muscles)?
- Any **problem with speech**, **swallowing** or **breathing** (bulbar and respiratory muscle weakness)?
- Any problem with **bladder or bowel control**?

Note: Loss of bladder and bowel control occurs in cord transection or cauda equina syndrome.

- Any **thinning of muscles** (lower motor neurone or long-standing upper motor neurone lesion) *or **rippling sensation*** (fasciculation due to anterior horn cell disease)?
- Does the **weakness fluctuate**, typically worsening towards the end of the day? Is the **weakness worse after exercise or repeated movements**?

Note: Fluctuation of weakness and fatiguability are features of neuromuscular junction disease (e.g. myasthenia gravis).

- Any **sensory symptoms**, like numbness or tingling?
- Any **pain** in her limbs, neck or back?

Note: Pain in the limb may be sharp and shooting like an electric shock sensation (nerve root pain) *or* continuous and burning (nerve pain). Neck or back pain may be caused by spinal pathology like degeneration, tumour, infection or fracture.

DOI: 10.1201/9781003430230-60

She denies weakness in her hands or feet, numbness, double vision, drooping of eyelids or problems with speech, swallowing, breathing, urination or defecation. She has not noticed thinning of her muscles or felt any rippling. The weakness is not related to activity, and it does not fluctuate through the day. She denies pain in her neck, back, shoulders and hips.

She has only motor symptoms and no numbness, so we can localise the lesion to the muscle, neuromuscular junction, motor nerve or anterior horn cell. Of these, a lesion at the neuromuscular junction is unlikely because of there is no fluctuation of weakness, fatiguability or oculo-bulbar involvement. A motor nerve lesion would not present with symmetrical, proximal weakness in all four limbs. An anterior horn cell lesion is unlikely, as her weakness is restricted to the proximal limbs and there are no other supporting features, like wasting or fasciculation. Her presentation is most likely due to myopathy, which indeed typically presents with symmetrical weakness, usually affecting the proximal upper and lower limbs (*see Box 60.1*).

It is important to ask about swallowing and breathing in all patients with suspected myopathy to screen for bulbar and respiratory muscle involvement. The differential diagnosis for breathlessness in a patient with myopathy includes aspiration pneumonia (in those with dysphagia), interstitial lung disease (seen in a subset of patients with inflammatory myopathy) and cardiac failure (due to cardiac muscle involvement). Patients with suspected respiratory muscle involvement should be closely monitored, with regular measurements of forced vital capacity or negative inspiratory force. For patients with dysphagia, it may be necessary to consider nasogastric tube or parenteral feeding to prevent aspiration.

The next set of questions should explore the features that may suggest an underlying cause of the myopathy. (*What is the lesion?*)

BOX 60.1   SOME UNDERLYING CAUSES OF PROXIMAL MYOPATHY

- *Toxic* (e.g. statins, fibrates, corticosteroids, alcohol).
- *Metabolic* (e.g. thyroid, parathyroid, adrenal and pituitary disease, osteomalacia, glycogen and lipid storage disorders).
- *Inflammatory* (polymyositis, dermatomyositis and inclusion body myositis).
- *Infection* (e.g. HIV, hepatitis B and C, cysticercosis, trichinosis).
- *Malignancy.*
- *Hereditary muscular dystrophies*.
- *Miscellaneous* (e.g. sarcoidosis).

- Ask about the *onset and temporal evolution* of weakness.

Hereditary myopathies and inclusion body myositis (IBM) begin insidiously and progress slowly over many years, while toxic or inflammatory myopathies begin acutely or subacutely and progress rapidly.

- Ask if her muscles are *painful*.

Muscle pain is a feature of infectious or inflammatory myopathy.

- Ask if she has *joint pain* or *skin rashes*.

Presence of these features may suggest idiopathic inflammatory myopathy (IIM) or myopathy secondary to a connective tissue disease like lupus.

- A *review of systems* (keep this brief) should help to pick clues that may suggest an endocrine disease, malignancy or infection.

Ask particularly about change in weight, bowel habits, palpitations, tremors, and heat or cold intolerance.

- Obtain a full *medication history*.

Also ask about *preparations taken across the counter*, use of *recreational drugs* (e.g. cocaine and heroin can cause myopathy) and *alcohol intake*.

Note: Prescription drugs are among the most common causes of myopathy, and there is potential for clinical improvement following discontinuation of the suspected agent.

- Obtain a *family history* of muscle disease.

Among the inherited muscle diseases, limb girdle muscular dystrophy, facioscapulohumeral dystrophy and Becker dystrophy can present for the first time in adult life. Family history is also relevant in patients with inherited metabolic problems like hypokalemic periodic paralysis, mitochondrial myopathies and inborn errors of glycogen or lipid metabolism.

*Review of systems is unremarkable. She denies muscle or joint pain, and skin rashes. There are no symptoms of thyroid disease. Her weight has been steady. Her medical history includes **hypertension** and **hyperlipidaemia**. She has never been diagnosed with cancer before. When she last had her mammogram five years ago, she was told that it was clear. She has never had colonoscopy before.*

*She has been on **lisinopril and simvastatin** for the last three years, with no recent change in dosages. She does not take 'over-the-counter' preparations or use recreational drugs. She has never smoked. Her usual **alcohol consumption is around 20 units a week** but she stopped drinking about four weeks ago on the advice of her GP, who told her that the '**liver tests were abnormal**'. She was also asked to discontinue the simvastatin at the time. Her family history is unremarkable. She is widowed and lives with her sister.*

Statins are associated with muscle toxicity, but true myopathy (proximal muscle weakness with elevated creatine kinase) is extremely rare. Moreover, the progression of weakness even after discontinuation of the statin should prompt a search for other causes of myopathy in this patient. Alcohol consumption of 20 units/week is unlikely to cause myopathy on its own, and she does not seem to be taking any other potential toxin. Although there are no clinical pointers in favour of an endocrine or metabolic problem, her thyroid function and vitamin D level should be checked. The onset at the age of 62, short duration of symptoms and absence of a positive family history would make it unlikely that her symptoms are due to an inherited muscle disease.

IIM is the most likely diagnosis. There are three discrete types of IIM, namely polymyositis (PM), dermatomyositis (DM) and IBM. Of these, IBM is least likely, as it usually occurs in elderly men and manifests as slowly progressive weakness of both proximal and distal muscles. PM or DM can present on its own, *or* in association with malignancy (especially DM) or another autoimmune connective tissue disease. IIM should be suspected if [a] toxic and metabolic problems have been excluded, [b] stopping the suspected drug does not lead to improvement in the muscle strength, [c] the typical skin rash of DM is present *or* [d] there is evidence of underlying malignancy.

WHAT SHOULD YOU LOOK FOR ON EXAMINATION?

You should

- Perform a focussed *neurological examination*.

Check the power in all four limbs to confirm the presence of neurological weakness.

- Look for *skin signs* that may suggest DM (*see Box 60.2*).

BOX 60.2   SKIN MANIFESTATIONS OF DERMATOMYOSITIS

- Heliotrope (meaning purplish) rash over upper eyelids.
- Erythematous rash over malar area of face and nasolabial folds.
- Erythematous rash over the anterior chest and shoulders.
- Erythematous, scaly papules over dorsum of metacarpophalangeal and interphalangeal joints of hands, extensor aspect of knees and elbows ('Gottron's papules').

- Listen to the *base of the lungs* for crepitations (interstitial lung disease).
- Offer to perform a detailed examination to check for *signs of malignancy* (e.g. lymphadenopathy, hepatomegaly, breast mass).

*Neurological examination reveals **grade 4 power in the proximal upper and lower limbs**. Distal power is preserved and there is no neck muscle weakness. There are **erythematous scaly papules over the dorsum of the metacarpophalangeal joints in both hands and behind her elbows**. Her lungs are clear.*

Examination has confirmed the presence of proximal symmetrical weakness in her upper and lower limbs. The presence of Gottron's papules over the dorsum of her metacarpophalangeal joints and elbows points to a diagnosis of DM.

HOW SHOULD THIS PATIENT BE INVESTIGATED?

You should request

- *Blood tests*, including full blood count, liver function tests, serum creatinine, creatine kinase, thyroid-stimulating hormone and vitamin D.

Note: Creatine kinase (CK) elevation occurs with most forms of myopathy. There are other causes of CK elevation, such as ethnicity (e.g. Afro-Caribbean), exercise, intramuscular injections, needle electromyography, hypothyroidism and motor neurone disease. Apart from CK, other enzymes such as aldolase, aminotransferases and lactate dehydrogenase may also be elevated. It is not necessary to ask for aldolase unless CK is normal.

- *Urine examination* (in patients with CK >10 times the upper limit of normal).

Presence of 'blood' in the absence of red blood cells would suggest myoglobinuria due to rhabdomyolysis (testing for myoglobin itself is expensive).

Specialist investigations may include

- *Myositis auto antibody panel*.

The different antibodies are associated with specific complications (e.g. interstitial lung disease with anti-Jo-1 antibody, cardiac involvement with anti-SRP, higher risk of cancer with anti-TIFF-γ and anti-NXP2).

- *Electromyography* (EMG) or *muscle imaging*.

EMG and MRI of the muscle are useful to identify inflammation and guide a suitable site for biopsy.

- *Muscle biopsy*.

Muscle biopsy is the definitive diagnostic procedure to confirm the diagnosis of myopathy.

- *Screening for malignancy* (once IIM is confirmed).

A positron emission tomography (PET)-CT scan is recommended for screening (or a CT scan of the thorax, abdomen and pelvis, if PET-CT is not available) in addition to age-appropriate screening tests such as colonoscopy and mammography. An ENT opinion should be sought, as there is an association between nasopharyngeal carcinoma and DM, particularly in Southeast Asian patients.

WHAT SHOULD YOU TELL THE PATIENT?

You should tell her that

- Her symptoms point to myopathy.

'You feel weak because of inflammation of the muscles in your arms and thighs. We call this myositis'.

- The underlying cause is most likely idiopathic inflammatory myopathy.

'A number of medical conditions can cause this kind of inflammation. In your case, I suspect the immune system is mistakenly attacking your muscles. We do not know why the immune system makes this mistake in some people. The skin rash on your hands is also related to the muscle problem'.

- You would arrange some blood tests.

'I'll first ask for a few blood tests. They will tell us if your muscles are inflamed and if this is due to the immune system attacking the muscles'.

- The abnormal liver function tests are most likely due to myositis.

'The abnormal liver tests are most likely related to the muscle problem. Some tests are common to both the liver and muscle'.

- You will seek an opinion from a rheumatologist (*'a specialist in muscle problems'*).
- The rheumatologist would probably suggest a muscle biopsy to confirm the diagnosis.

'The specialist might arrange a few more tests, including a biopsy of your muscle. A biopsy is a minor procedure in which a small piece of tissue is taken from the muscle in your thigh so that it can be examined under a microscope. This test will help to confirm the inflammation of muscles'.

- It is very likely that she *'would be treated with steroid pills'*.
- The statin is unlikely to be the cause of her weakness.

'I do not feel that the cholesterol pill is the cause of your weakness but I would suggest that you do not start taking it until we complete all the tests'.

- She can resume drinking alcohol, but it would be advisable to cut down the amount.
- You will update her once the results of the tests are back.

OUTCOME

The results of her initial investigations are as follows:

- Full blood count, serum creatinine and thyroid function are normal.
- **Aspartate aminotransferase 178 U/L** (normal 10–44) and **alanine aminotransferase 66 U/L** (normal 10–34).
- **Creatine kinase 9240 U/L** (normal <200).
- **Vitamin D 16 ng/mL** (normal >30).
- Urinalysis is negative for blood and protein.
- Myositis panel is negative.
- Chest X-ray normal.

The elevated CK is in keeping with our clinical impression of myositis. The 'abnormal liver function tests' are most likely due to myositis. The absence of myositis-related antibodies would not exclude IIM. Her low vitamin D is unlikely to be the cause of her muscle weakness because of the presence of Gottron's papules. A muscle biopsy should be organised to confirm the diagnosis of DM, and appropriate tests done to screen for malignancy and osteoporosis.

*Her **muscle biopsy shows features consistent with DM**. Her mammogram shows suspicious features and subsequent evaluation by the breast surgeon confirms **carcinoma of the right breast**. A CT scan of her thorax, abdomen and pelvis shows no evidence of metastases. She is treated with mastectomy of the right breast and referred to the oncologist.*

The rheumatologist commences her on high-dose prednisolone along with vitamin D replacement and co-trimoxazole for pneumocystis prophylaxis. He plans to gradually taper the dose of steroid and eventually commence a second-line immunosuppressive drug and a bisphosphonate as prophylaxis against steroid-induced osteoporosis.

The 68-Year-Old Man with Leg Weakness

Case 61

A 68-year-old man presents with a six-month history of leg weakness.

HOW SHOULD THIS PROBLEM BE APPROACHED?

---

*He tells you that he feels weak. He **drags his legs while walking** because they feel heavy. He recently had a **near fall on a couple of occasions** because of the leg weakness. This problem started about six months ago, and it seems to be **gradually worsening**.*

The first step is to establish the distribution of weakness and bracket the anatomical level of the lesion. (*Where is the lesion?*)

- Is he able to ***raise his arms*** to comb or wash his hair, put on his shirt or reach for objects above the level of his head?
- Is he able to ***turn the door handle or key*** without any difficulty?
- Does he struggle to ***rise from the seated position***?
- Does he ***slap his feet*** while walking?
- Any ***double vision*** or ***dropping of eyelids***?
- Any problems with ***speech***, ***swallowing*** ('*Do you choke when you eat?*') ***or breathing***?

Note: Patients with weakness due to polymyositis (muscle), myasthenia gravis (neuromuscular junction), Guillain-Barre syndrome (polyradiculoneuropathy) or motor neurone disease (MND) (anterior horn cell) may develop dysarthria, dysphagia or dyspnoea due to bulbar or respiratory muscle weakness.

*He says he **cannot rise from the seated position** without holding on to the arm rests. He also **finds it difficult to turn the tap or door handle** with his right hand. He keeps dropping plates and cups because of **poor hand grip**. He has no trouble raising his arms, and he does not slap his feet while walking. He denies double vision, dropping of eyelids or problems with speech, swallowing or breathing.*

 Patients with chronic infection or inflammation, cancer, anaemia, arthritis, depression and physical deconditioning may use the term 'weakness' to describe their fatigue or asthenia. It is therefore important to first clarify what the patient means by weakness. The weakness in this patient is clearly neurological, as he is describing *specific difficulties* with walking, rising from the seated position and turning the tap or door handle. His legs feel heavy, possibly because they are spastic.

 DOI: 10.1201/9781003430230-61

You should now check for the presence of other neurological symptoms to further help with the anatomical localisation of the lesion. Neurological weakness may be caused by a lesion anywhere along the motor tract from the cerebral cortex all the way down to muscle.

- Any *numbness*?

There are various patterns of numbness. Examples include (a) 'glove and stocking' sensory loss in peripheral neuropathy, (b) dermatomal sensory loss in radiculopathy, (c) loss of all modalities of sensation below a certain level in spinal cord transection (e.g. tumour, transverse myelitis) and (d) hemisensory loss in internal capsule infarct.

- Any *fluctuation in strength* or *fatiguability* (neuromuscular junction)?
- Any *thinning of muscles* (lower motor neurone or long-standing upper motor neurone lesion) or *rippling sensation* (fasciculation due to anterior horn cell disease)?
- Any *pain in the neck, back or limbs*?

Pain in the limb may be sharp and shooting like an electric shock (nerve root pain), *or* continuous and burning (nerve pain). Neck or back pain may be due to spinal pathology that compresses the cord or nerve roots (e.g. degeneration, tumour or infection).

- Any problem with *bladder or bowel control*?

Loss of bladder and bowel control occurs in cord transection or cauda equina syndrome.

- Any change in *higher mental functions* (memory, mood, behaviour or personality)?

*The weakness is not related to activity, and it does not fluctuate through the day. He thinks his **left leg is getting thinner**. He often feels a **rippling sensation in his thighs**. His **legs feel stiff and heavy**, but there is no pain or cramping. He denies numbness or tingling. He is able to control his bowels and bladder. There is no change in his mental functions.*

It appears that he has developed an asymmetrical weakness in his limbs, both proximally and distally. The absence of numbness would narrow down the anatomical level of the lesion to muscle, neuromuscular junction, motor nerve or anterior horn cell. Myopathy is unlikely, as this usually presents with symmetrical proximal limb weakness. The absence of fatiguability or fluctuation of weakness, involvement of fingers and stiffness of the legs would exclude a problem at the neuromuscular junction. Motor neuropathies predominantly present with distal weakness.

Hence, the lesion is most likely at the level of anterior horn cell (MND). This is supported by the combination of upper and lower motor neurone features in the same limb (stiffness and heaviness, wasting and fasciculations). However, before a diagnosis of MND is made, all possible treatable causes for a similar presentation should be excluded. Patients with MND may have involvement of the motor cranial nerve nuclei in the brain stem but the absence of dysphagia and dysarthria suggests that his disease is confined to the spinal cord.

The next set of questions should explore the features of possible underlying causes of weakness (*What is the lesion?*), which generally fall under one of the ten categories listed in *Box 61.1*. The questions should be tailored based on the clinical presentation.

*He has otherwise been well. Review of systems is unremarkable. His medical history is unremarkable except for **hyperlipidaemia** for which he takes a **statin**. He doesn't smoke and seldom drinks alcohol. He used to be a gardener until he stopped working three years ago. He lives with his wife.*

BOX 61.1   UNDERLYING CAUSES OF NEUROLOGICAL ILLNESSES

- *Congenital or hereditary* (e.g. muscular dystrophies, hereditary sensory-motor neuropathies).
- *Trauma* (e.g. subdural haematoma, spinal cord trauma).
- *Infection or inflammation* (e.g. human immunodeficiency virus, syphilis, tuberculosis, systemic lupus erythematosus).
- *Neoplasm* (e.g. brain or spinal cord tumour).
- *Vascular* (e.g. stroke, subarachnoid haemorrhage, vasculitis).
- *Degeneration* (e.g. motor neurone disease, Parkinson's disease).
- *Demyelination* (e.g. multiple sclerosis, Guillain-Barre syndrome).
- *Deficiency* (e.g. subacute combined degeneration due to vitamin B_{12} deficiency).
- *Toxic* (e.g. peripheral neuropathy due to alcohol, statin-induced myopathy).
- *Metabolic* (e.g. hypothyroidism, hepatic encephalopathy).

WHAT SHOULD YOU LOOK FOR ON EXAMINATION?

You should perform

- A *neurological examination*, focussing on the motor system (muscle bulk, fasciculations, strength in the limbs, deep tendon reflexes and plantar reflex).

*Examination of the limbs reveals **wasting of the small muscles of the right hand and left leg, fasciculations** in his thighs, **hypertonia**, **exaggerated deep tendon reflexes in all four limbs** and **bilateral extensor plantar response**. His **power is grade 4, both proximally and distally, in all four limbs**. His higher mental functions, cranial nerves and sensory examination are normal.*

 A diagnosis of MND is supported by (a) the combination of upper and lower motor neurone signs (brisk reflexes in a weak and wasted limb), (b) lack of sensory impairment, (c) fasciculations and (d) relentless progression of symptoms, with no improvement at all. MND is a clinical diagnosis that can be supported by electrophysiological studies. Further investigations to exclude treatable causes should always be done because of the grim prognosis of MND (although one is usually not found).

The presentation of MND depends on whether the brain stem or spinal cord is involved (*see Figure 61.1*).

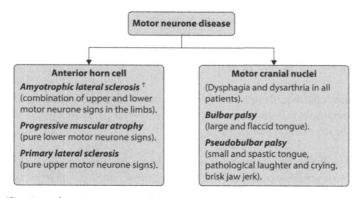

FIGURE 61.1   Classification of motor neurone disease.

[†] *Amyotrophic* means lack of nourishment to the muscle (resulting in atrophy) and *lateral sclerosis* refers to the involvement of the corticospinal tract.

HOW SHOULD THIS PATIENT BE INVESTIGATED?

The following investigations should be considered:

- *Magnetic resonance imaging* (MRI) scan of the brain and whole spine.

MRI scan will help to rule out lesions that compress the cord or nerve roots (an important differential diagnosis for MND is spondylotic cervical myelopathy and peripheral neuropathy).

- *Neurophysiological studies* (including electromyography and nerve conduction studies).
- *Blood tests*, including thyroid function, vitamin B_{12} and folate, creatine kinase, antinuclear antibody, human immunodeficiency virus test and test for syphilis.

The neurologist might ask for a muscle biopsy and lumbar puncture in some patients.

WHAT SHOULD YOU TELL THE PATIENT?

At this stage, there is no need to tell him that the most likely diagnosis is MND, as it would be good to rule out treatable causes and look for supportive evidence from neurophysiological studies. Moreover, it is best for the neurologist to break this news. You should tell him that

- His weakness is due to a neurological problem.

'Our muscles help us perform activities like walking, talking, swallowing, writing and so on. The muscles receive messages from the brain. I suspect you are feeling weak because of a problem with the brain sending messages to the muscles'.

- You will organise some tests.

'I will ask for scans of your brain and spinal cord, and also some blood tests. These tests will help us find out why your muscles are weak'.

- You will refer him to a neurologist (*'brain specialist'*).
- The neurologist might arrange further investigations.

'The brain specialist might arrange other tests to better understand the cause of your weakness. He will explain what the problem is once you have had these tests'.

- You will refer him to a physiotherapist, who can help to assess his walking and suggest measures to reduce his risk of falling.

OUTCOME

*The results of **EMG and nerve conduction studies are in keeping with motor neurone disease**. MRI scan of the brain is normal. MRI of the spine shows degenerative changes in the cervical and lumbar spine but there is no evidence of myelopathy or nerve root compression. His blood tests are all normal.*

The neurologist explains the diagnosis of MND to him and his wife (see Box 61.2). The consultation is challenging but he patiently answers all their questions. He commences him on riluzole. He and his team decide to closely follow him in the clinic and continue to offer their support. He is also seen by the physiotherapist and occupational therapist.

BOX 61.2   COMMUNICATING THE DIAGNOSIS OF MOTOR NEURONE DISEASE TO THE PATIENT

The challenge for the neurologist is that the patient has no idea what the problem is and he is hoping that the problem could be fixed. It has to be somehow tactfully conveyed to the patient that the weakness will continue to worsen, and his life span may be reduced. It is important to be honest with him and at the same time focus on the positive aspects.

Communication should be in lay terms (*'Your weakness is caused by damage of the nerve cells in the brain and spinal cord that help to convey messages to the muscles. We call this motor neurone disease'*).

It should be impressed upon the patient that although there is no cure for MND, a lot can be done to maximise his functional independence. This may include physiotherapy, occupational therapy, use of adaptive devices and speech and language therapy (for those with bulbar or pseudobulbar palsy). There are medications available to delay the onset of respiratory problems (riluzole), treat the cramping pain (e.g. baclofen) and relieve constipation. Two important aspects of therapy during the later stages of the illness are overnight ventilation for those with respiratory problems and percutaneous endoscopic gastrostomy feeding.

He should be provided with information booklets or referred to useful websites. A lot of kindness, empathy and support are essential (*'You don't have to fight this alone. Our entire team is here to help you manage this illness'*). If there are questions about the life span or end of life, he should be told that life span may be reduced but it is hard to predict by how much. If he brings up the topic of euthanasia, he should be politely discouraged and told that palliative measures can greatly help to maximise the quality of whatever life that remains.

The 46-Year-Old Man with Elevated Creatine Kinase

Case 62

A 46-year-old Chinese man is referred to the medical clinic for an opinion on his elevated creatine kinase.

HOW SHOULD THIS PROBLEM BE EVALUATED?

- Ask *why the creatine kinase (CK) level was checked in the first place*.
- Ask if he has *any symptoms*, like muscle pain or weakness.

To screen for weakness, ask if he has trouble raising his arms or getting up from the seated position.

*He tells you that he was **commenced on 40 mg of simvastatin six months ago**, as his cholesterol was found to be high during his annual health screening. His **muscles in the arms started aching about two months ago** but he did not feel weak.*

*His GP checked his CK along with a few other routine blood tests at the time, and the **CK was noted to be 824 IU/L** (normal <200 IU/L). He rechecked the CK a month later, and it was **still high at 866 IU/L**, hence this referral. He stopped the statin three weeks ago because of the persistently high CK but his muscle pain actually resolved even before he stopped the statin.*

- Ask if he has had a *heart attack or stroke before*, and check if has *other cardiovascular risk factors*.

Note: A history of heart attack or stroke, *or* the presence of other cardiovascular risk factors would lower the threshold for restarting lipid-lowering therapy at the earliest possible opportunity.

*He says he was diagnosed with **high blood pressure** about five years ago. He has since been getting his blood sugar and cholesterol checked annually. The blood sugar has been normal but the cholesterol was gradually creeping up, so the GP decided to start him on the statin. He has never had a heart attack or stroke. His kidney function is normal, there is no family history of premature cardiovascular disease and he has never smoked.*

Kinases are enzymes that transfer phosphate. Creatine kinase (CK) transfers phosphate from phosphocreatine to adenosine diphosphate (ADP) to form adenosine triphosphate (ATP). Thus, CK is present in tissues that have a high energy demand (e.g. muscle, brain and heart). There are two sub-units of CK: M type and

DOI: 10.1201/9781003430230-62

B type. The skeletal muscle contains two M sub-units (CK-MM), while the brain contains two B sub-units (CK-BB) and the heart contains one of each (CK-MB). The CK level depends on sex and ethnicity, with Black men having the highest level and Caucasian women the least. Thus, further evaluation may not be needed in Black men unless the CK is >1000 IU/L, but this may be required in White women with CK >300 IU/L.

Based on the chronology of events, it seems unlikely that the muscle pain was caused by statin, as his symptoms started more than four months after commencing the statin, and they resolved even before he discontinued it (the statin-associated muscle symptoms-clinical index [SAMS-CI] is useful to determine the likelihood of statin being the cause of muscle symptoms).

Having established that there is no muscle weakness or ongoing muscle pain, the next step is to consider other possible causes of elevated CK. The most common or important causes to consider (in the non-acute setting) are (a) strenuous physical activity, (b) toxins, (c) hypothyroidism, (d) idiopathic inflammatory myopathy, (e) familial muscle diseases and (f) the presence of macro-CK. Macro-CK is a complex of CK with immunoglobulin or an unidentified protein. Because of its high molecular weight, renal clearance is reduced, which results in the elevation of CK. Macro-CK is diagnosed by CK electrophoresis.

In the acute setting, elevated CK is encountered in patients with myocardial infarction, stroke, seizures, muscle injuries and prolonged immobilisation following a fall.

Further questions to ask:

- Ask about his level of ***physical activity*** during the week prior to the blood tests. Also ask if he regularly goes to the gym.
- Ask about his ***occupation*** to check if his work is physically demanding (e.g. construction work, heavy lifting, farming).

Physical activity can increase CK, especially if it is unaccustomed. CK levels should therefore be checked at least one week after the activity has ceased.

- Obtain a detailed ***medication history***.

Also ask about his ***alcohol intake, preparations taken across the counter*** (e.g. red yeast rice, a popular Chinese dietary supplement contains lovastatin) *and **use of illicit drugs*** (e.g. cocaine, heroin can cause myopathy) as well.

- Ask about symptoms of ***thyroid disease*** (e.g. weight gain, lethargy, constipation, reduced appetite, cold intolerance and lump in the neck).
- Ask if he has noticed any ***skin rashes*** (of dermatomyositis).
- Ask if there is ***anyone in his immediate family with muscle disease***.
- Ask about his ***urine output*** and ***colour of the urine*** (although not relevant in this patient, as the CK is usually >10–40 times the upper limit of normal in patients with rhabdomyolysis).

*He says he followed the advice of his GP and **started to exercise on a regular basis about six months ago**. He goes for a 30-minute brisk walk in the park about four to five times a week but has not been to the gym or done anything that would be considered strenuous. He works for an information technology firm, and his job is mainly desk-bound.*

*He takes lisinopril for his **high blood pressure**. He **stopped the simvastatin six weeks ago** after his CK was found to be high for the second time. He has not taken any other medication, including 'over-the-counter' preparations or supplements. He has never used illicit drugs. He drinks a glass of wine about two to three times a week and has never exceeded this amount ever. He has not noticed any skin rashes. There is no family history of muscle disease.*

 Up to 5–10% of patients taking statins might experience myalgia or have an asymptomatic elevation of CK, but true myopathy (muscle weakness with elevated CK) is very rare, with an incidence of only around 1.2 per 10,000 person years. See *Box 62.1* for factors that may increase the risk of statin-induced myopathy or muscle toxicity.

BOX 62.1 FACTORS THAT MAY INCREASE THE RISK OF STATIN-INDUCED MYOPATHY

■ Preparation.

Lipophilic statins like simvastatin, atorvastatin and lovastatin are more likely to cause muscle toxicity (as they are more permeable to muscle cells) than hydrophilic statins like pravastatin, fluvastatin or rosuvastatin.

■ Dose of the statin (higher dose >lower dose).
■ Genetic factors[†].
■ Older age.
■ Renal or liver dysfunction.
■ Hypothyroidism.
■ Alcoholism.
■ Heavy exercise.
■ Medications that inhibit cytochrome P450, which helps to metabolise statins (e.g. fibrates, colchicine, macrolide antibiotics, cyclosporine, protease inhibitors).

[†] Carriers of the SLCO1B1 gene have a higher risk of myopathy with simvastatin. Genetic testing is currently not recommended, as there is not enough evidence to show that this can identify patients at risk of myopathy. In the right patient, benefits of statins would still far outweigh the risks even in the presence of two abnormal SLCO1B1 alleles.

WHAT SHOULD YOU CHECK ON EXAMINATION?

You should

■ Examine the *muscle power* in the limbs, and check for *muscle tenderness*.

Motor neurone disease is a rare cause of elevated CK. If this is suspected, a more detailed motor system examination should be performed, particularly looking for the combination of upper and lower motor neurone signs (e.g. muscle wasting and fasciculation with exaggerated deep tendon reflexes and extensor plantar response).

■ Search carefully for the *rash of dermatomyositis* (*see Box 62.2*).

Patients with clinically amyopathic dermatomyositis may present with the typical skin rash and elevated CK, without muscle weakness.

BOX 62.2 CUTANEOUS MANIFESTATIONS OF DERMATOMYOSITIS

■ Heliotrope rash (means purplish) rash over the upper eyelids.
■ Erythematous rash over the malar area of the face and nasolabial folds.
■ Erythematous rash over the light exposed 'V area' of the chest and shoulders.
■ Erythematous scaly papules over the dorsum of the metacarpophalangeal and interphalangeal joints of the hands and extensor aspect of the elbows and knees (Gottron's papules).

- Check the **thyroid status**.

His motor system examination is entirely normal, with grade 5 power in all muscle groups, and no evidence of muscle wasting or fasciculation. There is no muscle tenderness. There are no skin rashes. He is clinically euthyroid.

HOW SHOULD THIS PATIENT BE INVESTIGATED?

You should ask for

- **Thyroid function tests.**
- **Vitamin D.**

You should look at his records to check the results of his lipid profile, liver and renal function.

Other tests (e.g. electromyogram, muscle biopsy, HMG-CoA reductase antibody) and specialist referral are indicated only if the CK continues to rise *or* the patient develops muscle weakness.

WHAT WOULD YOU TELL THE PATIENT?

You should tell him that

- Creatine kinase is a *'protein that is predominantly present in muscles. A small amount is also present in the blood'.*
- The elevation of CK is most likely due to statin therapy but there is no evidence of muscle disease.

'I suspect your CK level is high because of the statin. Statins can cause inflammation of muscles but I did not find any evidence of this when I examined you'.

- There are numerous causes for elevation of CK.

'Strenuous physical exercise, receiving an injection into the muscle, taking certain medications, consuming too much alcohol and thyroid problem can also cause the CK to go up'.

- You would ask for a few blood tests.

'I'll check your thyroid and vitamin D level. A low vitamin D level can increase the risk of getting side effects with statins, and it is easy to replace it if your level is found to be low'.

- You do not feel that the muscle aches were due to statins but he should stay off the statin for now because of the elevated CK.
- You would repeat the blood test after a month. He should not exercise for a week before the blood test.
- If the blood test shows that the CK level is coming down, he can restart the statin.

'Several different statin preparations are available. We could try a different statin in a smaller dose once your CK level starts to fall. Statins are effective in reducing the risk of heart attack and stroke, and they are generally safe'.

■ Further tests are necessary only if the CK level rises further or he develops weakness in his muscles.

OUTCOME

His thyroid function and vitamin D level are normal. His CK is repeated a month later, after a week without exercise, and it is found to be 372 IU/L.

He is commenced on 10 mg of atorvastatin, which he is able to tolerate well. He is told that the dose of atorvastatin could be gradually increased depending on his tolerance and results of his lipid tests.

Statin intolerance is defined as intolerance to at least two different statins. If the patient is truly intolerant of statin, options include (a) trying a long-acting statin like rosuvastatin one to three times/week, (b) ezetimibe, (c) bile acid sequestrants or (d) PCSK-9 inhibitor. Statins reduce co-enzyme Q10 levels but there is no evidence that replacing co-enzyme Q10 is beneficial.

If the CK level is more than ten times the upper limit of normal and there is evidence of muscle weakness, you should consider the possibility of autoimmune necrotising myopathy, and ask for a muscle biopsy and test for HMG-CoA reductase antibody (*see Figure 62.1*). Patients with necrotising myopathy should be managed with corticosteroids and immunosuppressive therapy.

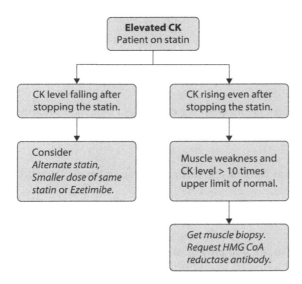

FIGURE 62.1   Management of patients with elevated CK on statin therapy.

The 56-Year-Old Man with Numbness in His Feet **Case 63**

A 56-year-old man presents with a four-month history of numbness and tingling in his feet.

HOW SHOULD THIS PROBLEM BE APPROACHED?

*He tells you that his **feet feel numb**. This is associated with a '**pins and needles**' sensation and **burning discomfort**, which is more or less constant. This problem started about four to five months ago, and it is gradually getting worse.*

You should first map the extent of numbness and ask about other neurological symptoms in order to bracket the anatomical level of the lesion.

- Ask **how far up the legs the numbness extends**, and if he has **numbness in the rest of his body**, especially hands.
- Ask if he feels **weak**.

Ask specifically if he has difficulty in turning the tap or key or slaps his feet while walking (due to distal limb weakness).

- Ask about his **vision**, **speech**, **swallowing**, and **bladder and bowel control**.

*The **numbness extends up to the mid part of the shins on both sides**. He has no numbness or tingling elsewhere and does not feel weak. He denies problems with his vision, speech, swallowing, urination or defecation.*

He has presented with sensory symptoms involving the distal legs and feet, with no weakness or other neurological symptoms. The absence of weakness would rule out a problem in the muscle, neuromuscular junction and anterior horn cell (unless there is a dual pathology). Spinal cord lesion can be ruled out, as it is unlikely to present without weakness, and the sensory loss would not be limited to the distal legs. Radiculopathy is also unlikely, as it would cause intermittent sharp and shooting pain radiating down to the foot, and symptoms are usually unilateral.

 DOI: 10.1201/9781003430230-63

A length-dependent sensory neuropathy is the most likely diagnosis (length dependent means the most distal fibres are affected first). The constant burning discomfort is also in keeping with this diagnosis. It is possible that there is subtle sensory loss in the hands *or* involvement of the motor component, which may be detected only on physical examination or nerve conduction studies.

Further questions to ask:

- Any **neck or back pain**?
- Any **postural giddiness** or **erectile impotence** (symptoms of autonomic neuropathy)?
- Does he experience **claudication** symptoms?

Patients with diabetes may have associated peripheral vascular disease.

- Any **sores or wounds in the feet**?

Trophic ulcers can develop in patients with sensory neuropathy.

- How are these symptoms **affecting his daily activities**, like walking or driving? Does the burning discomfort **disturb his sleep** at night?

*He denies neck or back pain, giddiness, problems with erection or pain in his legs while walking. He has not seen any sores on his feet. He is still able to walk without the use of any aids, although he says it **feels as if he is walking on cotton wool**. He does not drive. The burning discomfort **sometimes disturbs his sleep at night**.*

The rest of the history should explore the features that may suggest an underlying cause of his neuropathy (*see Box 63.1*). This should include a thorough review of systems, details of other medical problems, medications taken, alcohol intake, occupational history (for possible exposure to toxins), family history and sexual history.

BOX 63.1   UNDERLYING CAUSES OF PERIPHERAL NEUROPATHY[†]

- **Hereditary** (e.g. hereditary sensory-motor neuropathy).
- **Infective** (e.g. leprosy, human immunodeficiency virus disease, hepatitis B or C).
- **Inflammatory** (e.g. rheumatoid arthritis, systemic lupus erythematosus, sarcoidosis).
- **Vascular** (e.g. systemic vasculitis).
- **Neoplastic** (e.g. paraneoplastic neuropathy).
- **Demyelination** (e.g. Guillain-Barre syndrome, chronic inflammatory demyelinating polyneuropathy).
- **Deficiency** (e.g. vitamin B_{12} or folate, thiamine).
- **Toxic** (e.g. alcohol, lead poisoning, insecticides, drugs like isoniazid and vincristine).
- **Metabolic** (e.g. diabetes mellitus, thyroid disease, chronic liver or renal disease).

[†] The most common cause of peripheral neuropathy is diabetes in the Western world, and leprosy in countries like India, Indonesia, Congo and Brazil.

His medical history is blameless. He does not take any prescription drugs, 'over-the-counter' preparations or recreational drugs. Review of systems is unremarkable. He denies polyuria, polydipsia, weight loss and symptoms of thyroid disease or malabsorption. Apart from diabetes in his parents, the family history is unremarkable. He himself has not been tested for diabetes recently.

*He **drinks about two to three cans of beer every day**. He mostly drinks with friends in the evenings and has never experienced withdrawal symptoms. He has **smoked about 20 cigarettes a day** for the last 40 years. He is divorced and has been sexually inactive for more than ten years. He owns a pub.*

His excess alcohol consumption may be the cause of his peripheral neuropathy. However, the other causes of peripheral neuropathy should still be considered in the differential diagnosis. The relevant tests should be done to rule out common causes such as diabetes, thyroid disease, and vitamin B$_{12}$ and folate deficiency.

WHAT SHOULD YOU LOOK FOR ON EXAMINATION?

You should

- Perform a *general examination*.
- Ask for his lying and standing *blood pressure*.
- Examine the *nervous system*, particularly paying attention to the distal upper and lower limbs.
- Check the *pulses in the feet*, and inspect for *pressure sores or ulcers*.

*He is moderately built and well nourished. General examination is unremarkable. His **blood pressure is 134/82 mm Hg (lying) and 128/78 (standing)**.*

*In the limbs, there is **reduced perception of all modalities of sensation in the feet and lower legs in a stocking distribution**. There is no sensory loss elsewhere. **Ankle reflexes are lost bilaterally**. There is normal power in all muscle groups. All his peripheral pulses are felt, and there are no pressure sores or ulcers in his feet.*

The findings on examination have confirmed our suspicion of sensory polyneuropathy affecting the legs. The loss of ankle reflexes is also in keeping with neuropathy.

HOW SHOULD THIS PATIENT BE INVESTIGATED?

You should request

- *Blood tests*, including full blood count, liver function tests, serum creatinine, fasting glucose, HbA$_1$c, lipid panel, thyroid-stimulating hormone, vitamin B$_{12}$, folate and vitamin D.
- *Nerve conduction studies* are useful to confirm the presence of polyneuropathy and also detect the involvement of the nerves in the upper limbs.

WHAT SHOULD YOU TELL THE PATIENT?

You should tell him that

- The numbness in his feet is due to peripheral neuropathy.

'Our nerves are like wires that connect the brain and the rest of the body. These nerves run in two directions. The nerves that leave the brain help our muscles to work, and those that go towards the brain carry sensations like touch and pain. I suspect you are feeling numb because your nerves are not carrying the messages from the feet to the brain'.

- His excess alcohol consumption could be a possible cause of his neuropathy.

'The nerve problem may be due to alcohol'.

- You would like to arrange some blood tests to screen for medical conditions that are known to cause neuropathy.

'There are some medical conditions that can affect nerves, like diabetes, thyroid problem and deficiency of certain vitamins. I'll arrange some blood tests to check for these conditions'.

- You will organise nerve conduction tests (*'needle tests'*) and seek the opinion of a neurologist (*'nerve specialist'*) if there are no clear answers from the initial tests.
- He should cut down on his drinking.

'You should cut down your alcohol intake substantially. We may not be able to mend the damaged nerves but if you cut down the alcohol, we can stop further damage'.

- He should stop smoking.
- You would recommend amitriptyline (*'a medication to help the burning discomfort in the feet and improve your sleep'*).
- You would refer him to a podiatrist.

'I'll refer you to a podiatrist. A podiatrist is an expert on foot care. This is important because damage to the nerves can cause sores in the feet. The podiatrist will advise you on appropriate foot wear and how you can take care of your feet'.

- You will update him once the results of the tests are back.

OUTCOME

His blood test results are as follows:

- Hb 128 g/L, **mean corpuscular volume 102 fl** (normal 80–100 fl) and platelets 234×10^9/L.
- Liver function tests show **aspartate aminotransferase** (AST) **106 U/L** (10–44 U/L), **alanine aminotransferase** (ALT) **52 U/L** (10–34 U/L), alkaline phosphatase 114 U/L (40–150 U/L), **γ-glutamyl transferase** (γ-GT) **146 U/L** (12–64 U/L) and albumin 35 g/L (34–48 g/L).
- **Fasting blood glucose 8.4 mmol/L** and **HbA₁c 77 mmol/mol.**
- **Low-density lipoprotein 4.1 mmol/L** (target <2.7), **triglycerides of 3.8 mmol/L** (target <1.7) and high-density lipoprotein of 1.2 mmol/L (target >1.0).
- Thyroid-stimulating hormone, serum creatinine, vitamin B_{12} and folate normal.
- **Vitamin D 18 ng/mL** (optimal >30 ng/mL).

*Nerve conduction study confirms **axonal polyneuropathy in the lower limbs** and shows normal conduction in the upper limbs.*

The nerve conduction study has confirmed the presence of neuropathy. His blood test results have shown a number of abnormalities. The fasting blood glucose and HbA₁c results are in keeping with diabetes mellitus, which is another potential cause of his neuropathy. His urine albumin-creatinine ratio should be checked to detect albuminuria and his retinae examined for evidence of retinopathy. He would need appropriate dietary advice and oral hypoglycaemic agents.

The elevated AST, Υ-GT and MCV are in keeping with his excessive alcohol intake. An ultrasound scan of the liver should be arranged. He should be commenced on a statin, vitamin D replacement therapy and oral B vitamins. It may be a good idea to organise a bone density scan, as both alcohol and smoking increase the risk of osteoporosis.

Index

Note: **Bold** page numbers refer to tables and *italic* page numbers refer figures.

Printed in the United States
by Baker & Taylor Publisher Services